Patient Encounters

The Internal Medicine Work-Up

Patient Encounters

The Internal Medicine Work-Up

Brian T. Garibaldi, MD
Division of Pulmonary and Critical Care Medicine
The Johns Hopkins Hospital
Baltimore, Maryland

Series Editor

Alfa O. Diallo, MD, MPH
Department of Medicine
The Johns Hopkins Hospital
Baltimore, Maryland

Associate Editors

Susan Potter Bell, MBBS
Division of Cardiovascular Medicine Vanderbilt
University Medical Center
Nashville, Tennessee

D. Clark Files, MD
Division of Pulmonary and Critical Care Medicine
The Johns Hopkins Hospital, Baltimore, Maryland

Patrick J. Troy, MD
Division of Pulmonary and Critical Care Medicine
Harvard Medical School, Boston, Massachusetts

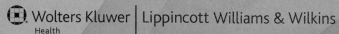
Wolters Kluwer | Lippincott Williams & Wilkins
Health

Philadelphia · Baltimore · New York · London
Buenos Aires · Hong Kong · Sydney · Tokyo

Acquisitions Editor: Susan Rhyner
Product Manager: Stacey L. Sebring
Marketing Manager: Christen Melcher
Compositor: Aptara, Inc.

Copyright © 2010 Lippincott Williams & Wilkins
351 West Camden Street
Baltimore, Maryland 21201-2436 USA
530 Walnut Street
Philadelphia, PA 19106

Printed in China

Library of Congress Cataloging-in-Publication Data

Patient encounters. The internal medicine work-up / editor, Brian T. Garibaldi ; associate editors, Susan Potter Bell, D. Clark Files, Patrick J. Troy.
    p. ; cm.
  Includes bibliographical references and index.
  ISBN 978-0-7817-9396-4
  1. Internal medicine—Handbooks, manuals, etc. 2. Clinical clerkship—Handbooks, manuals, etc. I. Garibaldi, Brian T. II. Title: Internal medicine work-up.
  [DNLM: 1. Internal Medicine—methods. 2. Diagnostic Techniques and Procedures. WB 115 P298 2010]
  RC55.P373 2010
  616—dc22
                                        2009035838

The publishers have made every effort to trace the copyright holders for borrowed material. If they have inadvertently overlooked any, they will be pleased to make the necessary arrangements at the first opportunity.

We'd like to hear from you! If you have comments or suggestions regarding this Lippincott Williams & Wilkins title, please contact us at the appropriate customer service number listed below, or send correspondence to **book_comments@lww.com.** If possible, please remember to include your mailing address, phone number, and a reference to the book title and author in your message. To purchase additional copies of this book call our customer service department at **(800) 638-3030** or fax orders to **(301) 824-7390.** International customers should call **(301) 714-2324.**

*To Mary, Violet, and Tyler—for allowing me
to pursue my dreams, while always reminding me
what's most important.*

Contributing Authors

Raja Abdulnour, MD
Fellow
Division of Pulmonary and Critical
    Care Medicine
Harvard Medical School
Boston, Massachusetts

Kia Afshar, MD
Fellow
Department of Cardiovascular
    Medicine
The Cleveland Clinic
Cleveland, Ohio

**Aimalohi A. Ahonkhai, MD,
MPH**
Fellow
Division of Infectious Disease
Massachusetts General Hospital
Boston, Massachusetts

Susan Potter Bell, MBBS
Fellow
Division of Cardiovascular Medicine
Vanderbilt University Medical Center
Nashville, Tennessee

Katharine Black, MD
Fellow
Division of Pulmonary and Critical
    Care Medicine
The Johns Hopkins Hospital
Baltimore, Maryland

Anupama Gupta Brixey, MD
Fellow
Department of Pulmonary and Critical
    Care Medicine
Vanderbilt University Hospital
Nashville, Tennessee

Lorrel E. Brown, MD
Resident
Department of Medicine
The Johns Hopkins Hospital
Baltimore, Maryland

Priscilla Brastianos, MD
Fellow
Dana-Farber Cancer Institute
Boston, Massachusetts

Elliott C. Dasenbrook, MD
Assistant Professor of Medicine and
    Pediatrics
Associate Director Adult Cystic Fibrosis
    Program
Division of Pulmonary, Critical Care
    and Sleep Medicine
Case Western Reserve University
Cleveland, Ohio

Neal W. Dickert, MD, PhD
Fellow
Division of Cardiology
Emory University School of
    Medicine
Atlanta, Georgia

Justin Dunn, MD
Resident
Department of Medicine
The Johns Hopkins Hospital
Baltimore, Maryland

Christine Durand, MD
Fellow
Division of Infectious Diseases
The Johns Hopkins Hospital
Baltimore, Maryland

D. Clark Files, MD
Fellow
Division of Pulmonary and Critical
    Care Medicine
The Johns Hopkins Hospital
Baltimore, Maryland

Joe C. Files, MD
Director, University of Mississippi
    Medical Center Cancer Institute
Director, Division of Hematology
Professor and Associate Chairman,
    Department of Medicine
University of Mississippi Medical Center
Jackson, Mississippi

Michael Fradley, MD
Fellow
Division of Cardiology
The Massachusetts General Hospital
Boston, Massachusetts

Brian T. Garibaldi, MD
Fellow
Division of Pulmonary and Critical
    Care Medicine
The Johns Hopkins Hospital
Baltimore, Maryland

Daniel Gilstrap, MD
Resident
Department of Medicine
The Johns Hopkins Hospital
Baltimore, Maryland

Sherita Hill Golden, MD, MHS
Assistant Professor
Department of Medicine
The Johns Hopkins University School
    of Medicine
Baltimore, Maryland

Todd M. Kolb, MD, PhD
Fellow
Division of Pulmonary and Critical
    Care Medicine
The Johns Hopkins Hospital
Baltimore, Maryland

James E. Lai, MD, MPH
Hospitalist
Atlanta Veterans Affairs Medical Center
Atlanta, Georgia

Peter J. Leary, MD
Fellow
Division of Pulmonary and Critical
    Care Medicine
The University of Washington
Seattle, Washington

Stephen C. Mathai, MD, MHS
Johns Hopkins Pulmonary
    Hypertension Program
Assistant Professor of Medicine
The Johns Hopkins University School
    of Medicine
Division of Pulmonary and Critical
    Care Medicine
Baltimore, Maryland

Thomas J. Mulhearn IV, MD
Fellow
Division of Cardiovascular Medicine
Duke University Medical Center
Durham, North Carolina

Santosh S. Oommen, MD
Fellow
Department of Cardiovascular
    Medicine
The Cleveland Clinic
Cleveland, Ohio

Shyam M. Parkhie, MD
Fellow
Department of Nephrology
The Johns Hopkins University School
    of Medicine
Baltimore, Maryland

Joanna Peloquin, MD
Resident
Department of Medicine
The Johns Hopkins Hospital
Baltimore, Maryland

Matthew R. Pipeling, MD
Fellow
Division of Pulmonary and Critical
  Care Medicine
The Johns Hopkins Hospital
Baltimore, Maryland

Robert Michael Reed, MD
Fellow
Division of Pulmonary and Critical
  Care Medicine
The Johns Hopkins Hospital
Baltimore, Maryland

M. Benjamin Shoemaker, MD
Resident
Department of Medicine
The Johns Hopkins University
Baltimore, Maryland

Marc Sonenshine, MD
Fellow
Division of Digestive Diseases
Emory University School of Medicine
Atlanta, Georgia

Patrick Sosnay, MD
Instructor
Division of Pulmonary and Critical
  Care Medicine
The Johns Hopkins Hospital
Baltimore, Maryland

R. Scott Stephens, MD
Fellow
Division of Pulmonary and Critical
  Care Medicine
The Johns Hopkins Hospital
Baltimore, Maryland

Brad Sutton, MD
Fellow in Cardiac Electrophysiology
The Johns Hopkins Hospital
Baltimore, Maryland

Emily Sydnor, MD
Fellow
Division of Infectious Diseases
The Johns Hopkins Hospital
Baltimore, Maryland

Patrick J. Troy, MD
Fellow
Division of Pulmonary and Critical
  Care Medicine
Harvard Medical School
Boston, Massachusetts

Tracy J. Wanner, MD
Fellow
Division of Pulmonary and Critical
  Care Medicine
Harvard Medical School
Boston, Massachusetts

Kevin E. Woods, MD
Fellow
Division of Gastroenterology
The Massachusetts General
  Hospital
Boston, Massachusetts

**Tinsay Ambachew Woreta,
MD, MPH**
Resident
Department of Medicine
The Johns Hopkins Hospital
Baltimore, Maryland

Baligh R. Yehia, MD
Fellow
Division of Infectious Disease
The University of Pennsylvania
Philadelphia, Pennsylvania

Series Reviewers

Rondeep S. Brar, MD
Stanford University
Stanford Hospital and Clinics

Doug Braucher
Iowa State University

Erica M. Fallon, MD
Harvard Medical School
Beth Israel Deaconess Medical Center

Olga Goldberg
Harbor UCLA Medical Center

Shreevidya V. Menon, BA, DO
Midwestern University
Cook County Hospital

Ahmed Mian
University of Ottawa Faculty of
  Medicine

Tung Ngo, DO, PhD
University of California Los Angeles
Kaiser Permanente, LAMC

John Ray
University of Texas Medical Branch

Jorge Rodriguez-Figueroa
Ponce School of Medicine

Shiwan K. Shah, DO
University of Texas Medical Branch at
  Galveston

Simant Shah
UMDMJ New Jersey Medical School

Stephanie C. Smith, MD
University of Minnesota

Niket Sonpal, MD
Brooklyn Queens Health Care

Anouar Teriaky
University of Ottawa Faculty of
  Medicine

Preface

The *Patient Encounters* series has been developed to provide a concise review of patient assessment and management. Each book in this series is organized logically and provides medical students with specialty-specific steps for managing patient care. The goal of this series is to remove the focus from "acing the shelf" to a focus on helping medical students become good doctors.

The books in this series provide a specialty-specific, step-by-step guide for managing a patient by candidly addressing, in a very practical fashion, a new clinical clerk's anxiety as well as hunger for learning. Each title within this series is a companion guide that candidly cuts to need-to-know info, directing medical students to what they need to do in each step of the patient encounter.

The books in this series discuss patient care from an overview of the disease or disorder, with brief pathophysiology information presented as necessary to support optimal patient assessment and care. It includes specific information that will help medical students from the point of reviewing the patient's chart to walking into the room and assessing the stability of the patient, including potential life threats. Each book then addresses acute management and workup, directing the student through the diagnosis, treatment, extended inhospital management, and discharge goals and outpatient care.

Each title provides students with the rationale for ordering appropriate diagnostic studies and allows clinical decision making that is consistent with the patient's disposition. The books provide an extended view of patient care so that the medical student can propose a well-informed choice of diagnostic studies and interventions when presenting his or her case to house staff and faculty.

The books use algorithms, tables, figures, icons, and a stylized design to support concise and easy-to-find patient management information. They also provide diagnosis-based, evidence-based information that includes peer-reviewed journal references.

Feedback from student reviewers gives high praise to this new series. Each of these new books was developed to provide practical information and to address the basics needed during a particular clinical rotation:

Patient Encounters: The Inpatient Pediatrics Work-Up
Patient Encounters: The Neurology and Psychiatry Work-Up
Patient Encounters: The Obstetrics and Gynecology Work-Up

How to Use This Book

Patient Encounters: The Internal Medicine Work-Up provides you with a concise, organized review of the most important patient assessment and management in internal medicine. This book is designed for you to quickly and efficiently review and enhance the knowledge you need to effectively manage patient care.

This book can help you ease the transition from the basic sciences to clinical medicine by providing you with a practical "how-to" guide for approaching a patient, including:

- Identifying pertinent positives and negatives in the patient history and physical exam
- Determining how to work up a patient by addressing pertinent diagnostic studies and procedures
- Explaining the rationale for clinical decision making

The 50 chapters in this text are divided into 9 sections. Each chapter features essential information related to patient assessment and management, supplemented with patient case studies that provide you with the opportunity to apply patient care principles and management goals to patient cases that are specific to each chapter's topic.

This book, as with all the books in the series, includes common features that will allow you to glean necessary information quickly and easily:

- **The Patient Encounter:** Each chapter begins with a patient case study that is followed up on at several intervals throughout the chapter. The patient encounter allows you the opportunity to see some of the common signs and symptoms with which a patient may present.
- **Overview:** This section provides an introduction to the chapter topic and includes the definition, epidemiology, and etiology of the disease or disorder. Brief pathophysiology information is included to support optimal patient assessment and care.
- **Acute Management and Workup:** This section includes the key information that you need to obtain in order to provide excellent patient care, addressing first what you need to do within the first 15 minutes through the first few hours. Topics include the initial assessment, admission criteria and level of care criteria, the patient history, the physical examination, labs and imaging to consider, and key treatment information.
- **Extended Inhospital Management:** This section provides information that you need to know when a patient needs extended inhospital management.

- **Disposition:** In this section, you will find the key discharge goals and outpatient care related to a patient with the specific condition or disorder addressed in the chapter.
- **What You Need to Remember:** This feature is a bulleted list of key points that are most helpful to remember about the chapter topic.
- **Suggested Readings:** Each chapter provides diagnosis- and evidence-based peer-reviewed journal references.
- **Clinical Pearl:** This feature presents clinical tips, statistics, or findings that will help you understand the patient's clinical presentation or help you better address diagnosis and management.

In addition to the features noted above, this text contains tables, line drawings, and photographs to supplement your learning.

I hope this text improves your knowledge of internal medicine, allowing you to feel confident that you're providing quality patient care. The ultimate goal of this book is to better prepare you to provide effective care to patients who you will encounter in your medical career.

Brian T. Garibaldi, MD
Division of Pulmonary and Critical Care Medicine
The Johns Hopkins Hospital
Baltimore, Maryland

Acknowledgments

I would like to recognize a number of individuals for helping to make this book become a reality. First and foremost I would like to thank Alfa Diallo for asking me to take the lead on the Internal Medicine book, and giving me the freedom to develop its content. I would also like to thank Julie Scardiglia for her insight, her thoughtfulness, and most importantly, her patience during this entire process.

Susan Bell was a constant inspiration to me throughout our residency training, and this book would never have gotten off the ground without her. Her keen insight into bedside physiology provided the main foundation for the cardiovascular section, and she was tireless in her efforts to help shape the style and content of the book. Patrick Troy is an exceptionally talented clinician-educator and joined the project at a time when we were in great need of his energy and his insight into medical student education. Clark Files' love of both music and medicine constantly reminded us why we embarked on this project in the first place. His practical approach to teaching helped to make the book accessible to medical students.

I would like to thank Dr. Charlie Wiener for encouraging me to take on this project. Over the last few years, he has shown me the kind of clinician, educator, and mentor that I hope to become during my career. I would also like to thank the Osler Housestaff for pushing me over the last 5 years to be the best doctor and person that I can be.

Finally, I would like to thank my family, especially my parents, Daniel and Kathleen Garibaldi, for giving me the unquestioning love and support that has helped me every step of the way.

Brian T. Garibaldi, MD

Contents

SECTION 9: Special Circumstances

Taking A History

INTRODUCTION

Obtaining a medical history from a patient interview can be one of the most difficult skills to grasp in medicine. Many physicians would argue that it is an art form in and of itself, and it can take years to become truly proficient. In this chapter, we will introduce you to key concepts that will expedite the learning curve when you come face to face with your first patient.

The two most important goals in obtaining a medical history are to gather all of the factual information that the patient has to offer and to do it in a way that is both comfortable for the patient and allows the patient to open up. These two parts are critically interrelated because the key to effective data gathering is allowing and encouraging the patient to speak. Beyond all laboratory tests and imaging, the medical history forms the cornerstone of diagnosing disease. In most situations, the patient himself or herself knows the cause of his or her symptoms. It is your job as the physician to enable the patient to express this knowledge in layman's terms and ultimately for you to translate this information into a medical diagnosis.

QUESTION TYPES

There are two broad types of questions that can be employed in a medical interview: the open-ended question and the direct question.

Open-Ended Questions

The open-ended question is one that can be answered in an infinite number of ways and allows the patient to lead the interview to wherever he or she desires. Examples of open-ended questions are:

"So, Mr. Brown, what brings you into the hospital today?"
"What do you think is the cause of your chest pain?"
"Tell me about how you have been feeling over the past week."

As illustrated by the last example, the "open-ended question" can also be a statement.

Direct Questions

The objective of the direct question is to obtain a specific piece of information; it generally only requires a few words to answer. A few examples of this type of question include:

"Where exactly is your chest pain?"

"Do you have any other symptoms when you get the chest pain?"
"Have you taken any medication for the pain?"

CONDUCTING THE PATIENT INTERVIEW

Every patient interview involves both open-ended and direct questions, but the key lies in knowing when to ask each type. Before starting the questioning in an interview, make sure you have introduced yourself and your role, and address the patient by his or her formal name. Then you should begin the interview with an open-ended question. This allows the patient to discuss what is most concerning to him or her, which is what should be most concerning to you, the physician. After asking a series of open-ended questions and allowing the patient to tell his or her story, it is appropriate to begin asking direct questions in order to "fill in the blanks." Even though direct questions seek to obtain specific information, it is important not to ask them in rapid-fire sequence. Often, the answer to one direct question will stimulate the next question. Ultimately, you must ask all of the necessary direct questions to obtain a thorough history, but you should ask them in a way that maintains the focus of the interview: helping the patient solve his or her problem, and *not* in a way that makes the patient feel he or she is answering questions to serve the doctor's agenda.

Questions Related to Patient Symptoms

In medical textbooks, you will commonly find lists of direct questions to ask that pertain to patient symptoms. These can be difficult to remember, so you may find the following mnemonic useful: *PPPQQRSST.* The following example uses pain as the symptom in question, but these questions can be applied to any symptom that the patient is having (e.g., shortness of breath, vomiting, etc.).

Presence: Where exactly is the pain located?
Provocation: What brings on the pain or worsens it?
Palliation: What relieves the pain or makes it abate?
Quality: How would you describe the pain?
Quantity: Using a scale of 1 to 10, how would you rate the pain?
Radiation: Does the pain spread anywhere?
Setting: What are you usually doing when the pain starts?
Symptoms associated: Do you have any other symptoms that occur when you have the pain?
Timing: Is the pain continuous or intermittent? How frequently do you experience the pain? How long does the pain last?

Always end a medical interview with an open-ended question so that the patient does not feel that he or she has left anything unaddressed. Examples of this type of question are:

"Are there any other concerns you have that we have not discussed?"
"Tell me what else you would like to talk about."

Remember to avoid medical jargon when asking patients questions, and gear your vocabulary to the patient's level of education. Even words that are considered part of layman's English, such as *constipation* or *incontinence*, are often not understood by patients, and a patient may incorrectly answer the question because of the embarrassment caused by admitting his or her lack of comprehension.

Observation

Although we have spent the majority of this chapter thus far discussing the type of information that needs to be gathered and the way in which questions should be phrased, there is an entire other side to the medical interview that does not involve words: body language. This is a two-way street in that the patient will be observing the physician while the physician is observing the patient.

Let's begin with the patient's perspective first. When taking a history, it is of the utmost importance to maintain good eye contact with the patient to show him or her that you are genuinely interested in what he or she is saying. Don't waste time taking extensive notes—if you pay attention, you will remember afterwards what the patient said. Maintain an appropriate distance with the patient (not too far to be standoffish and not too close to make him or her feel uncomfortable). Make sure to sit at the same eye level as the patient so that he or she doesn't feel as though he or she is being talked down to or lectured to. A recent study conducted in the United States showed that when patients were asked to recall medical encounters, they perceived the duration of the medical interview to be longer if the physician was seated than if standing. This is important because patient satisfaction has been correlated with perceived length of time spent doing a medical interview (1). If the situation is appropriate, feel free to touch the patient by placing your hand on his or her back or squeezing his or her hand. If you are still having trouble getting the patient to open up, oftentimes silence can be just what is needed to let a patient know that he or she can take his or her time and that you, the physician, are here to listen. This point takes on special significance in this age of high patient volumes and limited time slots per patient. One U.S. study found that physicians interrupted patients after a mean of 23.1 seconds, and once interrupted, patients rarely remembered to return to their original thought (2). Think of patient interruptions as missed chances to obtain valuable patient information.

From the physician's perspective, observing a patient plays a very large role in gathering information, particularly with patients who may not be able to give a history. Examples of this type of patient might include a nursing home resident with Alzheimer dementia or an asthmatic who is too short of breath to speak. Looking at the way the patient is dressed, observing his or her dental hygiene when he or she speaks, or taking note of the smells he or she exudes can all provide clues to his or her living situation and can help fill in the social history. The use of accessory muscles to breathe or a patient's level of anxiety can point to the severity of his or her respiratory distress. Listening to the manner in which a patient speaks and observing his or her affect can suggest the diagnoses of mania, depression, or even alcohol intoxication. Remember, anything affiliated with the patient (the presence of tattoos, medications hanging from an intravenous [IV] pole, family members sitting with the patient) should be noticed by you, the physician, and all of these things are fair game upon which to formulate more questions.

As a physician, you will assuredly be faced with difficult encounters due to a difference in cultural or social backgrounds between yourself and the patient. It is important to respect these differences, and to use whatever knowledge you have about the patient's background to facilitate the elicitation of information from the patient without causing him or her fear or embarrassment.

At the end of a medical interview, be sure to thank the patient for his or her time and shake the patient's hand.

Gathering the Patient's Medical History

For patients with a complicated medical history, or when interviewing a patient who is unable to provide much history, you will need to supplement your evaluation by gathering data from other sources. The "chart biopsy" (reviewing the patient's medical record to get a sense of his or her past problems) is daunting at first. Start by looking up information that is relevant to the patient's presenting complaint. You also will be able to fill in details that a patient would not likely know, such as the patient's last hemoglobin A1C level. For patients who are unable to provide a history, it is vital to assemble the story of what brought him or her to the hospital. Try to interview friends or family members who were with the patient when he or she became ill, even if it means calling them at home. Look at the emergency department record and the ambulance report to identify what the first responders could ascertain. If a patient is speaking a language you do not understand fluently, find a translator. Many hospitals employ translators that are available by telephone any time of the day or night. Just because a patient is unable to provide a history does not mean that this information should be excluded from your workup.

WHAT YOU NEED TO REMEMBER

The medical history is one of the most difficult skills to master. However, the benefits reaped from mastering this skill are arguably worth more than any other that you will learn in medicine. As you begin to conduct interviews for the first time, remember to sit down and show your patient that his or her time is important to you. Take notes if you have to, but make sure the patient knows that he or she is the center of your attention. Ask open-ended questions when possible, but do not be afraid to ask direct questions in order to gain important information. Be respectful and try not to interrupt your patient when he or she is speaking. Above all, observe your patient, and use this information to help refine your clinical impression when possible. Take your time learning this art; with practice comes perfection.

REFERENCES

1. Haney S, Lee D, Sur D, et al. Patient perception of physician position (4P study): does physician position influence patient perception of time? In Proceedings of UCLA Health Care, vol. 11. Los Angeles, CA: UCLA Department of Medicine; 2007.
2. Travaline JM, Ruchinskas R, D'Alonzo GE. *Patient-physician communication: why and how. J Am Osteopath Assoc.* 2005;105(1):13–18.

SUGGESTED READINGS

Marvel MK, Epstein RM, Flowers K, et al. Soliciting the patient's agenda: have we improved? *JAMA.* 1999;281(3):283–287.
Swartz MH. *Textbook of Physical Diagnosis.* 2nd ed. Philadelphia: W.B. Saunders; 1994.

The Physical Examination

INTRODUCTION

The key to the physical examination is to perform a thorough and organized assessment so that you do not miss pertinent findings and you gain the most information possible to help with your diagnosis and further management. One important component to developing strong physical examination skills is consistency: Perform your examination maneuvers in the same way each time. The other is practice. You will not appreciate subtle abnormalities on your physical exam until you have examined lots of "normal" patients. As medical students, take as much time as you need to examine your patients completely so that you begin to develop an idea of what is "normal" and what is "pathologic."

As you become more experienced, you will develop your own system for examining a patient that feels comfortable to you. This chapter will discuss the basic physical examination as it applies to all patients. The detailed assessment of each system is discussed in its corresponding chapter.

GENERAL OBSERVATION

General observation often gets overlooked during the examination but can provide extremely useful information. It includes a first impression from the moment you walk in the room as well as during your interview with the patient. Is the patient in any form of distress? Is he or she requiring oxygen therapy? What intravenous medications is he or she receiving? Is the patient placing himself or herself in a particular position to alleviate symptoms? Such questions may give you clues to the underlying diagnosis and the severity of the illness. These observations may also help to direct further questioning or even additional physical examination maneuvers during your time with the patient.

Take some time to think about your interaction with the patient, his or her body language, and any verbal cues from his or her communication. The patient's speech may be abnormal, as seen in neurologic disease, or muted and withdrawn, as seen in depression. The patient may even be confused and may not be able to communicate effectively; this can be a feature of central nervous system (CNS) disease or can even suggest poor perfusion to the brain, as can be seen in various forms of shock. You will be amazed by how much information you can gather about a patient just by carefully observing him or her during your interview and exam.

This is a good time to check the patient's vital signs, such as blood pressure, heart rate, respiratory rate, temperature, and oxygen saturation. The resulting measurements may change the way in which you manage a patient and help determine the level of care he or she will require once admitted.

SYSTEMATIC EXAMINATION

The importance of examining the patient without all of his or her clothes on cannot be overemphasized; if you don't take off the patient's shirt, you will be sure to miss the large thoracotomy scar the patient forgot to tell you about. This can be a very uncomfortable and personal experience for both you and your patient. Always remain courteous and try to respect the patient's privacy in a way that enables you to get everything you need from your patient. Never be afraid to ask for a chaperon when examining a patient, especially during breast, rectal, and genitourinary exams.

The Hands

A traditional place to start is the hands. Many disease processes manifest signs in the hands and nails. Examining the hands also provides a tactile contact with the patient that builds rapport. Take a look at the patient's nails, and observe the skin for rashes, swelling, color changes, and nodules (Table 2-1).

You also want to look for general skin changes, such as thinning, which can occur with steroid use; joint destruction and deformities, as are found in inflammatory arthritis; nodules (rheumatoid, tophaceous, xanthoma); and enlargement, as is seen in acromegaly.

The Head, Ears, Eyes, and Mouth

Every patient should undergo a thorough examination of the head and neck. Examine the hair for alopecia and hair thinning, often signs of autoimmune disease. Examine the face for rashes, deposits, or asymmetry. The examination should include an assessment of the eyes with funduscopy, if possible (see below). When examining the mouth, assess for the state of dentition, gum health, pigmentation, glossitis, mouth ulcers, and moistness of mucous membranes. The lips should be examined for pigmentation, puckering (i.e., systemic sclerosis), and telangiectasias.

The Neck

The carotid pulsation and the jugular venous pressure wave form will be discussed in the chapters corresponding to the cardiovascular system. Examination for lymph nodes should be done in a systematic way that includes the anterior and posterior triangle, as well as submandibular, occipital, preauricular, and supraclavicular areas. This is also a good time to examine the axillary lymph nodes so that these are not missed.

The thyroid is often not examined within a particular system, so it might be a good idea to include it in your general neck examination. Observe the neck to look for swelling, asymmetry, and thyroid movement; it is a good

TABLE 2-1
Physical Findings of the Hands and Nails

	Physical Finding	**Cause/Corresponding Disease**
Nails	Leuconychia (white nails)	Low albumin, liver disease/cirrhosis, protein-losing states
	Koilonychia (misshapen, concave nails)	Iron deficiency anemia—GI blood loss, malabsorption
	Clubbing (loss of angle at base of nail bed, soft tissue swelling, bogginess, and increased curvature of the nail)	Lungs—chronic hypoxia, carcinoma of the bronchus, chronic infection, bronchiectasis
		Liver—cirrhosis, Crohn disease, congenital
		Heart—congenital cyanotic heart disease, infective endocarditis
	Pitting of the nails	Poor health Psoriatic arthritis
	Onycholysis	Fungal infection of the nail bed
		Psoriatic arthritis
	Splinter hemorrhages	Infective endocarditis, septic emboli/vasculitis
Fingers	Tar stains	Smoking
	Osler nodes—red painful lumps on fingertips	Infectious endocarditis
	Janeway lesions—painless flat red papules on proximal fingers and palms	
	Heberden and Bouchard nodes—bony protuberances on DIP and PIP joints, respectively	Osteoarthritis

TABLE 2-1

Physical Findings of the Hands and Nails (Continued)

	Physical Finding	Cause/Corresponding Disease
Palms	Dupuytren's contracture—thickening of the palmar fascia with tethering of the fingers	Liver disease, drugs (phenytoin), occupational (vibrating tools), congenital/hereditary
	Palmar erythema—redness of palm that has central sparing	Chronic liver disease, pregnancy
	Muscle wasting	Neurologic compression, decreased innervation/use, protein or weight loss

DIP, distal interphalangeal; GI, gastrointestinal; PIP, proximal interphalangeal.

idea to observe while you ask the patient to swallow a sip of water. Palpation is most easily performed from behind, as you are able to use your fingertips to isolate nodules or enlargement. The thyroid should easily move as the patient swallows. Tethering or immobility may be a sign of malignancy. Percussion is not often performed, but in the setting of gross enlargement or anaplastic malignancy, the thyroid may extend retrosternally, causing compressive obstruction of the trachea. The last part of the examination should include auscultation for a bruit. In a hyperthyroid patient, a diffusely enlarged thyroid and a bruit are pathognomonic for Graves' disease.

The Chest

The pulmonary and cardiovascular examinations will be discussed in Chapters 4 and 16. In general, all patients should undergo a basic lung and heart examination. All women should undergo a yearly breast examination to assess for malignancy. This is often excluded during hospital assessment, but if malignancy is on your list of differential diagnoses, then a thorough examination is recommended.

The Abdomen

The abdominal examination can provide information about a wealth of organ systems, even in patients with no apparent abdominal complaints. The full gastrointestinal examination will be discussed in Chapter 31. As medical students, be sure to practice percussion and palpation of the liver and spleen.

Remember that, except in the thinnest of patients, a palpable spleen tip is abnormal and should warrant further investigation of either liver disease or infiltrative disorders such as malignancy. Always look for scars on the abdomen that can provide clues to prior surgical procedures and perhaps about ongoing medical conditions. The full abdominal examination should also include examination of the genitalia and rectum and a standing assessment for inguinal hernias. Remember to perform a pelvic examination in women with lower abdominal complaints, especially if they are sexually active.

The Nervous System

General observation is critical when assessing the neurologic system. Many neurologists will tell you that from the moment a patient walks down the hall to his or her clinical room, they are rapidly acquiring information from the patient's demeanor, walk, mobility, and speech. Higher cerebral functions such as cognition and memory will often have to be assessed by a specialist, but a simple Mini-Mental State Examination may provide crucial information. *Next Step: Patient Encounters in Neurology and Psychiatry* provides a more detailed assessment of the neurologic system.

Funduscopic Evaluation

Funduscopy is an important but extremely underutilized skill in the evaluation of the general medicine patient. The optic nerve and retina provide a window into the patient's microvasculature and central nervous system, and oftentimes provide invaluable information related to his or her underlying disease. If possible, funduscopy should be performed with the patient's pupils dilated. (Always let the nurse know that you are dilating your patient's eyes!) Start by standing several feet away from the patient to look for the red reflex (this may be obscured by cataracts). You should then focus on the disc. The edges should be crisp. Blurring of the disc edge suggests papilledema, which can be a sign of increased intracranial pressure. The disc should not be pale (optic atrophy) and the cup should be normal (deep cupping is seen in glaucoma). Follow the vessels from the disc starting with the arteries; look for narrowing, emboli, nicking of the veins, hemorrhages, and exudates. Dot and blot hemorrhages are characteristic of diabetes, whereas flame-shaped hemorrhages are seen with hypertension. Once you have looked at the vessels, check the background for pigmentation, deposits, or new vessels, as seen in proliferative diabetes. Lastly, ask the patient to look toward the light, at which point you will see the macula, a common area for significant degenerative disease. You should try to perform funduscopy on every patient you admit, but be especially vigilant in patients with hypertension, diabetes, and CNS complaints. Chapter 1 in *Next Step: Patient Encounters in Neurology and Psychiatry* discusses examination of the other cranial nerves in more detail.

Musculoskeletal Examination

All joints should be systematically examined, starting with inspection for swelling, erythema, nodules, and deformities. Take time to note every joint and the severity of how it is affected. Next, carefully palpate the joints to examine for tenderness, synovitis, and effusions. Many patients will have extremely painful joints, so be delicate and try not to hurt your patient. It is crucial to observe for rashes, including psoriasis, papules, and rheumatoid and tophaceous nodules; behind the ears or at the hairline are common places where they are likely to hide. Try to measure mobility and both passive and active movement. Patients may have restricted movement due to deformity, pain, or muscle weakness. Don't forget to examine the spine for curvature, tenderness, and restricted movement. A neurologic examination is also an integral part of any musculoskeletal examination, so you may find it helpful to combine the steps of each evaluation when assessing your patient.

 WHAT YOU NEED TO REMEMBER

The physical examination is one of the most important components of the medical encounter. Observation is critical to your physical exam and cannot be overemphasized. Remember that practice makes perfect—examining each patient in a meticulous and consistent manner will allow you to better understand the distinction between "normal" and "pathologic" and will help you to develop your own physical examination style.

SUGGESTED READINGS

Bickley LS, ed. *Bates' Guide to Physical Examination and History Taking*. 9th ed. Philadelphia: Lippincott Williams & Wilkins; 2007.

Fawcett RS, Linford S, Stulberg DL. Nail abnormalities: clues to systemic disease. *Am Fam Physician*. 2004;69(6):1417–1424.

Preparing the Write-up and Presenting on Rounds

In internal medicine, perhaps more than in any other specialty, communication of a patient's problem is vital to quality care. In medicine, the history, physical examination, and diagnostic tests all come together to provide information about a given patient with a given condition. No two patients are alike. Learning to communicate effectively is an important skill to be honed on your rotation, as it will be valuable in any medical specialty. The write-up of a medical admission will occupy a good portion of a medical student's time on the night he or she is admitting. As a student admitting fewer patients, your write-up should be the most thorough of all team members. As you progress to a subintern and eventually to a resident, the write-up may get shorter, but it should maintain key elements. Both the write-up and the oral presentation will be important to how the attending and residents evaluate your progress. The oral presentation will be limited in the information you can present in a reasonable amount of time. The write-up serves as a reference covering not only the most important features, but also all aspects of a particular case. The presentation is then your chance to sift through the myriad data and present a concise, clear case.

GENERAL INFORMATION ABOUT THE WRITE-UP AND PRESENTATION

The Write-up

The overall style of your write-up will in part depend on your hospital and even your attending physician's preference, but there are a few key elements that you should remember.

Write Legibly

It goes without saying that the write-up needs to be legible. Any review of a medical inpatient's chart will demonstrate that this is not always the case. If your handwriting is illegible, print. If that is still difficult to read, type. Even a medical student's write-up will become part of the permanent medical record.

Use Correct Spelling, Grammar, Punctuation, and Organization

The write-up is prepared as you are admitting a patient. You will not have the opportunity to proofread it the way you would a homework assignment or a manuscript. Do the best you can in the short time you have with spelling, grammar, and punctuation. The history of the present illness (HPI) and assessment and plan (A/P) sections should be written in complete sentences, with a logical flow of ideas through them. A sloppy write-up with poor grammar, spelling mistakes, and irrational organization will reflect poorly on the author.

Be Timely

Your attending or residents may have different requirements, but in general, the write-up of a patient you admit on call should be in the chart before rounds in the morning. If you want to use your write-up to present on rounds, make a copy of it and put the original in the chart.

Use Abbreviations Correctly

Medicine, internal medicine especially, contains a bewildering number of acronyms and abbreviations. These will creep into your lexicon as you progress through training. If you use an acronym or abbreviation in your write-up or presentation, make certain you know what it stands for and that it is presented correctly.

The Presentation

Your presentation style will also in part depend on your home institution, but there are a few general principles that should guide your organization.

Be Brief

Medicine rounds are notoriously too long. Even if your "rounds" are a card-flip while sitting in the office, word economy is an invaluable skill. This can be incredibly hard, especially at first and especially if you (as you should be) are obtaining a thorough history, performing a physical exam, and doing workups. An important idiom to keep in mind is the following: If you leave something out that you do not think is important but another person might, he or she can always ask you about it afterward.

Make a Case

Anyone can recite data. What you want to do with your presentation is support your assessment and plan for the patient. Begin with thinking about what you are going to say for your assessment and plan. Based on that, what case do you need to build in the HPI, past medical history (PMH), review of systems (ROS), physical examination, and tests to support your conclusions? If you conclude with an assessment that the patient has an ischemic coronary syndrome, you need to present in the HPI what it is about the patient's pain that makes you think so. You also need to present what historical features make you think that this is not a pulmonary embolism. You will need to mention when describing the physical exam that blood pressures were equal in both arms, making a case against aortic dissection. Now that you have an endpoint in mind, go through your presentation and pick out the important facts that led you to this conclusion. This will be how you choose what a *pertinent* positive and negative is. You want to present your conclusions like a lawyer trying a case. No one expects you to always be correct with your assessment, but what is expected of you is that you learn the thought and decision-making processes.

Do Not Read the Presentation

You have spent all night thoughtfully writing your history and physical (H&P). Now is not the time to read it verbatim. To effectively present on rounds, you need to engage your audience. Speak like you are telling your friends a story. This requires that you know the patient and the case extremely well. Some physicians may want you to present from memory. This is not to challenge your recall ability, but to make you organize the presentation in your head in digestible portions. As a student your load will be lighter; presenting from memory may be easier to try.

Be Respectful to the Patient

Bedside presentations used to be the norm. More and more, they are moving to the hallway or even to the conference room. That is unfortunate, because it removes the patient from the process. The level of respect and decorum should hold up regardless of where you are presenting. Speak as though your patient were in front of you. There is no place for complaining about the patient's complaints, the emergency department management, or the referring physician's oversights. You may see cynicism in your residents; this is unacceptable for anyone—especially a medical student.

Know Your Audience

If you present to three different attendings on your clerkship, undoubtedly you will be expected to present three different ways. Some attendings or residents will want you to be thorough and mention everything. Some might want a 1-minute bullet. You may be asked to read through all the labs so that the attending or resident can copy them down. As a trainee, all you can do is what they ask. The more you do, the more you will gain your own style. You will see residents and attendings who you feel communicate effectively, and you can adopt some of their techniques.

SPECIFIC INFORMATION ABOUT THE WRITE-UP AND PRESENTATION

Chief Complaint

In both the write-up and in the presentation the patient should be introduced with his or her chief complaint. This should ideally be in the patient's own words, and can usually be elicited by asking the patient why he or she came to the hospital or clinic today.

History of the Present Illness

The history of the present illness contains, in sentence format, the story of how your patient came to present, with his or her particular chief complaint. The narrative should follow a logical flow, whether you proceed temporally from the symptom or the problem's beginning or you organize it by level of importance. It is important to cover the qualifying factors for a given symptom (e.g., the "PQRST" mentioned in Chapter 1), but it is equally important to tell the story. You can mix in the patient's own descriptions with medical definitions; however, do not jump to make a diagnosis. The HPI will be the biggest piece of background evidence for the conclusions you will make in your assessment and plan. It is worth putting pertinent positive and negatives (i.e., those relating to the presenting symptom or problem) from the ROS in this section as well. When presenting the HPI on rounds, follow a logical flow and tell the story as opposed to making a series of disconnected factual statements.

The Past Medical History

The past medical history is usually written up in a list or bulleted format. For internal medicine patients, this may be extensive. The more PMH a patient has, the more important it is to provide the information in an organized fashion. The surgical history should also be added to the patient's PMH. Include items from your thorough interview, complemented with details (if available) from the medical record. For example, a patient you are admitting may have a chronic obstructive pulmonary disease (COPD) flare. You should look in the medical record for pulmonary function tests that document the severity of the patient's lung disease and for prior hospital admissions with COPD flares in which the patient may have required ventilatory support. For patients who are not able to provide a complete history, you may be able to ascertain parts of his or her medical history by looking at the patient's medication list. In addition to the presenting complaint, active features of the PMH will be included in the patient's ultimate problem list.

The Social and Family History

The relevance of a detailed social history will depend on the presenting problem. In general, the minimum that needs to be included is a statement about where the patient lives (and with whom) and what he or she does (or did) for a living, as well as the use of tobacco, alcohol, and illicit drugs. The family history should be included for any rare conditions, such as cystic fibrosis or sudden cardiac death, as well as for causes of death or major medical problems in first-degree relatives. This can be drawn out as a pedigree.

The Review of Systems

The review of systems is often included as a checklist and can be filled out as you are interviewing the patient. When presenting, you do not need to cover much ROS, if any. The pertinent positives and negatives should be included when you present the HPI.

Medications and Allergies

List all medications, including over-the-counter, as-needed medications, including the dosages, if possible. Also note any complementary or alternative treatments utilized by the patient. Medications should be recorded and presented by their generic names. All drug allergies should be documented, as well as the reaction (if known) when the patient is exposed to that allergen. *Relevant* food or environmental allergies should also be included.

Physical Examination

Document your complete physical exam. Record only findings that you appreciated, but also compare your exam with your resident's. It is acceptable to document portions of the exam that you did with your resident or attending. Include a description of the patient's general appearance. Spend the most time and "ink" with the portions of the exam that are relevant to the presenting complaint. Many preprinted H&P documents will not contain enough room for a detailed examination of any one organ system. On those preprinted documents, resist the temptation to simply check boxes. Describe only what you found in the portions of the exam that you did.

Diagnostic Tests

Include all admission labs, radiologic tests, electrocardiograms (ECGs), or other objective information. Mention also key tests that were done but the results of which are pending. For radiologic tests, distinguish between your interpretation and the radiologist's. Any abnormal lab deserves your consideration. In complicated patients in which there are often many abnormal labs, single out the most important (biggest change for the patient, biggest difference from a normal value) to consider in the patient's problem list (see below).

Assessment and Plan

There are several possible ways to organize the assessment and plan section of the write-up and presentation. You should check with your attending or clerkship director and use his or her preferred format. The way in which you organize this section may vary, depending on whether the case is a diagnostic dilemma or more of a management question. There are several key features that should be a part of any A/P section: (a) the summary statement or impression, (b) the problem list and, in certain cases, (c) the organization of problems by organ system.

Summary Statement or Impression

The A/P should start with a *one-sentence* summary of the patient's case. That statement should take into account all the information you have gathered and should communicate the most important features of the case. If you only had one sentence with which to present a patient, it should encompass everything you need to say. The impression will be the launching point for the discussion that will follow in the rest of the assessment and plan. Examples might include:

- "This is a 54-year-old man with cardiac risk factors presenting with chest pain and ECG changes."
- "This is a 75-year-old woman presenting with fatigue with renal insufficiency and electrolyte disturbances."

The summary statement or impression will usually not be the same as the patient's chief complaint, but instead is your interpretation of why the patient is admitted.

Problem List

For the write-up, the problem list should be comprehensive, encompassing all problems that you will evaluate, treat, or follow up on after hospitalization. Most often, each problem is the heading of a section of the A/P. Under each section/problem, you can write out what you plan to do to evaluate that problem and treat it. If the particular problem is a diagnostic uncertainty, you should provide a differential diagnosis. You should also reference back to the presenting problem and/or impression statement. For example, renal insufficiency as a problem in a patient presenting with heart failure needs to take into account that the kidney problem may be due to the heart failure, and that treatments for the heart failure may affect the patient's renal insufficiency. For your oral presentation, spend the most time on the most important problems. A thorough discussion of the differential of and plan for the patient's chest pain and ECG changes can be followed with a mere listing of their mild anemia, skin rash, and tinnitus.

Organization of Problems by Organ System

An alternative to organizing by problems and discussing each individually is to organize by organ system (e.g., pulmonary, cardiovascular, renal, neurologic, infectious disease, hematologic, gastrointestinal, endocrine). The headings of the A/P (after the impression statement) are each organ system. Under those headings, you discuss relevant problems and treatments. This is often done in the intensive care unit, where patients are likely to have multiple organ system pathology. It may be preferable in a general medicine patient to use a problem-based approach. However, it is worth going through a mental list of organ systems to ensure that you are not overlooking something.

In general, be as thorough in this section as possible. This is your chance to demonstrate how much information you have gathered and, more importantly, how well you organize it. A good example of the reasoning you should be using can be found in *The New England Journal of Medicine's* Clinical Pathologic Correlates.

WHAT YOU NEED TO REMEMBER

Communicating effectively is certainly a daunting task for a trainee. Just as it is impossible to learn all of medicine in your rotation, it is equally difficult to master the write-up and oral presentation. With more specialization and more transitions of care, these skills are vitally important to being a good physician, regardless of your specialty. Communicating well through the write-up and presentation are skills worth cultivating. In learning what to say and what not to say, you are learning the important distinguishing characteristics of a case.

SUGGESTED READINGS

Brancati FL. A piece of my mind. The generic H & P. *JAMA*. 1989;262(23):3338.
Brancati FL. Readers of the lost chart: an archaeologic approach to the medical record. *JAMA*. 1992;267(13):1860–1861.

Approach to the Cardiovascular Evaluation

In the chapters within this section, we will address conditions that fall into the category of cardiovascular disease that, together, represent the most common presentation of adult patients to the medical profession. The cardiovascular system does not include just the heart but the vascular system as well; together they are intimately linked to other organ systems, such as the kidneys, lungs, and brain. On first glance, the assessment of the cardiovascular patient may appear overwhelming. If you were asked to diagnose a patient with mitral stenosis just from listening to his or her heart sounds, then you would probably not get the diagnosis right or be able to understand the physiologic consequences of the valvular lesion. Alternatively, if you start with the patient and the history of his or her symptoms and then follow through with a full examination, the auscultation of the precordium will just serve as confirmation of the diagnosis that you already suspect.

Cardiovascular Physiology

The heart and vascular system in their simplest form consist of a pump with chambers and corresponding tubes. This system carries blood around the body with the ultimate goal of delivering oxygen and nutrients to the tissues.

The cardiac cycle is continuous but, for simplicity, is divided into two parts:

1. *Systole* is the phase in the cardiac cycle during which the ventricle contracts, and by increasing pressure (isovolumic contraction), ejects blood from the ventricle into the arterial system. This period starts with isovolumic contraction and ends when the left ventricle relaxes, causing pressure to fall in the ventricular chamber. At the end of systole, forward flow ceases due to equalization of pressures between the ejecting ventricle and the receiving vasculature. At this point, the aortic and pulmonary valves close and diastole begins.
2. *Diastole* makes up about two thirds of the cycle and encompasses the relaxation and then the filling of the ventricular chambers with blood from the atrium. The coronary arteries are also perfused during diastole.

The previous description defines cardiologic systole and diastole; however, true physiologic systole and diastole occur at the time points of initiation of contraction and relaxation. These are very difficult to measure in vivo, so the borders of the cycle are taken from the first and second heart sounds using closure of the valves as a surrogate.

The function of the ventricle is composed of three separate components—contractility, preload, and afterload—that you will hear mentioned frequently whenever a patient with cardiovascular disease is discussed.

Contractility

Contractility refers to the intrinsic ability of the myocardium to contract and generate force independent of any loading factors.

Preload

Preload is the load on the ventricle prior to contraction. It is a function of the volume already within the ventricle at the end of systole and primarily a function of filling from the atrial cavity during diastole. It is a difficult concept to understand, but you can think of it as similar to the volume and load of all your groceries on a grocery bag. The myocardium, however, is not like a fixed sack—it is made up of an intrinsic network of filaments that together orchestrate shortening and thickening of the myocardial tissue and therefore ejection. What is interesting about the impact of preload on the ventricle as described by Frank and Starling is that increased filling, and therefore increased volume in diastole, leads to increased inotropy as evidenced by increased stroke volume and force of contraction. In other words, the more you fill the normal healthy heart in diastole, the greater the stroke volume and the force at which blood is ejected. However, there comes a point during which the stretch of the heart by increased filling is greater than the ability of the actin and myosin to remain connected in their architectural harmony; they struggle to contract against the increased volume and pressure. At this point on the left ventricle (LV) filling versus stroke volume curve, the Frank-Starling relationship no longer holds true and the result of increased preload is a reduction in LV function (Fig. 4-1).

Afterload

The concept of afterload is difficult even for a cardiologist to understand. Afterload, just like preload, is independent of the intrinsic contractility of the heart. One way of thinking of afterload is that it is the load the ventricle has to overcome to perform its job during systole. This load is essentially the column of blood located just after the aortic valve. It is determined by the intrinsic pressure within the arterial system, which is generated by the size of the vessel, the compliance of the vessel, the volume of fluid within the system, the wave of pressure that is generated during systole, and the reflection of that wave during diastole.

Compliance

Compliance is the change in volume for a given change in pressure of a system. In a normal healthy individual, the compliance of the heart and vessels is extremely adaptive due to the natural elasticity of the substrate. For a change in volume, the increase in pressure is low. The walls of the system are able to withstand and absorb the change without increasing the pressure. However, as cardiovascular disease progresses, the heart chambers and the arterial vessels become stiff and noncompliant due to changes in architecture,

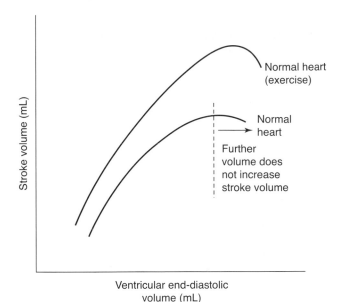

FIGURE 4-1: The Frank-Starling curve illustrates the relationship between ventricular end-diastolic volume (preload) and stroke volume in the normal heart.

increased collagen deposition, reduced and fragmented elastin, and hypertrophy and fibrosis that occurs as an adaptation to stress. Changes in volume that previously were hemodynamically less significant now have a large impact on pressure. The result is rapidly increasing pressures for the same given volume previously encountered as seen in disease states such as hypertension, ischemia, and diastolic heart failure.

Pressure–Volume Relationship Curves

You will see disease processes that refer back to the relationship between the pressure and volume that occurs in the ventricle. This is especially true when discussing heart failure and valvular disease. If you can learn to draw a pressure volume loop for the normal heart, then you can translate a pressure–volume curve for each disease as it relates to the normal heart. This will help you to understand the differences in hemodynamics and how they impact on symptoms and clinical signs (Fig. 4-2).

PATIENT EVALUATION

The history, physical examination, and electrocardiogram are the most important components of the cardiovascular evaluation.

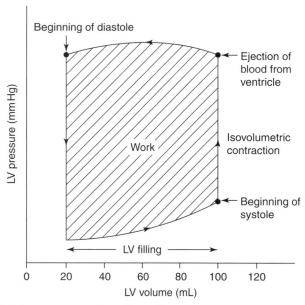

FIGURE 4-2: Pressure–volume loop illustrating normal left ventricular (LV) function. The area inside the loop represents "work" for the left ventricle.

History

The history of the presenting complaint is critical in cardiovascular disease. The characteristics of pain caused by ischemic heart disease can be very different from pain caused by inflammation of the pleural space. Therefore, when taking a history of chest pain, try to listen to the patient as he or she describes the character, severity, position, relief, exacerbation, and timing of the pain. It is helpful to ask about chest pain in several ways, including asking the patient to describe his or her pain as discomfort, squeezing, or pressure; patients may not describe ischemic symptoms as pain and, in certain circumstances, such as with older female or diabetic patients, their main symptom could be shortness of breath or nausea. Other important points in the history should focus on cardiac disease in family members, including premature coronary artery disease and congenital disease, including sudden death. The patient's social history should focus not only on his or her smoking and alcohol use, but also on daily activities and limitations as these items will help classify the severity of his or her disease.

Physical Examination

When examining the patient with cardiovascular disease, the following areas deserve particular attention: the peripheries and pulse, jugular venous pressure, the precordium, and auscultation.

The Peripheries and Pulse

First, touch the patient and get a quick assessment of the temperature of the peripheries. This will give you a sense of the cardiac output—cool extremities in a cardiovascular patient tend to mean a low cardiac output. The pulse can give you a wealth of information about the flow of blood from the ventricle to the vasculature. Try to take a moment to feel the radial pulses and then the radial and femoral pulses simultaneously, as these pulses may be an important sign to diagnose aortic or subclavian stenotic disease. The character of the pulse should be measured at the carotid. When assessing the carotid pulse, get a sense of the timing of maximum pulsation, the force, and the waveform, as if your fingers are tracing out a plot.

Jugular Venous Pressure

The art of examining the jugular venous pressure is difficult to master; however, some time spent examining the height of the pulsation at 45 degrees, the waveform, and timing with the carotid pulse will help you to notice abnormalities when they are present. The importance of this becomes clear when you examine a patient who has a cardiomyopathy or pericardial disease (especially tamponade), as the estimate of mean atrial pressure by jugular venous pressure height and characteristics of the waveform in these diseases can help with immediate management.

Precordial Examination

The precordial examination should start with inspection for heaves, thrills, or other chest wall findings, such as a sternotomy scar, which is suggestive of a prior surgery. Next, palpate the apex checking its exact position; a normal apex beat should be palpated with one to two fingers and lie in the fifth intercostal space in the midclavicular line. Left and right ventricular heaves can be palpated over the point of maximal impulse and at the left sternal edge, respectively. Thrills may be palpated over their respective valvular areas.

Auscultation and the Evaluation of Other Organs

By this point, you should already have some idea of what you may hear on auscultation. Carefully listen to the heart sounds in each area with the diaphragm and also with the bell at the apex. At each area, first listen for the first and second heart sounds and their timing in the cycle, trying to get a sense of the rhythm. Next, listen for added sounds, rubs, or murmurs. Extra heart sounds occur between the second and first heart sound and can be characteristic of ventricular pathology. A rub tends to run through the systolic component of the cycle but has a harsher, rough sound and is not confined by the borders of the heart sounds. In comparison, a murmur should be defined by its character, its place in the cardiac cycle (i.e., systolic or diastolic, or early, midcycle, or late), the area where it is heard loudest, and the area to which it radiates. The exam should include all other areas related to the cardiovascular system, including the lungs, the liver, central vessels, peripheral vasculature, and, finally, the retina.

Key Diagnostic Evaluations

Laboratory investigation should be directed to diagnosis and management.

Laboratory Tests

Cardiac enzymes and brain natriuretic peptide in the correct setting are appropriate. A basic metabolic panel will also provide information about electrolyte abnormalities and renal function and may be especially important in patients with heart failure who are on diuretic therapy.

Imaging

In most cases of cardiovascular disease, an electrocardiogram (ECG) is useful for both its negative and positive findings.

CLINICAL PEARL

If a prior ECG, even from a different source/hospital, can be made available, then try to compare the data—subtle changes may only be evident with comparison.

A chest radiograph, although often normal, can provide evidence of congenital disease, anomalies, cardiac silhouette, and chamber size, and can provide evidence of a noncardiac pathology. Further investigations, such as echocardiography and cardiac catheterization, will be discussed in specific chapters.

WHAT YOU NEED TO REMEMBER

- A thorough understanding of a normal flow–volume loop will greatly help when you encounter patients with heart failure or valvular heart disease.
- The history is one of the most important components of the cardiovascular evaluation.
- Practice evaluating the jugular venous pulsation in all of your patients, because this often provides invaluable information about a patient's hemodynamics.
- Auscultation should be the last part of your examination and oftentimes will confirm what observation, percussion, and palpation have already suggested.
- The ECG is critical and, when possible, should be compared to previous studies.

SUGGESTED READINGS

Bickley LS. The cardiovascular system. In: *Bates' Guide to Physical Examination & History Taking*. Philadelphia: Lippincott Williams & Wilkins; 2007.

Braunwald E, Zipes D, Libby P, et al., eds. *Braunwald's Heart Disease: A Textbook of Cardiovascular Medicine*. 7th ed. Philadelphia: Elselvier Saunders.

Dubin D. *Rapid Interpretation of EKG's: An Interactive Course*. Tampa, FL: Cover Publishing Company; 2001.

Acute Coronary Syndromes

THE PATIENT ENCOUNTER

A 62-year-old man is brought to the emergency department by ambulance after experiencing chest pain at home. The pain began 45 minutes prior while watching TV and is described as a dull but severe substernal pressure that radiates to his left arm and jaw. He states he became very sweaty and short of breath when the pain began. His blood pressure on presentation is 160/100 mm Hg, his pulse is 98 bpm, his temperature is 37.1°C (98.7°F), his respiratory rate is 20 breaths per minute, and his oxygen saturation is 98% on room air. The patient appears anxious and diaphoretic, and his hand is clenched over his chest. He has mild crackles at both lung bases, and his cardiac exam is unremarkable except for an S_4 gallop.

OVERVIEW

Definition

The term *acute coronary syndrome* (ACS) refers to a continuum of myocardial ischemia that ranges from unstable angina to non–ST-elevation myocardial infarction (NSTEMI, sometimes called *non–Q-wave myocardial infarction*) to ST-elevation myocardial infarction (STEMI, sometimes called *Q-wave myocardial infarction*). More than 90% of cases of ACS result from an acute disruption of an atherosclerotic plaque in a coronary artery with subsequent platelet aggregation and formation of an intracoronary thrombus, which leads to an imbalance between myocardial oxygen supply and demand. The form of ACS that results depends on the degree of coronary obstruction and the resulting ischemia. Unstable angina and NSTEMI are closely related and are typically caused by a partially occlusive thrombus. They present with similar symptoms, with NSTEMI being distinguished from unstable angina by the presence of cardiac biomarkers of myocardial necrosis. A STEMI is typically caused by a completely occluded coronary artery and results in more severe ischemia and a potentially large amount of necrosis.

Pathophysiology

Atherosclerotic plaque rupture leads to thrombus formation via two major mechanisms: (a) platelet aggregation via exposure of subendothelial collagen and (b) activation of the coagulation cascade via exposure of tissue factor from the atheromatous plaque core. Once platelets are activated they release their granule contents, causing further platelet aggregation, further activation of the coagulation cascade, and release of vasoconstrictors such as thromboxane and serotonin. In addition to the two major mechanisms described previously, another contributing mechanism of thrombus formation is coronary endothelial dysfunction due to atherosclerosis. This dysfunction impairs the release of nitric oxide and prostacyclin, both potent vasodilators. Vasodilatation helps prevent thrombus formation by augmenting blood flow (which minimizes contact between procoagulant factors) and by reducing shear stress (an inducer of platelet activation).

Thrombus formation causes ischemia and infarction of myocardial tissue, and this can have a devastating impact on cardiac function. Infarction quickly leads to impaired ventricular contraction and systolic dysfunction, which compromises cardiac output. Depending on the size, location, and extent of the infarction, certain types of ventricular wall motion abnormalities can result. A localized region of reduced contraction is termed *hypokinetic*; a segment that does not contract at all is called *akinetic*; and a *dyskinetic* region is one that bulges outward during contraction of the remaining functional portions of the ventricle. Ischemia and infarction can also impair diastolic relaxation, which is an energy-dependent process, leading to diastolic dysfunction and elevated ventricular filling pressures. If the dysfunction of the myocardium is caused by transient ischemia and infarction does not result, the period of dysfunction is sometimes reversible and is referred to as *stunned myocardium*. Stunned myocardium is tissue that demonstrates prolonged systolic dysfunction after a discrete episode of severe ischemia, despite restoration of adequate blood flow, and gradually regains contractile force days to weeks later.

Epidemiology

Cardiovascular disease is the leading cause of death in the United States, and coronary artery disease (CAD) significantly increases the risk of developing ACS. Approximately 1.7 million people are hospitalized for ACS each year. Roughly 30% of these patients will have a STEMI, resulting in an estimated 500,000 STEMI events in the United States each year (1).

Etiology

Some significant risk factors for coronary heart disease include age (over 80% of patients who die of CAD are older than 65 years of age), male sex, a family history, smoking, high cholesterol, hypertension, physical inactivity, obesity, and diabetes. As mentioned previously, more than 90% of ACS is caused by rupture of an atherosclerotic plaque; however, the exact mechanism of atherosclerosis that leads to plaque rupture and ACS has not been fully elucidated. The general causes of plaque disruption appear to be chemical factors that destabilize atherosclerotic lesions and physical stresses to which the lesions are subjected. ACS can sometimes occur in the setting of certain triggers, such as physical or emotional stress. The activation of the sympathetic nervous system in these situations increases the blood pressure, heart rate, and force of ventricular contraction, actions that may stress the atherosclerotic lesion, thereby causing the plaque to fissure or rupture. ACS is more likely to occur in the early morning hours, which may be related to the tendency of key physiologic stressors such as systolic blood pressure, blood viscosity, and plasma epinephrine levels to be most elevated during that time of day.

In addition to plaque rupture, ACS has some much less frequent alternative causes. These causes include significant coronary vasospasm (primary or cocaine induced); severe narrowing alone (e.g., progressive atherosclerosis or restenosis after stent placement); coronary trauma, aneurysm, or dissection; coronary emboli (often from endocarditis or artificial valves); vasculitic syndromes; significantly increased blood viscosity (e.g., polycythemia vera, thrombocytosis); and congenital anomalies of the coronary arteries.

ACUTE MANAGEMENT AND WORKUP

Time is myocardium! The initial assessment of chest pain should focus on quickly determining if the patient is truly suffering from an ACS.

The First 15 Minutes

Whether the patient is having unstable angina, a NSTEMI, or a STEMI, the initial management is essentially the same.

Initial Assessment

Before Coming to the Hospital

Patients in the community with symptoms of possible ACS, including chest discomfort with or without radiation to the arm(s), back, neck, jaw, or epigastrium; shortness of breath; weakness; diaphoresis; nausea; and lightheadedness should be instructed to call 911 and should be transported to the hospital by ambulance rather than by friends or relatives. This is especially true if the patient complains of chest discomfort or other ischemic symptoms at rest for >20 minutes, has hemodynamic instability, or has recent syncope or presyncope. Patients for whom nitroglycerin (NTG) tablets have been previously prescribed may take *one* dose of the NTG sublingually at home. If the chest discomfort is not improved or worsens, the patient should call 911 and be brought to the emergency department (ED). In patients with chronic *stable* angina, it is appropriate if the patient repeats the sublingual NTG every 5 minutes for a maximum of three doses and then calls 911 if symptoms don't resolve. Prior to arriving at the hospital, emergency medical service (EMS) providers should administer 162 to 325 mg of aspirin (chewed) unless contraindicated or already taken by the patient. In addition, EMS providers may obtain and evaluate a 12-lead electrocardiogram (ECG), if available, to help in the early triage of the patient.

In the Emergency Department

If a patient shows up in the ED with chest pain, it is important to triage the patient quickly, categorizing the patient as having a low, intermediate, or high risk of obstructive coronary disease. The patient in our vignette has a concerning story for an acute coronary syndrome and should be evaluated immediately. A 12-lead ECG should be obtained and presented to an experienced emergency physician *within 10 minutes* of arrival for all patients with chest discomfort or other symptoms suggestive of ACS. This can be a major branch point in the management of ACS. In unstable angina or NSTEMI, ST-segment depression and/or T-wave inversions are most common on ECG. These abnormalities may be transient, occurring just during chest pain episodes in unstable angina, or they may persist in patients with NSTEMI. If the ECG shows ST elevations consistent with a STEMI or a *new* left bundle branch block, the ED should have a specific protocol in place to initiate immediate reperfusion therapy for the patient if he or she is determined as being eligible (Fig. 5-1). Typically, these protocols involve an immediate cardiology consult. If you are the first provider to evaluate a patient who you suspect is having a STEMI, notify an ED attending or a cardiologist *immediately*. The management of STEMI is beyond the scope of this book, but the basic approach will be discussed below.

Admission Criteria and Level of Care Criteria

The history, physical exam, 12-lead ECG, and initial cardiac biomarker tests should be integrated to categorize patients with chest pain into one of four categories: (a) a noncardiac diagnosis, (b) chronic stable angina, (c) possible ACS, and (d) definite ACS. Patients with probable or possible ACS but whose initial 12-lead ECG and cardiac biomarkers are normal should be observed in a facility with cardiac monitoring, and repeat ECG and repeat cardiac biomarker measurements should be obtained, often for 24 hours if all are negative. In patients with suspected ACS in whom ischemic heart disease is present or suspected, if the follow-up ECG and biomarkers are normal, a stress test to provoke ischemia should be performed in the ED, in a chest pain unit, or on an outpatient basis within 72 hours as an alternative to inpatient admission.

CLINICAL PEARL

An alternative to stress testing that is gaining utility in this type of patient is a noninvasive coronary imaging test such as coronary computed tomography (CT) angiography.

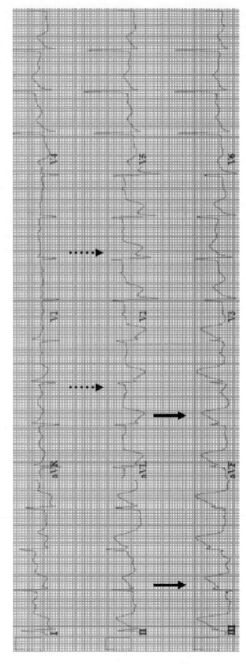

FIGURE 5-1: 12-lead electrocardiogram showing inferior ST-segment elevations (solid arrows) and reciprocal changes (dotted arrow) in a patient with an acute ST-elevation myocardial infarction. (Courtesy of Andrew DeFilippis, MD, Division of Cardiology, The Johns Hopkins Hospital.)

Patients with definite ACS and ongoing ischemic symptoms, positive cardiac biomarkers, new ST-segment deviations, new deep T-wave inversions, hemodynamic abnormalities, or a positive stress test should be admitted to the hospital. Admission to the cardiac intensive care unit is recommended for those with active, ongoing ischemia and hemodynamic or electrical instability. Otherwise, admission to a telemetry step-down unit is reasonable.

The First Few Hours

In a patient with chest pain that is suspicious of ACS, after the first 15 minutes, the patient should have undergone an ECG and received initial treatments to halt platelet aggregation and thrombus growth, as well as have received medications to decrease the oxygen demand of the heart (discussed below). STEMI patients should be on their way to immediate reperfusion, while patients with ST depressions or T-wave inversions require further evaluation to determine if urgent reperfusion is warranted. If the initial ECG is nondiagnostic but the patient remains symptomatic and there is high clinical suspicion for ACS, serial ECGs, initially at 15- to 30-minute intervals, should be performed to detect the potential for development of ST-segment elevation or depression. Cardiac biomarkers (creatine kinase [CK], CK-MB, troponin) should be measured in all patients who present with chest discomfort consistent with ACS, with troponin being the preferred marker. Patients with negative cardiac biomarkers within 6 hours of the onset of symptoms should have biomarkers remeasured within 8 to 12 hours after symptom onset. It is reasonable to measure positive biomarkers at 6- to 8-hour intervals two to three times or until levels have peaked.

History

The patient history is critical when evaluating a patient with chest pain. Noncardiac chest pain is very common, and incorrectly diagnosing a patient with ACS can lead to potentially harmful medications and procedures. The five most important factors in the initial history are (a) the nature of the anginal symptoms, (b) a prior history of CAD, (c) sex (especially male), (d) age older than 65, and (e) the presence of coronary risk factors such as diabetes, hypercholesterolemia, hypertension, and a family history of coronary disease. Patients with unstable angina/NSTEMI may have discomfort typical of chronic angina except that the episodes are more severe, are prolonged, occur at rest, or are precipitated by less exertion. The chest discomfort is typically substernal and is described more as pressure than as pain. Some patients have no chest discomfort (especially women and diabetics) but present solely with jaw, neck, arm, shoulder, back, or epigastric discomfort; unexplained dyspnea without discomfort; or, occasionally, nausea. Unstable angina presents as an acceleration of stable angina symptoms (e.g., longer, more frequent, and/or more intense), angina that now occurs at rest, or new-onset angina in a patient without known CAD. NSTEMI and STEMI present with more crushing substernal chest pain that is prolonged and with more radiation (typically to the left arm and jaw). If the pain is sharp, very transient (a few seconds), reproducible with movement or palpation, or radiates to the lower extremities, it is likely not ACS.

Physical Examination

The physical examination of a patient with chest pain is often used to assess the hemodynamic impact of the ischemia, to search for precipitants of ischemia, or to rule out other noncardiac causes of the chest pain. Some precipitants of ischemia include uncontrolled hypertension, thyrotoxicosis, or gastrointestinal bleeding. On examination, listen for an S_3 or S_4 gallop (a dilated or stiff ventricle, respectively) and pulmonary rales (congestive heart failure). Jugular venous distention suggests right heart failure. Many patients with ACS become diaphoretic, cold, and clammy. If the patient has unequal pulses, think of aortic dissection; if you hear a friction rub, think acute pericarditis—both are important diagnoses as providing anticoagulation to these patients can be detrimental. Cardiogenic shock manifested by hypotension and evidence of end-organ hypoperfusion can occur in patients with NSTEMI or STEMI and constitutes a medical emergency.

The Killip classification of heart failure signs and symptoms in this setting provides a helpful prognostic evaluation: (a) Killip Class 1 is the absence of rales on examination; (b) Killip Class 2 is the presence of rales, an elevated jugular venous pressure, and an S_3 gallop; (c) Killip Class 3 is the presence of frank pulmonary edema; and (d) Killip Class 4 is cardiogenic shock. Mortality from myocardial infarction increases as the Killip class increases.

Labs and Tests to Consider

Cardiac biomarkers and an ECG are the most important tests in your evaluation of a patient with suspected ACS.

Key Diagnostic Labs and Tests

As discussed previously, the most important labs to draw early in your evaluation are the cardiac enzymes CK, CK-MB, and troponin (and sometimes myoglobin). These can help you determine if a patient is having an ACS, and if so the time frame and extent can often be elucidated. Any positive troponin should be concerning and fully worked up. The earliest rising biomarkers are myoglobin and CK, detectable at 2 hours but not cardiac specific. They are usually undetectable after 24 hours. Troponin and CK-MB are detectable at 2 to 4 hours, but can be delayed for up to 8 to 12 hours. CK-MB returns to normal in 2 to 3 days, but troponin often remains elevated for 7 to 12 days. Other initial labs to order include a comprehensive metabolic panel (look specifically at the creatinine level and liver function tests), complete blood count, coagulation studies, and thyroid-stimulating hormone. If the patient appears to be in cardiogenic shock, check a lactate. A brain natriuretic peptide can also be helpful to evaluate for congestive heart failure and can provide prognostic information. Given recent evidence, checking C-reactive protein (a marker of inflammation) may be useful.

Imaging

A chest radiograph should be obtained in all patients who present with chest pain. If aortic dissection or pulmonary embolism is suspected, a CT with intravenous (IV) contrast may be warranted. In patients with suspected cardiogenic shock, an immediate bedside echo may be useful to determine a rough estimate of ejection fraction and to rule out a pericardial effusion.

Treatment

The treatment of ACS depends in part on the severity of the presentation (i.e., NSTEMI vs. STEMI), but there are several general principles that apply to patients with ongoing coronary ischemia.

The General Initial Treatment of Acute Coronary Syndrome

Supplemental oxygen should be administered to patients with an arterial oxygen saturation level <90% or respiratory distress, although it is reasonable to administer oxygen to all ACS patients during the first 6 hours of presentation. Sublingual nitroglycerin 0.4 mg every 5 minutes for three doses should be given to all patients with ongoing ischemic discomfort, and if the pain is not relieved, consider an IV nitroglycerin drip, especially in patients with heart failure or hypertension, as in our patient from the encounter. NTG should *not* be given to patients with systolic blood pressure <90 mm Hg or 30 mm Hg below baseline, severe bradycardia (<50 bpm), tachycardia (>100 bpm), or suspected right ventricular infarction; in patients who have received phosphodiesterase inhibitors for erectile dysfunction in the past 24 to 48 hours; or in patients with critical aortic stenosis. IV morphine can also be given to help relieve ischemic pain. Aspirin (162–325 mg) should be chewed by all patients with ACS as soon as possible if they did not receive it at home or in transport. Oral or IV beta-blocker therapy should be promptly initiated in all patients unless they have signs of heart failure, evidence of a low-output state, an increased risk of cardiogenic shock, or other relative contraindications to beta-blocker therapy, such as a PR interval >0.24, second- or third-degree heart block, or reactive airway disease. Of note, if the patient is borderline hypotensive and you must choose between NTG and a beta-blocker, the beta-blocker should be given first.

Treatment of Unstable Angina and Non–ST-Elevation Myocardial Infarction

Two treatment pathways have emerged for treating patients with unstable angina and NSTEMI—the "early invasive" strategy and the "conservative" strategy. Patients treated with the early invasive strategy undergo coronary angiography within 4 to 24 hours of admission. The conservative strategy calls for invasive evaluation only with symptomatic failure of medical therapy or other objective evidence of recurrent or latent ischemia. The cardiology team should typically be involved to discuss the management strategy, because the patient's condition is often complicated. In general, higher-risk patients with recurrent symptoms, elevated troponin levels, ECG changes, hemodynamic instability, or an ejection fraction <40% are typically managed with the invasive strategy. Regardless of the strategy chosen, all patients with unstable angina or NSTEMI should be admitted and placed on a cardiac monitor. Patients should initially be placed on bedrest and mobilized once they are symptom-free. Most patients benefit from clopidogrel, an antiplatelet therapy, in addition to aspirin unless there is some reason to suspect the patient may need urgent coronary artery bypass grafting (CABG); clopidogrel should be held for 5 to 7 days prior to CABG (CABG is often used for patients with multivessel disease, especially in diabetics). Anticoagulant therapy, typically with unfractionated heparin or low-molecular-weight heparin, should be added to antiplatelet therapy as soon as possible after presentation to prevent further thrombus formation. More recently, the alternative use of bivalirudin has been added to the American College of Cardiology guidelines. It is important to note that fibrinolytic therapy is *not* indicated in unstable angina or NSTEMI and can be harmful.

The Treatment of ST-Elevation Myocardial Infarction

The key to achieving good outcomes in patients with a STEMI is rapid diagnosis and immediate reperfusion. The two primary ways of opening up occluded coronary arteries are with fibrinolytics and percutaneous coronary intervention (PCI). In general, the goal is to facilitate rapid recognition and treatment so that (a) the door-to-needle time for initiation of fibrinolytic therapy can be achieved within 30 minutes or (2) the door-to-balloon time for PCI can be kept under 90 minutes. If the presentation is <3 hours from the onset of symptoms and there is no delay to PCI, there is no real preference for either strategy. Fibrinolysis is generally preferred if it is 3 hours or less from symptom onset, PCI is not an option, or there is a delay to invasive strategy (door-to-balloon minus door-to-needle time >1 hour). PCI is generally preferred if a skilled PCI laboratory is available with a door-to-balloon minus door-to-needle time <1 hour, the patient is in cardiogenic shock, there are contraindications to fibrinolysis, the symptom onset was >3 hours prior, or the diagnosis of STEMI is in doubt.

EXTENDED IN-HOSPITAL MANAGEMENT

All patients with ACS should be on aspirin 81 to 162 mg, a beta-blocker, an angiotensin-converting enzyme inhibitor (ideally started within the first 24 hours of presentation), a statin, and possibly clopidogrel. Exercise testing should be performed either in the hospital or early after discharge in patients with unstable angina, NSTEMI, or STEMI who are not selected for cardiac catheterization to assess for the presence and extent of inducible ischemia. An echocardiogram should also be performed to assess left ventricular function and to allow for further risk stratification.

DISPOSITION

Discharge Goals

Patients with unstable angina or NSTEMI who have undergone successful PCI with an uncomplicated course can usually be discharged the next day. Post-CABG patients are often discharged in 4 to 7 days. STEMI patients are at high risk for dangerous ventricular arrhythmias, especially in the first 48 hours, and should be observed on a cardiac monitor. All patients who received a bare metal stent *must* take clopidogrel every day for at least 1 month, and all patients who received a drug-eluting stent *must* take clopidogrel every day for at least 1 year. This is *critical* in order to prevent in-stent thrombosis, which can be rapidly fatal. Patients with ACS who did not receive a stent should still take clopidogrel for 1 month and ideally up to 1 year.

Outpatient Care

Secondary prevention is very important in patients with ACS, as having one ACS event places patients at very high risk of having another event. Patient education, lipid lowering, weight management with diet and exercise, blood pressure control, and diabetes control are all very important. Cardiac rehab has been shown to improve exercise tolerance without increasing cardiovascular complications and may have a benefit on long-term outcomes. Patients should follow up with a health care provider 1 to 2 weeks after an ACS episode. Close follow-up is critical to continually reassess cardiovascular risk, assess for new symptoms, and work toward lipid, blood pressure, blood glucose, and weight management goals.

WHAT YOU NEED TO REMEMBER

- Patients with chest pain should be assessed immediately for possible ACS.
- An ECG, cardiac biomarkers, and the initial history and physical examination should be obtained as soon as possible, with the ECG shown to an attending within 10 minutes of presentation.
- Unless contraindicated, *all* patients with suspected ACS should receive aspirin 162 to 325 mg at the first signs of ACS, and the patient's heart rate, blood pressure, and pain should be controlled with NTG, beta-blockers, and morphine.
- ACS can quickly cause fatal ventricular arrhythmias or cardiogenic shock, both of which are medical emergencies.
- Patients with a STEMI should be evaluated for reperfusion therapy immediately. Do *not* wait for cardiac biomarkers to become positive if STEMI is highly suspected.
- Patients who receive a bare metal stent *must* take clopidogrel daily for 1 month, and those who received a drug-eluting stent *must* take clopidogrel for 1 year.

REFERENCES

1. Antman E, Anbe DT, Armstrong PW, et al. ACC/AHA guidelines for the management of patients with ST-elevation myocardial infarction—executive summary: a report of the American College of Cardiology/American Heart Association Task Force on Practice Guidelines. *Circulation.* 2004;110:588–636.

SUGGESTED READINGS

Antman E, Hand M, Armstrong PW, et al. 2007 Focused update of the ACC/AHA 2004 guidelines for the management of patients with ST-elevation myocardial infarction: a report of the American College of Cardiology/American Heart Association Task Force on Practice Guidelines: developed in collaboration with the Canadian Cardiovascular Society endorsed by the American Academy of Family Physicians: 2007 Writing Group to Review New Evidence and Update the ACC/AHA 2004 guidelines for the management of patients with ST-elevation myocardial infarction, writing on behalf of the 2004 Writing Committee. *Circulation.* 2008;117:296–329.

Anderson J, Adams C, Antman E, et al. ACC/AHA 2007 guidelines for the management of patients with unstable angina/non-ST-elevation myocardial infarction: executive summary. *Circulation.* 2007;116:803–877.

Lilly LS. *Pathophysiology of Heart Disease.* 4th ed. Baltimore: Lippincott Williams & Wilkins; 2007.

Nilsson K, Piccini J. *The Osler Medical Handbook.* 2nd ed. Philadelphia: Saunders Elsevier; 2006.

Systolic Heart Failure

THE PATIENT ENCOUNTER

A 61-year-old man presents to the emergency room with a 1-month history of worsening fatigue and dyspnea on exertion. He has also noted a 25-pound weight gain and swelling of his lower extremities. He has a past medical history of hypertension, type II diabetes, and two prior myocardial infarctions. His blood pressure is 95/70 mm Hg, heart rate is 115 bpm, respiratory rate is 22 breaths per minute, and SaO_2 is 90% on room air. The physical exam reveals an elevated jugular venous pressure at 14 cm, a laterally displaced sustained point of maximal impulse with an audible S_3, and a 3/6 holosystolic murmur at the apex. On auscultation of his lungs, there are coarse bilateral inspiratory rales in the mid- and basal zones. His extremities are warm with 2+ pitting edema of his lower extremities. A chest radiograph shows bilateral alveolar infiltrates. Electrocardiography reveals sinus tachycardia and anteroseptal Q waves. Echocardiography is notable for a dilated hypokinetic left ventricle, an ejection fraction of 35%, and moderate mitral regurgitation.

OVERVIEW

Definition

Heart failure is the inability to deliver adequate blood to meet the body's metabolic demands at normal cardiac filling pressures. Clinically, when we speak of systolic heart failure, we are referring to a constellation of signs and symptoms that result from a low left ventricular ejection fraction ($\leq$50%). These include those symptoms that are caused by increased filling pressures or preload that leads to hepatic congestion and peripheral and pulmonary edema, and those that are caused by poor cardiac output and therefore reduced perfusion, including confusion, anorexia, and renal failure.

Pathophysiology

The major determinants of left ventricular forward flow are preload (venous return and end-diastolic volume), myocardial contractility (stroke volume at a given fiber length), and afterload (arterial vascular impedance and wall stress).

In normal ventricles, increasing filling pressures result in increasing cardiac output. When systolic dysfunction occurs, cardiac output can be maintained

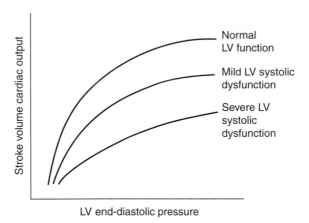

FIGURE 6-1: The Frank-Starling curve in congestive heart failure. The Frank-Starling pressure–volume relationship in normal, mild, and severely depressed left ventricular (LV) function. In normal LV function, an increase in LV filling results in a marked increase in contractility and cardiac output. This relationship deteriorates in LV systolic dysfunction, resulting in a smaller increase in cardiac output for each incremental increase in volume.

by several compensatory mechanisms. As the left ventricle fails and cardiac output drops, these protective mechanisms become maladaptive. Concentric left ventricular hypertrophy (LVH) ensues, which serves, at first, to unload individual muscle fibers and thereby decrease wall stress as defined through Laplace's law. As it progresses, LVH can impair ventricular relaxation and filling, facilitating myocardial ischemia. The Frank-Starling curve plots left ventricular end-diastolic pressure or wedge pressure against stroke volume or cardiac output (Fig. 6-1). In systolic heart failure, the curve is shifted to the right and a higher filling pressure is required to achieve the same cardiac output. The pressure–volume loop consequently changes to maintain cardiac output (Fig. 6-2). Eventually, the ventricle dilates, further increasing wall stress and reducing myocardial fiber shortening at the expense of reducing stroke volume.

Neurohormonal activation follows, causing increased sympathetic activity and activation of the renin-angiotensin-aldosterone system. This serves to augment both contractility and heart rate to maintain cardiac output but comes at a cost to the cardiovascular system with progressive salt and fluid retention and peripheral vasoconstriction.

CLINICAL PEARL

The majority of patients with systolic heart failure also have some degree of diastolic dysfunction.

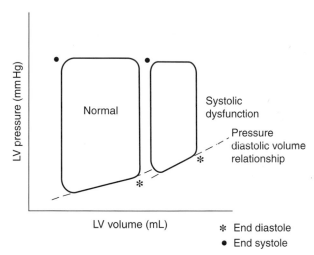

FIGURE 6-2: Pressure–volume loop of systolic heart failure. In left ventricular (LV) systolic dysfunction, the end-systolic and end-diastolic volumes are considerably larger with a reduced stroke volume and a significantly reduced ejection fraction.

Epidemiology

The scope of the problem is enormous. Heart failure affects 5.7 million people in the United States. In addition, the incidence of heart failure increases with age, with an incidence of 10 cases per 1,000 over the age of 65 (http://www.americanheart.org/presenter.jhtml?identifier=1486). Consequently, as the general population ages, the burden of heart failure and its cost to our health care system will increase.

Etiology

Systolic heart failure is the final common pathway for a host of disease states, both cardiac and systemic. The most frequently encountered is ischemic heart disease, the most common cardiovascular problem in the United States. Other common causes include hypertension; valvular heart disease; familial or genetic diseases; toxins; infections; inflammatory diseases; high-output states, such as hyperthyroidism and severe anemia; and infiltrative diseases.

ACUTE MANAGEMENT AND WORKUP

Patients with systolic heart failure will often present with symptoms of volume overload, including shortness of breath, dyspnea on exertion, lower extremity edema, and possible chest tightness or discomfort. The first step in your evaluation is to identify heart failure as the cause of the patient's complaints (as opposed to other processes such as acute ischemia, pulmonary embolism, and pneumonia).

The First 15 Minutes

Once heart failure has been identified as the cause of the patient's presentation, it is important to assess the severity of his or her heart failure in order to decide on the timing and appropriateness of specific therapies.

Initial Assessment

When examining a patient in heart failure, it is helpful to determine whether the patient is "warm" or "cold." This refers to a clinical estimate of cardiac output and corresponding vascular resistance (i.e., cold = low cardiac output and high vascular resistance). Skin examination is useful in this regard, as is a quick bedside assessment of the patient's mental status. A cold, clammy, and confused patient is likely in a low-output state and needs urgent hemodynamic interventions.

It is also important to determine if the patient is "wet" or "dry" as a marker of the patient's preload status (i.e., wet = increased preload; Fig. 6-3). An accurate assessment of volume status is the hallmark of a good heart failure doctor. This allows you to guide initial decisions regarding diuresis and the need for inotropic support. Serial assessment of jugular venous pressure

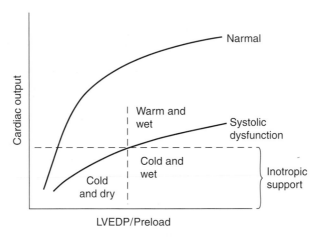

FIGURE 6-3: Classifying patients according to preload and cardiac output. When assessing a patient with left ventricular (LV) systolic dysfunction and decompensation, a general review of which category the patient falls into will help with management. Patients who are cold have a low cardiac output and high systemic vascular resistance and may require inotropic support to increase contractility.

(JVP), urine output, weight, and renal function will dictate further care along these lines. The patient in our encounter is a good example of someone who is "warm" and "wet."

Following your initial assessment, you should begin treatment with the goal of hemodynamic optimization and symptom relief.

Admission Criteria and Level of Care Criteria

For patients who have an established relationship with their doctor, a trial of increased diuretic dosing and a careful monitoring of weights at home can often avoid an inpatient stay. Patients with new-onset heart failure and those with dyspnea at rest require an inpatient stay for intravenous diuretics, careful monitoring of fluid balance, and, often, heart failure education. Inpatients undergoing heart failure management should be placed on continuous cardiac monitoring. Patients with evidence of severe end-organ hypoperfusion, hypotension, or significant hypoxia should be admitted to a coronary care unit for closer monitoring and evaluation.

The First Few Hours

A careful but focused history and physical exam are essential to be able to quickly glean details about the patient's symptoms and their cause.

History

Inquire about which, if any, of the patient's symptoms are new and how they compare to the patient's chronic condition. Asking pointed questions designed to determine classic left heart failure symptoms can be helpful. For example, ask, "Do you ever wake up at night gasping for air?" (paroxysmal nocturnal dyspnea), "Can you lay flat comfortably?" and "How many pillows do you sleep on at night?" (orthopnea). Classic right heart failure symptoms include lower extremity edema and abdominal fullness and distention. The trajectory of symptoms often clues you in about the cause of the heart failure exacerbation. Dietary habits and medication compliance are an essential component of the history. The prevention of recurrent hospitalizations can be as simple as careful education about appropriate dietary and fluid restrictions (e.g., low-salt foods, no canned soup, 1.5-liter fluid restriction, etc.).

Physical Examination

In heart failure, the physical exam is key to the management of the patient, both on initial presentation and in daily follow-up to assess efficacy of therapy. There are several parts to the exam on which to focus.

Careful inspection of the JVP can provide a tremendous amount of information regarding a patient's overall volume status, response to heart failure therapy, right-sided cardiac performance, and even cardiac rhythm disturbances. An astute clinician can estimate JVP within a couple centimeters of water pressure. But perhaps more important is the ability to identify the JVP in a given patient and follow it serially as the patient undergoes diuresis and other interventions. At the bedside, differentiating carotid artery from venous pulsations can be tricky. Here are a few tips that may help:

1. The primary deflection of the JVP is inward and bi- or triphasic, while the carotid pulse is primarily an outward deflection.
2. Move the patient's head of the bed up and down. The jugular meniscus will fall and rise but the carotid pulsations won't change.
3. Abdominal pressure will elevate the JVP as venous return is augmented. In a normal heart, abdominal pressure will make JVP rise and fall within a few seconds. In decompensated congestive heart failure (CHF), the right heart cannot augment output much further, so an increase in venous return causes a prolonged elevation of JVP. This is referred to as a positive *hepatojugular reflux sign*.

CLINICAL PEARL

Despite the term hepatojugular reflux, *you should try to avoid pressing directly over the liver because doing so may be painful if the patient is volume overloaded and has hepatic congestion.*

Focusing on respiratory effort and the use of accessory respiratory muscles will help determine the amount of distress the patient is experiencing. Listening to the lungs can identify cardiac wheezing or crackles suggestive of pulmonary edema and percussion of dullness suggestive of infiltrate or effusion.

Careful palpation of the point of maximal impulse can provide information about cardiac chamber enlargement or left ventricular hypertrophy. A right ventricular (RV) heave is suggestive of RV pressure or volume overload. Occasionally, a thrill can be felt, which suggests turbulent flow across an abnormal valve.

Listen to the heart in several locations, including over each valve area and at the cardiac apex. Characteristic findings in systolic heart failure include an S_3, a low-pitched sound best heard with the bell of the stethoscope as passive ventricular filling begins after relaxation is completed. Having the patient lay in the left lateral decubitus position may aid in identifying this left ventricular gallop. It coincides with the Y descent of the atrial pressure tracing and typically occurs 0.14 to 0.16 seconds after S_2. It should be noted, however, that a fair amount of provider variability exists when it comes to identifying extra heart sounds.

A quick inspection of the extremities can yield a wealth of information. Edema can be grossly characterized based on its pitting characteristics and extension up the leg. If a patient is bed bound or spends time reclined, then this edema may be found at the sacrum or other dependent areas. An often neglected but important component of the extremity exam is the assessment of perfusion. Are the patient's legs warm or cold? What is the capillary refill time? Do the patient's legs appear to be chronically edematous or is this relatively acute? Chronic skin changes and even secondary infection can be a common finding.

Labs and Tests to Consider

A basic metabolic panel to assess electrolyte status and renal function is essential. Classically, patients with decompensated heart failure have a low sodium level and elevated blood urea nitrogen and creatinine levels. Poor perfusion may also manifest as elevated liver enzymes and a lactic acidosis. It is important that magnesium and potassium levels be followed closely during diuretic therapy. Try to maintain a magnesium level ≥ 2 mg/dL and a potassium level ≥ 4 mg/dL as lower levels may predispose to arrhythmia. Brain natriuretic peptide (BNP) has been shown to be elevated in instances of increased myocardial distension and correlates well with heart failure. It may be useful in instances in which the etiology of shortness of breath is unclear. In chronic management of heart failure, baseline BNP values, which may be chronically elevated when the patient is clinically stable, have been shown to correlate with episodes of decompensation.

Key Diagnostic Labs and Tests

For new diagnoses of systolic heart failure, a thorough evaluation is necessary to identify the cause. It is becoming increasingly clear that many cases of systolic heart failure that were previously thought to be idiopathic are actually familial in nature. Thus, a careful family history is warranted to identify possible genetic patterns of disease and to allow the screening of potentially affected family members. In less-clear cases, a broader serologic workup may be undertaken, including thyroid-stimulating hormone, human immunodeficiency virus, rapid plasma reagin (RPR), serum ferritin, serum protein electrophoresis/urine protein electrophoresis, and an evaluation for connective tissue disorders.

Imaging

Chest radiography may show an enlarged cardiac silhouette, which suggests cardiomegaly, evidence of increased pulmonary vascular congestion, and possibly bilateral pleural effusions (usually right greater than left) (Fig. 6-4). An echocardiogram is an essential tool in the assessment of heart failure. It provides an estimate of the left ventricular systolic function in the form of the ejection fraction, as well as atrial and ventricular chamber size and characteristics, valvular heart disease, and regional wall motion abnormalities.

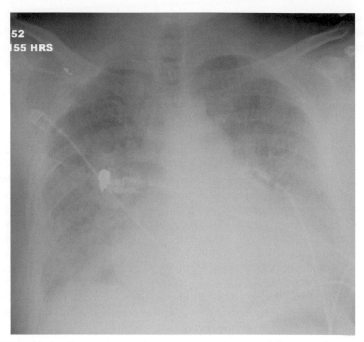

52
55 HRS

FIGURE 6 4: Chest radiograph of a patient with severe left ventricular systolic dysfunction that shows cardiomegaly, pulmonary vascular congestion, and small bilateral pleural effusions. (*Courtesy of Brian T. Garibaldi, MD, Division of Pulmonary and Critical Care Medicine, The Johns Hopkins Hospital.*)

All patients should be evaluated for ischemic heart disease as the cause of the systolic heart failure. Left heart catheterization can be used to evaluate the coronary arteries and assess the need for possible coronary revascularization. The improvement of myocardial perfusion in ischemic coronary disease can lead to improvement in systolic function and therefore improvement in clinical symptoms and prognosis. Left ventricular end-diastolic pressure can also be measured with a pressure-transducing catheter in the left ventricular cavity to allow the assessment of left ventricular diastolic pressure as a surrogate of left ventricular volume status. Right heart catheterization is particularly useful to measure right atrial filling pressures and pulmonary artery pressures, and to estimate left heart filling pressures and cardiac output.

Treatment

The mainstay of pharmacologic therapy for chronic systolic heart failure includes beta-blockers, hydralazine/nitrates, angiotensin-converting enzyme (ACE) inhibitors or angiotensin receptor blockers (ARBs), and, in selected patients, a potassium-sparing diuretic. Each of these portends a mortality benefit to the patient. In addition, drugs like digoxin may improve symptoms and decrease hospitalizations but have no mortality benefit. Loop diuretics are often introduced first for symptom benefit and fluid control. ACE inhibitors or ARBs can be started at a low dose and titrated to achieve afterload reduction. The patient from our encounter should be given intravenous furosemide and, if his creatinine will allow, a short-acting ACE inhibitor. Beta-blockers should be initiated once the patient is stable on the above regimen. If a patient presents in decompensated heart failure, you should not initiate beta-blockade until he or she is approaching euvolemia. If the patient is already on a beta-blocker, then you might consider reducing the dose on initial presentation. Digoxin may be added for symptom benefit in patients otherwise on optimal therapy. In African American patients, an additional benefit has been demonstrated with the combination of hydralazine and long-acting nitrates added to the regimen noted previously. This combination may be used in all patients in lieu of ACE inhibitors or ARBs when drug intolerance or renal failure precludes their use.

Certain drugs should be avoided or used cautiously in heart failure. Nonsteroidal anti-inflammatory drugs can worsen existing CHF, thiazolidinediones can cause fluid retention and exacerbate CHF, and metformin increases the risk of lactic acidosis in heart failure patients. Antiarrhythmic agents often have negative inotropic effects and many are potentially proarrhythmic.

EXTENDED IN-HOSPITAL MANAGEMENT

Patients with acute decompensated heart failure require prompt attention and rapid transfer to an intensive care unit. The use of vasodilators and positive inotropes can sustain the hemodynamics of a subset of critically ill patients when awaiting pump function recovery, the placement of a mechanical support device, or cardiac transplantation. In rare instances in which a patient is not a suitable candidate for destination left ventricular assist devices (LVADs) or cardiac transplantation, discharge to home with inotropes may be undertaken as a palliative measure.

Several kinds of mechanical support devices are available. Most commonly used are counterpulsation devices such as intra-aortic balloon pumps (IABPs) and LVADs. IABPs reduce afterload and improve coronary perfusion pressure. They are temporary devices, require anticoagulation, and carry a risk of arterial complications. LVADs are currently approved by the U.S. Food and Drug Administration as a bridge to transplantation. Recent data suggest that this form of aggressive unloading may favorably remodel the left ventricle, allowing explantation of the device. LVADs have been shown to improve survival relative to optimal medical therapy in patients with severe disease who are not eligible for transplantation. Cardiac transplantation is the only definitive therapy for end-stage cardiomyopathy.

DISPOSITION

Discharge Goals

Ideally, patients are euvolemic, are symptom-free, and have appropriate education and follow-up before discharge. Correction of systemic contributors (e.g., thyroid dysfunction, infection, and glycemic and blood pressure control) and lifestyle modification (e.g., alcohol and illicit drug cessation, limiting salt and fluid intake, daily weights, and an exercise regimen) are key to preventing future heart failure exacerbations.

Outpatient Care

Patients should see their primary care physician or cardiologist within 2 weeks of discharge. A heart failure specialist can follow the patient's functional status, ejection fraction, and response to discharge medications. If the patient is able, monitoring daily weights is often a useful way to adjust a patient's diuretic regimen on an outpatient basis.

WHAT YOU NEED TO REMEMBER

- Many heart failure admissions are preventable with good medical compliance and appropriate outpatient follow-up.
- The rapid assessment of the patient's hemodynamic and volume status is essential and allows for appropriate triage and treatment.
- Medications known to improve mortality include ACE inhibitors, beta-blockers, aldosterone antagonists, and nitrates/hydralazine in selected patients.
- Education about diet and lifestyle modification is one of the most important ways to prevent future heart failure exacerbations.
- Ischemic heart disease is the most common cause of systolic dysfunction and should be assessed in all patients.

SUGGESTED READINGS

Bonow RO, Bennett S, Casey DE Jr, et al. ACC/AHA clinical performance measures for adults with chronic heart failure. *Circulation*. 2005;112;1853–1887.

Bozkhurt B, Mann D. Dilated cardiomyopathy. In: Willerson J, Cohn J, Wellens H, et al., eds. *Cardiovascular Medicine*. 3rd ed. London: Springer; 2007:1233–1259.

Carson P, Ziesche S, Johnson G, et al. Racial differences in response to therapy for heart failure: analysis of the vasodilator-heart failure trials. Vasodilator-Heart Failure Trial Study Group. *J Card Fail*. 1999;5(3):178–187.

Cook D, Simel D. Does this patient have abnormal central venous pressure. The rational clinical exam. *JAMA*. 1996;275:630–634.

The effect of digoxin on mortality and morbidity in patients with heart failure. The Digitalis Investigation Group. *N Engl J Med*. 1997;336(8):525–533.

Effect of enalapril on survival in patients with reduced left ventricular ejection fractions and congestive heart failure. The SOLVD Investigators. *N Engl J Med*. 1991;325(5):293–302.

Effect of metoprolol CR/XL in chronic heart failure: Metoprolol CR/XL Randomised Intervention Trial in Congestive Heart Failure (MERIT-HF). *Lancet*. 1999;353:2001–2007.

Effect of ramipril on mortality and morbidity of survivors of acute myocardial infarction with clinical evidence of heart failure. The Acute Infarction Ramipril Efficacy (AIRE) Study Investigators. *Lancet*. 1993;342:821–828.

Heerdt P, Holmes J, Cai B, et al. Chronic unloading by left ventricular assist device reverses contractile dysfunction and alters gene expression in end-stage heart failure. *Circulation*. 2000;102:2713–2719.

McCullough P, Nowak R, McCord J, et al. B-type natriuretic peptide and clinical judgment in emergency diagnosis of heart failure: analysis from Breathing Not Properly (BNP) Multinational Study. *Circulation*. 2002;106(4):416–422.

Mortality and morbidity reduction with candesartan in patients with chronic heart failure and left ventricular systolic dysfunction: results of the CHARM Low–Left Ventricular Ejection Fraction Trials. The Candesartan in Heart Failure Assessment of Reduction in Mortality and morbidity (CHARM) Investigators and Committees. *Circulation*. 2004;110:2618–2626.

Packer M, Coats A, Fowler M. Effect of carvedilol on survival in severe chronic heart failure. *N Engl J Med*. 2001;344:1651–1658.

Rose E, Gelijns A, Moskowitz A, et al. Long-term use of a left ventricular assist device for end-stage heart failure. *N Engl J Med*. 2001;345:1435–1443.

Heart Failure with Preserved Ejection Fraction

THE PATIENT ENCOUNTER

A 67-year-old woman with a history of poorly controlled hypertension presents to the emergency room with increased shortness of breath over the last day. Two days ago she was in her normal state of health and attended a family cookout without any problems. However, that evening she started to notice difficulty sleeping flat and by the next day her shortness of breath was becoming a problem. On examination, she is sitting upright in bed, her respiratory rate is 30 breaths per minute, her blood pressure is 184/92 mm Hg, and her heart rate is 108 bpm. Her jugular venous pressure is elevated at 14 cm above the right atrium at 45 degrees.

OVERVIEW

Definition

Heart failure with preserved ejection fraction (HFPEF) or, as it has previously been known, *diastolic dysfunction*, relates to the increasingly common syndrome of heart failure symptoms experienced by patients with normal or near-normal ejection fractions. This chapter will focus on HFPEF as an entity separate from systolic heart failure and will review the approach to medical inpatients with HFPEF.

Pathophysiology

During diastole, auto-relaxation of the ventricle facilitates a fast passive filling phase similar to a vacuum. The long-term exposure of the heart to high pressures in the systemic vasculature during systole or from left ventricular outflow obstruction (i.e., aortic stenosis or hypertrophic obstructive cardiomyopathy) leads to hypertrophy of the myocardium. This results in a thickened ventricular wall with a reduced ability to relax as well as a smaller ventricular cavity. The loss of this relaxation leads to the impairment of diastolic filling and a greater dependence on the active atrial filling phase. The resulting pressures in the left ventricle (LV), left atrium (LA), pulmonary capillaries, and venous system during diastole are all increased. This phenomenon becomes even more pronounced with exercise as the reliance on increased stroke volume and cardiac output is dampened, producing marked symptoms as patients exert themselves. Other less common causes of restricted relaxation may result in similar pathology (Table 7-1).

TABLE 7-1
Causes of Restricted Relaxation with Preserved Ejection Fraction

Cause of Restricted Relaxation	Examples of Disease States
Left ventricular hypertrophy: concentric or eccentric	Hypertension Hypertrophic cardiomyopathy Aortic stenosis prior to systolic dysfunction
Myocardial infiltrative processes	Amyloid: primary, secondary, and senile Hemochromatosis Sarcoidosis Idiopathic
Abnormal filling secondary to right ventricular disorders	Pulmonary hypertension Right ventricular myocardial infarction Congenital heart disease with shunt
Pericardial diseases	Constrictive pericardial disease Cardiac tamponade
Myocardial edema	Ischemic heart disease

Epidemiology

HFPEF is estimated as the cause of heart failure in 50% to 60% of patients presenting with heart failure symptoms. It is more common in the elderly, women, and patients with hypertension. As a result, the incidence of diastolic dysfunction is on the rise as the population ages and hypertension becomes more prevalent.

Etiology

Any process that results in reduced relaxation of the ventricular cavity can result in symptoms consistent with diastolic heart failure. The pressure–volume relationship in this condition is much steeper when compared with the relationship seen in systolic heart failure and the normal heart. This means that any change in volume results in a significant change in pressure within the left ventricle as shown in the corresponding pressure–volume curve and vice versa. This pressure–volume change can be the result of even a one-time excess sodium load, missed medications, ischemia, or an arrhythmia (Fig. 7-1).

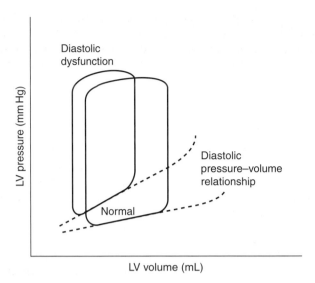

FIGURE 7-1: Pressure–volume loops in normal left ventricular (LV) function and diastolic dysfunction. In diastolic dysfunction, the diastolic pressure–volume relationship is much steeper than in normal LV function. The result is that any change in volume causes a much higher increase in pressure than is seen in normal LV diastolic function.

ACUTE MANAGEMENT AND WORKUP

The first part of the workup should focus on recognizing heart failure as the cause of a patient's symptoms. Patients with HFPEF often present in the same manner as patients with systolic dysfunction, and it may not be possible to tell the two apart from the initial presentation alone.

The First 15 Minutes

As always, first impressions are very important. Take a few moments to carefully observe your patient.

Initial Assessment

A patient who is severely unwell may exhibit rapid, shallow breathing and may require supplemental oxygen due to poor gas exchange secondary to pulmonary edema. He or she may be pale secondary to poor perfusion and may be diaphoretic due to an increased sympathetic drive. Patients with poor cardiac output often have a gray, waxy, or dusky look that should prompt rapid intervention. A patient who feels cool with poor capillary refill and a low-volume pulse likely has a poor cardiac output and poor perfusion of the tissues; such a patient needs careful and experienced clinical management.

A patient is often the best judge of how he or she is feeling. Listen to what the patient says; it will help you assess his or her level of consciousness, responsiveness, and distress, and will also build a good rapport with the patient, which will facilitate good communication through his or her hospital stay.

A patient who has been chronically ill may on occasion look and feel "not too bad" but may actually have very unstable blood pressure and oxygenation levels.

Admission Criteria and Level of Care Criteria

Most patients who present to the emergency department with a heart failure exacerbation will require admission to the hospital for evaluation and management. Because arrhythmias are a common cause of heart failure exacerbations and patients may experience electrolyte abnormalities secondary to diuretic therapy, most, if not all, heart failure patients should be placed on continuous telemetry.

Patients in decompensated heart failure may benefit from noninvasive positive-pressure ventilation. Positive end-expiratory pressure serves to both decrease preload and improve afterload while at the same time improving oxygenation. Any patient who requires noninvasive ventilation or who has blood pressure that is either low or difficult to control is classified as seriously unwell and should be monitored in an intermediate-care or intensive care unit setting. Occasionally, patients may require invasive mechanical ventilation if their mental status or hemodynamics do not allow for safe administration of noninvasive ventilation. Patients may also require intravenous vasodilator or inotropic therapy. Such patients should be managed aggressively in the intensive care unit.

The First Few Hours

Once you have addressed the hemodynamic stability of the patient, you can begin to gather further information that may help you distinguish HFPEF from systolic heart failure.

History

The symptoms of HFPEF may be indistinguishable from systolic heart failure. However, the time course of the symptoms may provide important clues. Patients with HFPEF will often report a very rapid onset over a period of hours to a day and may also describe previous presentations in which he or she felt better after just a short time of treatment in the emergency room. Recent illness, pneumonia, missing medications such as blood pressure tablets, or even a small indiscretion in dietary compliance, such as a very salty meal, may be enough to cause the patient's present exacerbation. The family cookout from the encounter was probably a significant salt load that led to our patient's heart failure exacerbation.

Ask about palpitations and a history of atrial fibrillation. The stiff ventricle relies heavily on the active "kick" of the atrium during filling, so any loss or disturbance of this mechanism can lead acutely to a loss in filling and therefore to reduced cardiac output, increased retrograde pressures, and marked pulmonary symptoms.

Compare the patient's current level of activity to what he or she was able to do a month ago or when he or she was last feeling well. This can help you to assess the severity of the patient's current illness in the setting of baseline comorbidities that may impair exercise tolerance and functional status.

Physical Examination

After assessing the vital signs of the patient, perform a full cardiovascular examination. Look carefully for evidence of end-organ damage secondary to hypertension, as it is the leading cause of HFPEF. When assessing the pulse, assess for abnormalities in rhythm, such as atrial fibrillation that could be caused by increased atrial size. A weak, thready pulse could indicate poor cardiac output. The jugular venous pressure wave should be assessed as previously discussed. The precordium may be quite active with a heaving left ventricle due to marked hypertrophy. There is often no displacement of the apex as found in systolic heart failure. Listen for an S_3 and more commonly an S_4 gallop. Listen carefully for murmurs suggestive of aortic stenosis or outflow obstruction; don't forget radiation and enhancing maneuvers. On percussion of the lungs, "stoney dullness" suggests pleural effusions. On auscultation, wet crackles or wheezing from increased left atrial pressures may be heard. Abdominal examination can illicit right-sided heart failure signs, such as an increased pulsatile liver and ascites. Your examination should also include assessment for peripheral edema, funduscopy to assess for hypertensive disease, and microscopic examination of the urine.

Labs and Tests to Consider

There are a number of key laboratory and imaging studies that will aid in the diagnosis and further management of patients with HFPEF.

Key Diagnostic Labs and Tests

Laboratory evaluation should search for signs of damage to vital organs, including blood urea nitrogen and creatinine levels to assess for acute renal failure, liver enzymes to assess for hepatic congestion, and cardiac enzymes, including troponin, to assess for myocardial ischemia. Plasma pro–B-type natriuretic peptide (pro-BNP) is widely used and when elevated can be used for diagnosis and prognosis but will not distinguish the type of heart failure. A one-time measurement in a patient with known chronic heart failure can often be unhelpful, whereas a trend related to other hospitalizations and out-patient visits may help in management. A hemoglobin should also be sent as anemia is a more unusual but important trigger of disease.

Imaging

The electrocardiogram should always be personally reviewed and a comparison should be made with any previous studies. Look for evidence of left ventricular hypertrophy by voltage criteria, increased chamber size due to constant back pressure, and evidence of cardiovascular strain in the form of ST/T-wave changes (Fig. 7-2). As described previously, atrial fibrillation may also be present either as a consequence of the high atrial pressure or as a cause of the acute decompensation. Although true coronary atherosclerotic ischemia is less common in diastolic failure as compared to systolic heart failure, it is always important to rule out an acute coronary event. There may also be poor filling of the coronary arteries due to high-end diastolic pressures.

A chest radiograph may show evidence of increased back pressure, which results in increased pulmonary vascular markings and evidence of pulmonary edema, such as Kerley B lines, bilateral interstitial infiltrates, and pleural effusions. Echocardiography is often useful to document a normal ejection fraction and exclude structural abnormalities. However, frequent repetition of this exam, unless there is a clear question, is expensive and will not help with in-hospital management. The definitive diagnosis is made by cardiac catheterization to assess chamber pressures. This is rarely performed but is part of the formal diagnostic criteria.

Treatment

Patients with diastolic dysfunction will often maintain normal blood pressures or even present with hypertension. Blood pressure control is therefore critical as the overwhelming force needed to match the intense pressures in the vasculature may be causing a large part of the problem. Nitroglycerin-derived medications in a patient with adequate pressures can provide fast-acting blood pressure control by reducing afterload and decreasing venous return. Loop diuretics are the drugs of choice to remove fluid. A patient may improve after a small amount of diuresis because a small drop in preload translates to a large drop in end-diastolic pressure in the stiff, noncompliant left ventricle. Afterload reducers such as angiotensin-converting enzyme (ACE) inhibitors and angiotensin receptor blockers are key components of acute blood pressure management and will also aid in the prevention of ventricular remodeling over time, although neither has been shown to improve mortality. Our patient in the encounter should be administered intravenous furosemide and a short-acting oral ACE inhibitor to decrease preload and reduce afterload, respectively. Further doses should be determined based on her initial response in terms of symptoms and blood pressure. In the acute setting of decompensated heart failure, beta-blockers are not usually tolerated. However, if a patient is given a beta-blocker as an outpatient, the beta-blocker should be continued to avoid increased sympathetic drive on already up-regulated adrenergic receptors. As discussed previously, patients in

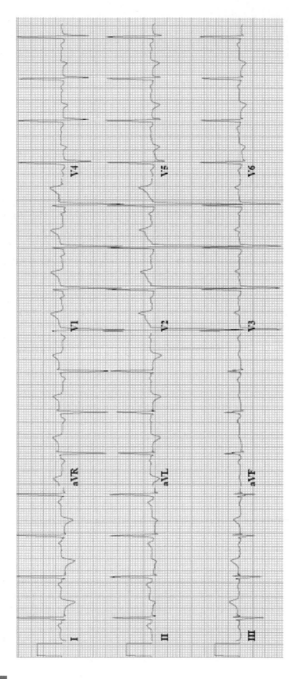

FIGURE 7-2: Twelve-lead electrocardiogram demonstrating left ventricular hypertrophy with a strain pattern in a patient with long-standing, poorly controlled hypertension. (Courtesy of Brian T. Garibaldi, MD, Division of Pulmonary and Critical Care Medicine, The Johns Hopkins Hospital.)

respiratory distress or with decompensated heart failure may benefit from noninvasive positive-pressure ventilation while diuretics and afterload-reducing medications begin to take effect.

EXTENDED IN-HOSPITAL MANAGEMENT

During the next few days, the goal of care is to remove the extra pressures that have been placed on the stiff ventricular system. Diuretics should be used to remove fluid and therefore reduce the increased ventricular filling pressures.

> ## CLINICAL PEARL
>
> *Diuresis should be undertaken a little less aggressively than in a patient with systolic heart failure, as overdiuresis can lead to prerenal kidney dysfunction, a common cause of a protracted hospital stay in patients with diastolic dysfunction.*

Every day it is important to check that blood pressure control is optimal, to record accurate intake and output, and to measure daily standing weights yourself on the same scale. Take time to educate your patient on his or her heart and how to manage his or her fluids and diet at home. Remember to remove unnecessary Foley catheters as soon as possible. A patient who is immobile due to his or her symptoms or comorbidities should receive deep vein thrombosis prophylaxis. All patients should be evaluated by physical and occupational therapy, and eligibility for cardiovascular rehabilitation programs should be assessed.

DISPOSITION

Discharge Goals

Patients should have a marked reduction in symptoms and should not require any supplemental oxygen prior to discharge. Once their peripheral edema has resolved, their jugular venous pressure has returned to normal, and they are able to tolerate their usual activities, they are ready to return home with follow-up.

At discharge, all patients should receive vaccination against influenza if it is during the influenza season, and should also receive a pneumococcal vaccination. The transition to home, especially for elderly patients, can often be hazardous and can result in readmission unless careful education and planning is undertaken. This should include assessment of the ability to pay for often highly priced cardiovascular medications, the complexity of the regimen, and the ability to follow up in the outpatient setting soon after discharge.

Outpatient Care

The goal of long-term care is to maintain fluid balance status, prevent progression of heart failure, and improve modifiable risk factors. On discharge, a dry weight should be recorded and the patient should be educated about its importance. Education on blood pressure control, diet, exercise, and regular physician follow-up is crucial.

WHAT YOU NEED TO REMEMBER

- Heart failure with preserved ejection fraction is common and its prevalence increases with age.
- Chronic hypertension leading to left ventricular hypertension is the most common cause of HFPEF, but other causes should be considered and assessed.
- Blood pressure control is a key factor in both inpatient and outpatient management.
- The inpatient time course for diastolic heart failure is often short and patients tend to feel better quickly.
- Daily standing weights and fluid balance are essential in management, and a "dry weight" should be noted prior to discharge.
- Patients require education about daily measurements of weight, following a low-salt diet, fluid intake, and the importance of compliance with medications to prevent readmission.

SUGGESTED READINGS

Borlaug BA, Kass DA. Ventricular-vascular interaction in heart failure. *Heart Fail Clin.* 2008;4(1):23–36.

Das A, Abraham S, Deswal A. Advances in the treatment of heart failure with a preserved ejection fraction. *Curr Opin Cardiol.* 2008;23(3):233–240.

Hess DM, Carroll JD. Clinical assessment of heart failure. In: Braunwald E, Zipes D, Libby P, et al., eds. *Braunwald's Heart Disease: A Textbook of Cardiovascular Medicine.* 8th ed. Philadelphia: Elsevier Saunders; 2007.

Mann DL. Alterations in ventricular function: diastolic heart failure. In: *Heart Failure: A Companion to Braunwald's Heart Disease.* Philadelphia: Elsevier; 2004.

Pulmonary Hypertension and Right Heart Disease

THE PATIENT ENCOUNTER

A 28-year-old woman presents to the emergency department with complaints of shortness of breath for the past 2 years. She states that previously she exercised on a daily basis, running several miles. Over the past 18 months, she noted dyspnea on exertion that has progressed to shortness of breath while walking up more than one flight of stairs. She has been treated with inhaled bronchodilators without any improvement in her symptoms. She has a normal lung exam with a prominent second heart sound and marked peripheral edema.

OVERVIEW

Definition

Pulmonary hypertension (PH) is a progressive disease of the pulmonary vasculature that leads to right heart failure and eventually death. Pulmonary hypertension is defined as a mean pulmonary artery pressure (mPAP) >25 mm Hg at rest or 30 mm Hg with activity. PH may result from a wide number of diseases.

The World Health Organization (WHO) recognizes five distinct categories of PH (Table 8-1).

Pulmonary arterial hypertension (PAH) has a more specific definition than PH: mPAP >25 mm Hg, pulmonary capillary wedge pressure (PCWP) <15 mm Hg, and pulmonary vascular resistance (PVR) >3 Wood units. PAH includes idiopathic PAH (IPAH, formerly known as primary pulmonary hypertension), familial PAH (FPAH), and associated PAH (APAH). This last form of PAH includes PAH associated with collagen vascular disease, human immunodeficiency virus (HIV), hemoglobinopathies, congenital left-to-right shunting, portal hypertension, and drugs or toxins such as anorexigens. Importantly, this classification system distinguishes between diseases that primarily affect the pulmonary vasculature and diseases that affect the pulmonary vasculature through other interactions with the cardiopulmonary system. It is of utmost importance to properly classify patients with elevated pulmonary pressures in this schema because treatment varies greatly between groups. Treatments that may be appropriate for patients in one group (e.g., Group I) may be deleterious to those in another group (e.g., Group II or III).

TABLE 8-1

Categories of Pulmonary Hypertension (PH)

Group I: Pulmonary arterial hypertension (PAH)—includes idiopathic, human immunodeficiency virus, portopulmonary hypertension, and connective tissue disease, such as scleroderma

Group II: PH that is caused by left-sided heart dysfunction or pulmonary venous hypertension

Group III: PH associated with lung disease (chronic obstructive pulmonary disease) and/or chronic hypoxemia

Group IV: PH as a result of chronic thrombotic and/or embolic disease

Group V: Miscellaneous—includes sarcoidosis and eosinophilic granuloma

Adapted from Simonneau G, Galié N, Rubin LJ, et al. Clinical classification of pulmonary hypertension. *J Am Coll Cardiol.* 2004;43(12 Suppl S):5S–12S.

Pathophysiology

In large part, the pathophysiology of PH depends on the underlying cause. For example, the increased pulmonary vascular resistance in PAH is thought to be related to three main processes: hypoxic vasoconstriction, in situ thrombosis, and pulmonary vessel wall remodeling. Alveolar hypoxia directly affects vasoconstriction through smooth muscle contractility mediated by calcium channels. In situ thrombosis in the distal pulmonary arterioles also contributes to the increased PVR seen in PAH and is thought to be related to the low-flow state that results from progressive increases in pulmonary artery pressures and subsequent right heart dysfunction. Abnormal proliferation and contraction of pulmonary artery smooth muscle cells are also integral to the development of PAH. Imbalance between endothelial-derived vasoconstrictors, such as endothelin-1 (ET-1), and vasodilators, such as nitric oxide (NO) and prostacyclin, has been implicated in the pathogenesis of the disease.

Regardless of the underlying etiology, progressive increases in pulmonary artery pressures and resistance cause right heart strain. While the right ventricle can adapt to increased pressure and resistance by increasing muscle mass (hypertrophy), it is not able to adapt as well as the left ventricle in response to increased afterload.

Epidemiology

The epidemiology of PH is dependent on the underlying cause. For example, PAH is a rare disease. The estimated incidence of IPAH in the

United States is 1 to 2 cases per million persons per year, with a prevalence of 15 cases per million (1). In general, the disease tends to affect women more than men, and may have a bimodal age distribution with many cases diagnosed in patients in the third decade and fifth or sixth decade of life. The incidence of other forms of PAH is unknown.

The prevalence of PH in chronic obstructive pulmonary disease (COPD) is not clear, but it increases as the degree of severe airflow obstruction worsens. Obstructive sleep apnea (OSA) is generally associated with mild PH, but obesity hypoventilation syndrome may result in right heart failure. Chronic thromboembolic-induced PH occurs in approximately 4% of patients who experience a thromboembolic event. Pulmonary venous hypertension is increasing in frequency as the number of patients with left heart disease and poorly controlled systemic hypertension increases.

Etiology

The etiologies of PH are best outlined in the WHO classification system (see Table 8-1). The most common cause of PH overall is left-sided heart failure (previously referred to as secondary pulmonary hypertension). The etiology of PAH is unknown. A small proportion of patients have a familial form of PAH in which most demonstrate a mutation in the bone morphogenetic receptor type II pathway. Environmental factors, such as exposure to drugs or toxins, have also been implicated. Specifically, exposure to derivatives of fenfluramines, such as the diet agent Fen-Phen, is associated with the development of PAH. Patients with liver disease, hemolytic disorders, HIV, or thyroid disorders are also at higher risk of developing PAH.

ACUTE MANAGEMENT AND WORKUP

Recognition of pulmonary hypertension is difficult; the definitive diagnosis can only be established with right heart catheterization. However, the general principles of acute management can be applied in situations in which the diagnosis has yet to be confirmed.

The First 15 Minutes

Most patients with PH present with complaints of progressive dyspnea on exertion. Many processes can lead to this symptom, and some, such as pulmonary embolism or right heart failure, may be life-threatening (and also cause PH). Specific interventions and diagnostic tests may need to be completed urgently, depending on this assessment.

Initial Assessment

As with many clinical situations, assessing the mental status of the patient is an important determinant of severity of illness. An unarousable or confused patient might suggest hypoxia or poor cerebral perfusion, both of which may be related to PH and right heart failure. If the patient is unable to respond in full sentences due to shortness of breath or tachypnea, uses accessory muscles while breathing, or demonstrates paradoxical breathing, respiratory failure may quickly ensue. Because PH is often only recognized later in the course of the disease, patients may present with "unexplained" shortness of breath with signs of right heart failure, including elevated jugular venous pressure, ascites, and peripheral edema. The young woman in our vignette likely already has right heart failure as evidenced by her dyspnea and lower extremity edema.

CLINICAL PEARL

Patients with PAH are unlikely to develop pulmonary edema as this is caused by elevations in pulmonary venous pressure.

Admission Criteria and Level of Care Criteria

Patients who present with signs and symptoms of right heart failure and who have suspected pulmonary hypertension should be admitted for further evaluation and treatment. Patients with hypotension, tachycardia, new-onset hypoxia, and/or chest pain should be evaluated by the intensive care unit. Patients who present with syncope or near syncope should be admitted to the intensive care unit as this suggests hypotension related to severe right heart failure.

The First Few Hours

Once the patient has been properly triaged, it is important to obtain a detailed history to help ascertain the etiology of his or her pulmonary hypertension.

History

Because several disorders can predispose to the development of PAH, it is important to focus the history on details that are suggestive of these disorders. A detailed medication history is necessary, including the use of any prescription anorexigens or amphetamines. Persistent arthralgias may suggest connective tissue disease. A history of a hemoglobinopathy, such as sickle cell disease, warrants further evaluation for pulmonary hypertension. Risk factors for sexually transmitted diseases, especially HIV and hepatitis C, should be reviewed. Symptoms of liver disease, such as jaundice, persistent nausea, vomiting, or easy bruising or bleeding, can suggest portopulmonary hypertension. Patients with palpitations, heat intolerance, nervousness, hair loss, or other symptoms suggestive of hyperthyroidism are at risk for PAH.

Several more common pulmonary disorders are associated with pulmonary hypertension. Tobacco use in an older patient should raise the possibility of COPD. Pulmonary hypertension can be associated with interstitial lung disease (ILD) and likely results from chronic hypoxic vasoconstriction. Similarly, patients with sleep-disordered breathing can develop pulmonary hypertension. Symptoms of excessive daytime somnolence, disruptive snoring, awakening with headaches or sore throat, and/or the need for frequent daytime naps are suggestive of a sleep disorder and should be further evaluated by a sleep specialist.

A history of pulmonary embolism or deep vein thrombosis is important to elicit. Pulmonary hypertension in the setting of acute pulmonary embolism results from elevations in pulmonary artery pressures related to obstruction from the clots. This tends to resolve over time with resorption of the embolus. However, a small percentage of patients will develop chronic thromboembolic pulmonary hypertension.

As previously mentioned, the most common cause of pulmonary hypertension in the United States is pulmonary venous hypertension related to left heart disease. Left ventricular dysfunction, both systolic and nonsystolic, and mitral or aortic valvular disease can cause pulmonary hypertension. Risk factors for coronary disease or a personal history of coronary artery disease predisposes patients to left ventricular dysfunction and pulmonary venous hypertension. A detailed history focusing on cardiac disease should be obtained.

Physical Examination

Cyanosis suggests hypoxemia that may be related to a chronic right-to-left cardiac shunt. An elevated jugular venous pressure can be caused by many processes, including pulmonary hypertension, cardiac tamponade, constrictive pericarditis, restrictive cardiomyopathy, heart failure, and pulmonary embolism. Signs on cardiac exam, such as a left-sided S_3 or S_4 gallop; a laterally displaced point of maximal impulse; or the murmurs of mitral regurgitation, stenosis, or aortic regurgitation, suggest left-sided heart failure. A pronounced second heart sound suggests pulmonary hypertension, though it is not specific for this diagnosis. A right-sided S_3 or right ventricular heave suggests right-sided heart failure, which can be found in patients with decompensated PH. The murmur of tricuspid regurgitation is common in PH, but is not necessarily reflective of disease severity. Increased intensity of the murmur with inspiration in patients with tricuspid regurgitation (Carvallo sign) can be helpful to distinguish right-sided from left-sided murmurs.

The lung exam in patients with PAH is usually unremarkable. Velcro-like crackles suggest interstitial lung disease, wheezing suggests reactive airway disease, and rales suggest pulmonary edema; all of these findings are unusual in PAH. A prolonged expiratory phase and/or barrel chest can be seen in COPD. Ascites can be present in volume overload related to liver, renal, or left heart failure, although it may also occur with severe right heart failure. Peripheral edema is commonly seen in volume overload and thus in PH. Swollen and erythematous joints suggest possible connective tissue disease as a cause of PAH.

Labs and Tests to Consider

As discussed previously, it is imperative to determine the underlying cause of elevated pulmonary pressures to appropriately categorize patients according to the WHO classification.

Key Diagnostic Labs and Tests

A complete blood count is helpful to evaluate for anemia. Serum creatinine can be used to screen for renal disease. Liver function tests along with hepatitis serologies, especially hepatitis C, are important to screen for possible underlying liver disease. Additional testing should include HIV antibody, antinuclear antibodies, and thyroid-stimulating hormone if there is clinical suspicion or the underlying cause of PH is unclear.

Pulmonary function testing is essential to identify both obstructive (COPD) and restrictive (ILD) forms of lung disease. Arterial blood gas analysis is also recommended, especially in patients with hypoxemia at rest.

For obese patients or in those with symptoms of sleep-disordered breathing, overnight polysomnography is important. Overnight pulse oximetry is an alternative screening test, but will only identify those patients with more severe obstructive sleep apnea.

Finally, an electrocardiogram, although not sensitive, may reveal evidence of right ventricular hypertrophy, right atrial enlargement, or right axis deviation, or may suggest left-sided heart disease.

Imaging

There are a number of imaging modalities to consider. A chest radiograph may reveal prominence of the pulmonary arteries or other hilar vessels. It may also demonstrate evidence of ILD. A chest computed tomography (CT) scan with intravenous contrast is an essential component of the evaluation to assess for pulmonary embolism. Additionally, subtle interstitial disease not seen on a chest radiograph may be identified by a CT scan. A ventilation–perfusion scan can be useful to exclude pulmonary embolism and chronic thromboembolic disease, especially when trying to avoid the use of contrast.

Transthoracic echocardiography (TTE) is a noninvasive screening tool for PH. It provides an estimate of right ventricular systolic pressure (RVSP). The RVSP is determined from the Doppler-acquired tricuspid regurgitation jet velocity and the estimation of the right atrial pressure using a modified Bernoulli equation:

$$4 \times (\text{tricuspid regurgitant jet velocity})^2 + \text{estimated right atrial pressure}$$

In addition, TTE can also evaluate for left-sided ventricular or valvular dysfunction as a cause of PH.

The definitive diagnostic test for pulmonary hypertension is right heart catheterization. During right heart catheterization, the measurements of right atrial pressure, right ventricular systolic and diastolic pressure, pulmonary artery systolic and diastolic pressure, PCWP, and cardiac output can be made. As mentioned previously, a mean pulmonary pressure >25 mm Hg at rest or >30 mm Hg with exercise is diagnostic of pulmonary hypertension. Because PCWP is an estimate of left atrial pressure, an elevated PCWP (>15 mm Hg) suggests left heart disease as the cause of the pulmonary hypertension. Additionally, oxygen saturations from the large veins, right-sided chambers, and pulmonary arteries can be obtained to assess for possible shunt.

Treatment

Treatment, when possible, should be directed to the underlying cause of PH. If the patient presents with signs and symptoms of right heart failure, as in our patient from the encounter, treatment with diuretics should be initiated, usually with a loop diuretic.

Administering diuretics to patients who are hypotensive seems counterintuitive as this may worsen hypotension; intravascular volume expansion with intravenous fluids would seem more appropriate. However, given the pathophysiology of pulmonary hypertension and right heart failure, a patient's hypotension will likely be exacerbated by a fluid challenge as right and left ventricular function is further compromised by volume and pressure overload. Diuresis will "decompress" the right ventricle and improve left ventricular function. As long as the patient maintains an appropriate mental status and does not develop symptoms or signs of hypoperfusion, diuresis can be undertaken while under close clinical observation. Occasionally, hypotension may be accompanied by changes in mental status or other signs of hypoperfusion. In these situations, the maintenance of blood pressure with the use of intravenous vasopressors is recommended.

Supplemental oxygen should be given to patients who are hypoxemic as this may alleviate some hypoxic pulmonary vasoconstriction and thus improve pulmonary pressures.

Therapies Specific to Pulmonary Arterial Hypertension

As discussed previously, hypoxic vasoconstriction plays a role in pulmonary vascular tone, likely through smooth muscle contractility mediated by calcium channels. However, only a minority of patients with PAH (about 10% of IPAH patients) demonstrate vasodilator responses to calcium channel blockers and less than half of these initial responders will continue to have a long-term response. Thus, a vasodilator challenge should be performed during right heart catheterization in patients with suspected IPAH to identify patients who may benefit.

A general prothrombotic state likely exists in PAH. Although there are no prospective, randomized, placebo-controlled trials of anticoagulation in PAH, many pulmonary hypertension experts recommend lifelong treatment with warfarin, with a goal international normalized ratio between 2.0 and 2.5.

Abnormal proliferation and the contraction of pulmonary artery smooth muscle cells are central to the development of PAH. Imbalance between vasoconstrictors, such as ET-1, and vasodilators, such as NO and prostacyclin (PGI2), has been implicated in the pathogenesis of the disease. Prostacyclin analogs (e.g., intravenous epoprostenol and inhaled iloprost), endothelin receptor antagonists (e.g., bosentan and ambrisentan), and phosphodiesterase type 5 inhibitors (e.g., sildenafil) are designed to restore the balance between vasoconstrictors and vasodilators in the pulmonary vasculature.

The only cure for PAH is lung transplantation. Patients who present with severe PAH should be referred for lung transplantation immediately. However, despite curing PAH, survival following lung transplantation remains poor, with a 70% 1-year survival rate and a median survival of 5 years.

Therapies for Non–Pulmonary Arterial Hypertension Pulmonary Hypertension

In general, the use of pulmonary vasodilators in other causes of PH has not been well studied and should not be attempted without consulting a PH expert. In addition to the management of right heart failure, other therapies will be dictated by the underlying cause of the patient's PH. For example, oxygen therapy may be helpful in patients with hypoxemia, nocturnal continuous positive airway pressure for patients with OSA, corticosteroids for patients with sarcoidosis, etc. Patients with left-sided heart disease or valvular disease should be managed accordingly. Patients with chronic thromboembolic PH should be on lifelong anticoagulation and, in some circumstances, may benefit from surgical removal of their chronic clot burden with pulmonary endarterectomy at a specialized center.

EXTENDED IN-HOSPITAL MANAGEMENT

Patients may deteriorate despite aggressive diuresis and supportive care. Sudden changes in cardiopulmonary status, such as increased shortness of breath, increased oxygen requirement, or a drop in blood pressure, warrant evaluation for other processes such as pulmonary embolism, acute coronary syndrome, or pericardial effusion.

It is imperative that the patient be maintained on a diuretic regimen to sustain euvolemia. The combination of a loop diuretic combined with an aldosterone antagonist (Aldactone) may be used to minimize the need for potassium supplementation if a loop diuretic is used alone.

Recovery from right heart failure can be prolonged. Thus, physical and occupational therapy evaluations and interventions are important to facilitate functional improvements.

DISPOSITION
Discharge Goals
Once a patient with PH achieves euvolemia, he or she may be ready for discharge. Additional factors include proper understanding of medications and their side effect profiles, as well as arranging for home oxygen and a physical therapy regimen if needed.

Outpatient Care
The patient will need to see a specialist in pulmonary hypertension—either a cardiologist or pulmonologist—within 1 week of discharge. If the patient is receiving intravenous or subcutaneous infusion of a prostacyclin analog, he or she will need to have 24-hour access to a health care provider familiar with the management of these PAH medications. The patient's primary care physician should be contacted and updated regarding the diagnosis, treatment plans, and follow-up.

WHAT YOU NEED TO REMEMBER

- The WHO classification of pulmonary hypertension provides a framework to approach patients with newly diagnosed PH.
- The initial evaluation of a patient with suspected PH should focus on the treatment of right heart failure with diuresis. Once stabilized, the patient should undergo an extensive workup to identify the etiology of elevated pulmonary pressures.
- The diagnosis of PH can only be established with right heart catheterization.
- PAH is a rare disease characterized by nonspecific symptoms that may be attributed to other more common processes. Because of this, patients may present with advanced disease and right heart failure.
- Vasodilator challenge during right heart catheterization should be performed in all patients with suspected idiopathic PAH, but <10% of these patients will demonstrate a positive response.
- The treatment of a patient with PH will in part depend on the underlying cause of the patient's disease; PAH-specific therapy should be reserved for patients with established PAH.
- The only cure for PAH is lung transplantation.

REFERENCES
1. Gaine S. Pulmonary hypertension. *JAMA*. 2000;284(24):3160–3168.

SUGGESTED READINGS

Badesch DB, Abman SH, Simonneau G, et al. Medical therapy for pulmonary arterial hypertension: updated ACCP evidence-based clinical practice guidelines. *Chest.* 2007;131:1917–1928.

Barst RJ, McGoon M, Torbicki A, et al. Diagnosis and differential assessment of pulmonary arterial hypertension. *J Am Coll Cardiol.* 2004;43:40S–47S.

Humbert M, Sitbon O, Simonneau G. Treatment of pulmonary arterial hypertension. *N Engl J Med.* 2004;351:1425–1436.

Simonneau G, Galie N, Rubin LJ, et al. Clinical classification of pulmonary hypertension. *J Am Coll Cardiol.* 2004;43:5S–12S.

Tuder RM, Marecki JC, Richter A, et al. Pathology of pulmonary hypertension. *Clin Chest Med.* 2007;28:23–42.

Hypertensive Crisis

THE PATIENT ENCOUNTER

A 68-year-old man is brought to the emergency room by his wife with increasing shortness of breath, headaches, and confusion that have progressed over the last 24 hours. His wife reports that he has a history of high blood pressure but ran out of his medications 4 days ago. His pulse is 105 bpm, his blood pressure is 224/125 mm Hg, and his oxygen saturation is 90% on 2 liters nasal cannula. On examination, the patient is drowsy and confused and has inspiratory rales bilaterally to the mid-lung fields.

OVERVIEW

Definition

Hypertensive crisis is characterized by the presence of dangerously elevated blood pressure (typically, systolic blood pressure [SBP] >180 mm Hg or diastolic blood pressure [DBP] >110 mm Hg) and is typically divided into two categories. *Hypertensive emergency* is defined by evidence of acute end-organ damage and an immediate need for blood pressure reduction. *Hypertensive urgency* is defined by blood pressure elevation placing patients at risk for acute end-organ damage and a need to reduce blood pressure (typically over 24 to 48 hours) in order to prevent such damage from occurring. Acute end-organ damage typically does not occur unless DBP exceeds 130 mm Hg, but it can occur with DBP closer to 100 in patients who are not normally hypertensive. Because patients tolerate blood pressure elevation differently, the treatment of hypertensive crisis requires significant clinical judgment and, above all, an ability to recognize the signs of end-organ damage.

Pathophysiology

Hypertensive crisis occurs in two stages: (a) an initial rise in blood pressure and (b) an ensuing cascade of events that leads to further escalation of blood pressure and end-organ damage. Within the normal range of blood pressure, arterioles are able to regulate flow to vital organs to ensure adequate perfusion. In the setting of rapid and significant increases in pressure, however, vascular stress results in endothelial damage, increased permeability, the activation of coagulation cascades and platelet aggregation, and fibrin deposition. These events lead to arteriolar fibrinoid necrosis, vascular leak,

TABLE 9-1
Common Types of End-organ Damage by System

System	Type of End-organ Damage
Central nervous system	Hypertensive encephalopathy, ischemic and hemorrhagic stroke, intracerebral and subarachnoid hemorrhage, and eclampsia in pregnant and peripartum women
Cardiac	Acute myocardial infarction, acute-onset ventricular failure
Vascular	Acute aortic dissection
Pulmonary	Pulmonary edema (typically secondary to left ventricular failure)
Renal	Acute renal failure
Hematologic	HELLP syndrome in peripartum women, microangiopathic hemolytic anemia

and, ultimately, the failure of autoregulation mechanisms. Unfortunately, the resulting ischemia further amplifies the problem by activation of the renin-angiotensin system and increased release of vasoactive substances. Furthermore, elevated blood pressure induces a natriuresis that can cause severe volume depletion and worsened ischemia.

Multiple organ systems can be compromised by this cascade (Table 9-1). Ischemia can lead to myocardial infarction and heart failure (also caused by increased wall stress), acute renal failure, and ischemic stroke. Vascular leak is thought to be responsible for cerebral vasogenic edema and central nervous system (CNS) hemorrhage, as well as glomerular injury.

Epidemiology

The epidemiology of hypertensive crisis mirrors hypertension itself (higher among older patients, men, and African Americans, for example), and most patients who experience hypertensive crises carry a diagnosis of hypertension at baseline. It has been estimated that 1% to 2% of patients with hypertension will experience hypertensive emergency, making this a very common condition given the enormous percentage of the population that suffers from hypertension. Far more patients experience hypertensive urgency. Many of these patients are often treated appropriately by primary doctors, particularly if the reason for their elevated pressure is simply running out of medication or missing doses.

Etiology

Poorly controlled baseline hypertension and running out of medication and other forms of medication nonadherence are the leading causes of hypertensive crises. Studies suggest that more than half of patients with hypertensive emergency have not been compliant with their home medications in the week preceding admission. However, illicit drug use, particularly cocaine and methamphetamine, represents a precipitant that is particularly important to consider in patients who are not normally hypertensive. Finally, other causes of hypertension that tend to be associated with precipitous rises in blood pressure include pheochromocytoma, renal artery stenosis (RAS), and other causes of acute renal failure.

CLINICAL PEARL

Alcohol withdrawal can be associated with rises in blood pressure (particularly DBP) and significant mental status changes. As a result, it can be confused with hypertensive emergency but warrants different treatment to prevent morbidity.

ACUTE MANAGEMENT AND WORKUP

The proper early management of hypertensive crisis is critical to preventing, minimizing, and reversing end-organ damage. Identifying the evidence of acute end-organ damage is the key to proper disposition, the establishment of treatment goals, and the choice of pharmacologic therapy.

The First 15 Minutes

The first decision that must be made is whether a patient has evidence of end-organ damage and is thus having a hypertensive emergency. In addition to reviewing any laboratory or radiographic data that may already be available, the first few minutes of your evaluation should be designed to identify major organ system dysfunction, particularly CNS involvement, heart failure, aortic dissection, and myocardial infarction. These conditions are life-threatening but may not be obvious, and their presence indicates the need for immediate intensive care unit (ICU)–level care.

Initial Assessment

As soon as you walk into the room, pay careful attention to the patient's mental status, the presence of obvious focal neurologic deficits such as a facial droop or gaze deviation, evidence of respiratory distress, and any other signs of obvious cardiac discomfort. You then must review the patient's vital signs, paying careful attention to the blood pressure measured both on arrival and at present. You should immediately ask what medications the patient has already received in the emergency department, and you should screen for triggers of hypertensive crisis, with a particular emphasis on substance abuse, current home medications, and lapses in taking home medications. Finally, your focused but thorough physical examination, directed primarily toward identifying neurologic or cardiovascular failure, will be instrumental in making your decision about whether the patient needs to be admitted and whether he or she should be sent emergently to an ICU. The patient at the beginning of the chapter has evidence of altered mental status as well as signs of heart failure on exam and will likely require ICU management of hypertensive emergency.

Admission Criteria and Level of Care Criteria

After your initial assessment, you should be in a position to decide whether the patient has severe hypertension that warrants treatment but does not require admission, hypertensive urgency that requires admission to a telemetry unit for controlled blood pressure reduction over a 24- to 48-hour period, or a hypertensive emergency that necessitates immediate admission to an intensive care unit.

Importantly, patients with hypertensive emergency need ICU-level care even if their blood pressure has been lowered to the target range in the emergency department. The clinical challenge is not lowering the blood pressure, but doing so in a controlled fashion and monitoring the patient for progressive organ failure. Only rapid-acting, easily titratable intravenous medications and very aggressive monitoring will allow you to do this safely.

CLINICAL PEARL

If a patient presents in hypertensive emergency and achieves a near-"normal" blood pressure in the emergency department, he or she may be in more serious need of ICU-level care than on arrival because of potential overcorrection of blood pressure and subsequent end-organ hypoperfusion. Such overaggressive lowering of blood pressure can lead to stroke, myocardial infarction, renal failure, and even death in extreme cases.

If the patient is not in distress, has no evidence of other systemic illness or of acute end-organ damage, and has a history of significant hypertension, the patient can likely be safely treated by resumption of his or her home medication regimen, particularly if the rise in blood pressure appears to have been precipitated by one or several missed doses of regular medication. In fact, this patient will likely be better off lowering his or her pressure over days to weeks rather than making quick adjustments. Reviewing outpatient clinic notes, when available, can be particularly helpful in making this determination.

Patients with hypertensive urgency who do not fall into one of the two categories listed previously should be admitted to a telemetry bed, hopefully for a 1- to 2-day admission, during which you can slowly lower their blood pressure, monitor for the development of end-organ failure, and develop a treatment regimen that will allow them to be successfully discharged.

The First Few Hours

Your first few hours with a severely hypertensive patient will be focused on implementing a controlled blood pressure–lowering strategy and monitoring for signs of new or worsening end-organ damage.

History

Your history should focus on two questions: (a) Why is the patient having a hypertensive crisis? and (b) Does the patient have evidence of acute end-organ damage?

In determining why a patient is having a hypertensive crisis, focus first on identifying whether the patient is hypertensive at baseline, has comorbidities that predispose him or her to hypertension (such as end-stage renal disease), has been prescribed antihypertensive medications, and has been taking those medications. You may ask if he or she knows what his or her blood pressure typically runs in the physician's office or at home and whether he or she has had significant elevations prior to this presentation. A patient who has poorly controlled very elevated blood pressure for several months needs to be managed differently; this patient has had time to equilibrate to elevated perfusion pressures and therefore the rate of reduction should be more gradual and less aggressive.

Similarly, it is critical to identify any other important triggers, such as whether the patient is pregnant, has recently used illicit drugs, or may be withdrawing from alcohol. A young patient without obvious comorbidities who is suddenly hypertensive and has no recent substance use raises immediate concern for unusual, secondary causes of hypertension (such as pheochromocytoma or RAS) and is at high risk for suffering acute end-organ damage with a high blood pressure reading. When available, history from the patient's primary care physician and/or family may be helpful to get a good overview of compliance and access to care.

Physical Examination

The neurologic exam is important to identify stroke, hemorrhage, or hypertensive encephalopathy. A funduscopic exam should be performed to identify retinal hemorrhage or papilledema (the latter being indicative of increased intracranial pressure). The cardiopulmonary exam will help to identify the presence of heart failure. Abdominal pain and tenderness on examination may suggest the presence of bowel ischemia, and abdominal bruits may be suggestive of renal artery stenosis as a precipitant. On examination of the extremities, discordant blood pressure or pulses between both arms is an important clue for aortic dissection or coarctation of the aorta, and edema may suggest heart failure. Bruising or petechiae suggest hematologic complications.

Labs and Tests to Consider

Lab tests and imaging studies should focus on identifying evidence of end-organ damage.

Key Diagnostic and Lab Tests

At the outset, you should request basic labs that focus on renal dysfunction (urinalysis with microscopic analysis, protein/creatinine ratio, and basic chemistries) and cardiac involvement. It is imperative that all patients with hypertensive crisis have an electrocardiogram (principally for evidence of ischemia) and, where warranted, you should consider imaging (noncontrast head CT, chest radiograph, thoracic CT with contrast if there is concern for dissection, and renal artery magnetic resonance angiogram or duplex if you suspect RAS). If possible, you should also spin the patient's urine and examine it directly for the presence of red blood cells and red cell casts, an important indicator of acute hypertensive injury.

Treatment

Treatment choices are most critical for patients who require ICU admission for hypertensive emergency. These patients must have an arterial catheter placed for invasive blood pressure monitoring. Most will also need a central line placed for the secure delivery of medications and potentially for central venous pressure monitoring. Most importantly, all of these patients should be started on an appropriate intravenous drip medication. Although oral medications can lower blood pressure quickly, the risk of overcorrection is much greater.

There are a variety of medications available for the treatment of hypertensive emergency, many of which are listed in Table 9-2. The ideal agent is one that acts quickly and has a short half-life so that you can make rapid adjustments. However, there are insufficient data to suggest the superiority of any particular agent for treatment. In general, your target blood pressure reduction should be to reduce the mean arterial pressure (MAP) 10% to 15% or to a DBP of 110 mm Hg in the first hour, generally not more than 20% over the first few hours, and then very gradually over the next 12 hours.

There are several forms of end-organ failure that are treated uniquely in terms of blood pressure goals and appropriate agents. If your patient has an acute aortic dissection, you should aim to lower the SBP to <120 mm Hg (and MAP to 80 mm Hg) as fast as possible, and the first agent must be a beta-blocker (typically labetalol or esmolol) in order to decrease strain on the aorta. If you need a second agent, nitroprusside can be added to the beta-blocker. For patients with acute congestive heart failure, focus on vasodilatory

TABLE 9-2

Common Intravenous Medications Used in Hypertensive Emergencies

Medication	Notable Characteristics and Indications
Sodium nitroprusside	• Most rapid onset (seconds) and offset (3- to 4-min half-life) • May limit cerebral blood flow • Cyanide toxicity
Fenoldopam	• No reflex tachycardia or rebound hypertension • Rapid onset (5–15 min) and offset (<1 hr)
Nicardipine	• Minimizes cerebral ischemia • Rapid onset but longer half-life (4–6 hr)
Labetalol	• Beta-blockers are the first line in aortic dissection • Rapid onset but longer half-life (2–4 hr) • May want to avoid if cocaine ingestion suspected
Esmolol	• Very rapid onset/offset • Effective (often with nitroprusside) in aortic dissection
Enalaprilat	• Contraindicated in acute renal failure
Nitroglycerin	• Particularly useful in coronary ischemia and pulmonary edema • Tachyphylaxis occurs in about 12 hr

agents, such as nitroglycerin or nitroprusside with the addition of intravenous loop diuretics. If your patient has increased intracranial pressure or a cerebral infarct, the target blood pressure will be higher (blood pressure should not be reduced more than 20% acutely), and nicardipine may help to avoid cerebral ischemia. Finally, if your patient has acute renal failure, ACE inhibitors should be avoided, and nitroprusside should be used as briefly as possible, if at all, with close monitoring of thiocyanate levels. The patient in our initial encounter would likely benefit from intravenous nitroprusside and a loop diuretic since he has evidence of both hypertensive encephalopathy and congestive heart failure.

In addition to lowering the blood pressure appropriately, you must keep a close eye on your patient's fluid status. Many patients with hypertensive emergency are severely dehydrated from pressure-induced natriuresis and may require intravenous fluids in order to prevent ischemic injury and close observation of urine output as an indicator of renal perfusion. If your patient has end-stage renal disease and hypertensive emergency, ask about missed hemodialysis sessions and be ready to call in the renal fellow. The patient almost certainly will need emergent dialysis and may dramatically improve following such treatment.

If your patient is in hypertensive urgency and is admitted to a telemetry unit for monitoring, your goal should be to use oral medications to reduce the blood pressure slowly into a more acceptable range over 24 to 48 hours. The best place to start in choosing a medication regimen is the patient's home regimen—particularly if the hypertensive crisis was precipitated by missing medications—while also paying careful attention to the patient's comorbidities. If the patient has significantly reduced renal function or suspected renal artery stenosis, you will need to be careful with ACE inhibitors, and if the patient is a cocaine abuser, you should avoid beta-blockers. Some popular agents for effective blood pressure control in the inpatient setting are long-acting nifedipine, hydralazine, and captopril. Captopril in particular can be easily titrated because it is a relatively short-acting oral medication. Other classes of medications can also be used easily in this setting; the key is to make adjustments gradually, avoid precipitous drops in blood pressure, and work toward a reasonable medication regimen for discharge.

EXTENDED IN-HOSPITAL MANAGEMENT

After achieving your initial blood pressure goals, you can transition patients to oral blood pressure regimens and monitor them closely to ensure resolution of organ damage. For patients in whom a secondary cause of hypertension is suspected, this is the time to pursue the workup further.

DISPOSITION

Discharge Goals

Once the acute issues have been tackled, the primary goal ought to be to develop, with the patient, a plan for sustainable treatment of his or her hypertension. This includes ensuring follow-up, developing a medication regimen that the patient can afford as an outpatient, minimizing pill burden to maximize adherence, educating the patient on the importance of blood pressure control, enlisting the help of ancillary providers such as dieticians, and working with family members and other caregivers. Particularly if your patient is chronically and profoundly hypertensive, your goal for the admission is not to "normalize" his or her blood pressure—it is to stabilize the blood pressure and develop a plan to lower it over a long period as an outpatient.

Outpatient Care

Regular outpatient care will be the cornerstone of treatment for patients with hypertension. Establishing outpatient follow-up prior to discharge is crucial, and the patient should ideally be seen within 1 to 2 weeks of discharge. It is also critical to outpatient success that the patient is discharged on a medication regimen that is as simple as possible (i.e., long-acting and once per day when possible) and affordable to the patient. Lifestyle changes such as weight loss, salt restriction, and exercise should also be emphasized.

WHAT YOU NEED TO REMEMBER

- Hypertensive emergency is defined by the presence of acute end-organ damage; recognizing that end-organ damage is the most important task in assessing a patient in hypertensive crisis.
- The most common precipitants of hypertensive crisis are untreated hypertension and medication nonadherence.
- Hypertensive emergency requires aggressive treatment in an ICU with invasive blood pressure monitoring and intravenous medications.
- Aggressive lowering of blood pressure in patients with hypertensive urgency and chronic severe hypertension can cause more harm than benefit. Go slowly with these patients when they are stable.

SUGGESTED READINGS

Marik PE, Varon J. Hypertensive crises: challenges and management. *Chest.* 2007;131:1949–1962.

Perez M, Musini V. Pharmacological interventions for hypertensive emergencies. *Cochrane Database Syst Rev.* 2008;1:CD003653.

Vaughan CJ, Delanty N. Hypertensive emergencies. *Lancet.* 2000;356:411–417.

Pericardial Disease

THE PATIENT ENCOUNTER

A 45-year-old woman with no significant past medical history presents to the emergency room with 2 days of sharp, retrosternal chest pain and a low-grade fever. She states that the pain is worse with deep inspiration and seems to improve when she leans forward. An electrocardiogram reveals 1 mm of ST elevation inferolaterally, no reciprocal changes, and PR depression best seen in lead II.

OVERVIEW

Definition

The pericardium is a well-innervated fibrous sac that surrounds the heart. It is composed of two layers, a thin visceral layer adherent to the epicardium and a parietal layer composed of collagen and elastin. These layers are separated by a potential space that normally contains 15 to 35 mL of serous fluid. Pericardial disease can roughly be divided into three major categories: (a) acute pericarditis, (b) cardiac tamponade, and (c) pericardial constriction. The presentation, evaluation, and management of the first two categories will be reviewed in this chapter.

ACUTE PERICARDITIS

Pathophysiology

Pericarditis can occur in isolation or as part of a systemic disease. Inflammation of the heavily innervated pericardium produces a classically sharp pain that is often relieved by sitting forward. The pain may also be worsened with movement or respiration. In some cases, the inflammation may progress to cause a simultaneous myocarditis.

Epidemiology

Acute pericarditis may account for up to 5% of presentations to the emergency room for nonischemic chest pain. However, this is likely an underestimate because many cases of pericarditis go unrecognized.

TABLE 10-1
Causes of Acute Pericarditis and Pericardial Effusions

Infectious—viral, bacterial, mycobacterial, fungal, human immunodeficiency virus related

Immune mediated—connective tissue disease, postmyocardial infarction, medication related

Traumatic—blunt trauma, cardiac surgery

Malignancy—primary or metastatic to pericardium

Postradiation

Uremia

Thyroid disease

Etiology

There are a number of potential causes of acute pericarditis (Table 10-1), but about 80% to 90% are termed *idiopathic*. The vast majority of cases are likely caused by viral infections.

ACUTE MANAGEMENT AND WORKUP

The first part of your assessment should focus on confirming the diagnosis of pericarditis.

The First 15 Minutes

Acute pericarditis may mimic an acute coronary syndrome, aortic dissection, or pulmonary embolus. Therefore, an evaluation for life-threatening causes of chest pain is critical. This should include a careful history that assesses the risk of coronary artery disease and characteristics of the pain or other cardiovascular symptoms. The physical exam should focus on a careful cardiopulmonary assessment but should also search for clues of a systemic process that may be the cause of the pericarditis.

Initial Assessment

The electrocardiogram (ECG), as in our patient encounter, will help to confirm the suspicion of pericarditis and to exclude other causes of chest pain, such as ongoing coronary ischemia. The characteristic pattern on an ECG initially will show PR depression in all leads except aVR, which commonly has PR elevation. This is then followed by diffuse ST elevation that is often saddle shaped (Fig. 10-1). Reciprocal ST depressions are not usually seen in

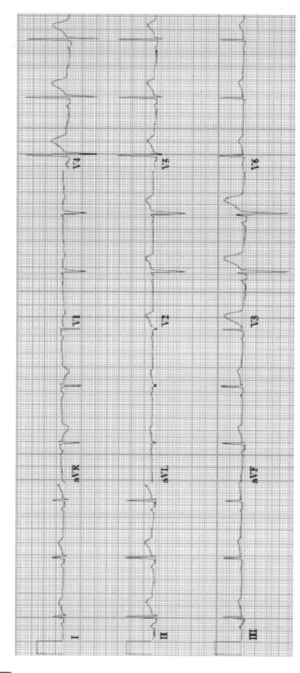

FIGURE 10-1: Twelve-lead electrocardiogram showing diffuse ST-segment elevation and PR depression. (Courtesy of Brian T. Garibaldi, MD, Division of Pulmonary and Critical Care Medicine, The Johns Hopkins Hospital.)

pericarditis and should prompt urgent evaluation for an ST-elevation myocardial infarction. Over time, the ECG then evolves with normalization of the ST and PR segments, followed by T-wave inversions and then normalization of the T waves.

Admission Criteria and Level of Care Criteria

If the diagnosis is clear and the patient is relatively comfortable, an outpatient trial of nonsteroidal anti-inflammatory drugs (NSAIDs) may be reasonable. In most instances, however, a short hospital stay is recommended to fully evaluate the cause of the chest pain and to initiate therapy. Patients with known malignancy, with evidence of heart failure or tamponade, with suspected myocarditis (i.e., elevated biomarkers of cardiac necrosis), or on anticoagulation should be admitted for management and careful observation. Hemodynamics will determine if a patient is best served on a cardiac telemetry floor or in the coronary care unit.

The First Few Hours

Once the diagnosis is made and the patient is hemodynamically stable, you can turn your attention to the cause of the pericarditis.

History

A careful review of the patient's past medical and surgical history should be performed, including screening for malignancies and systemic diseases such as systemic lupus erythematosus that may cause pericarditis. While chest pain is the most common symptom, patients may presents with dyspnea, fever, and malaise as their predominant complaints. A prior viral illness may precede the onset of chest pain by several days. Pericarditis can also be seen in the setting of acute bacterial infections such as pneumonia, so a good review of systems will also be helpful.

Physical Examination

About 85% of patients with acute pericarditis have an audible friction rub that is typically described as scratchy or high pitched and is best heard at the left sternal border as the patient leans forward. The classic rub consists of three components thought to correlate to ventricular contraction, ventricular filling, and atrial contraction. It tends to be present earlier in the disease when the two inflamed pericardial surfaces are in contact. As the inflammation progresses and inflammatory cells encourage pericardial fluid production, the surfaces will separate and the rub may no longer be heard. Rubs frequently come and go, so if your suspicion for pericarditis is high, be sure to listen to your patient on multiple occasions. It is important to also perform a thorough hemodynamic assessment to exclude heart failure from a concurrent myocarditis, or cardiac tamponade from a new or rapidly enlarging pericardial effusion.

CLINICAL PEARL

To differentiate a pericardial rub from a pleural rub, ask the patient to hold his or her breath at peak inspiration. A pericardial rub will still be audible, whereas a pleural friction rub will disappear.

Labs and Tests to Consider

As discussed previously, the ECG is the most important diagnostic test.

Key Diagnostic Labs and Tests

A complete blood count may reveal a mild leukocytosis with a lymphocytic predominance. A markedly elevated white blood cell count should raise the suspicion of a more fulminant infection, such as bacterial pericarditis. Elevated biomarkers of necrosis, such as troponin I, should raise the question of a concurrent myocarditis.

Imaging

Echocardiography may reveal a pericardial effusion, provide information about the hemodynamic significance of the effusion, and also assess for ventricular dysfunction from either a recent myocardial infarction or myocarditis. Chest radiography may reveal an underlying pneumonia or an enlarged cardiac silhouette. Routine screening for viral etiologies is of little benefit. Likewise, pericardial biopsy is generally low yield and is not routinely recommended.

Treatment

NSAIDs such as aspirin or indomethacin are the cornerstone of management for acute pericarditis for both pain and reduction of inflammation and should be tried as empiric treatment in the patient from our encounter. The Colchicine for Acute Pericarditis Trial (COPE) randomized patients with a first episode of pericarditis to acetylsalicylic acid (ASA) versus ASA plus colchicine (1 to 2 mg for the first day followed by 0.5 to 1 mg/day for 3 months). Colchicine significantly reduced symptoms at 72 hours and recurrence at 18 months and on this basis is a reasonable addition to ASA as first-line therapy (1). Refractory disease may require a longer course of NSAIDs with a slow taper. While steroids generally rapidly improve symptoms, they are associated with an increased likelihood of relapse and are not recommended as first-line therapy.

EXTENDED IN-HOSPITAL MANAGEMENT

The primary goal of hospitalization for acute pericarditis is to achieve pain control and to rule out potential life-threatening conditions such as cardiac tamponade and myopericarditis. Because most cases are likely viral in etiology, an extensive inpatient diagnostic workup is usually not indicated.

DISPOSITION

Discharge Goals

Patients are ready for discharge once their pain is adequately controlled and life-threatening conditions have been ruled out.

Outpatient Care

Patients can follow up with their primary care provider shortly after hospitalization to ensure the resolution of symptoms. Patients with persistent symptoms or recurrent episodes should be referred to cardiology for further evaluation and management.

CARDIAC TAMPONADE

Pathophysiology

The hallmark of cardiac tamponade is external compression of the cardiac chambers due to transmitted increased pericardial pressure. The pericardial space can accommodate even a moderate amount of fluid if it increases slowly over time. However, larger volumes or fluid that accumulates quickly in a vulnerable area such as adjacent to the right ventricular free wall can impair filling of the chamber and consequently can reduce cardiac output. The more rapidly pericardial fluid accumulates, the less total volume is required to impact hemodynamics.

Because total cardiac volume is limited by the effusion, volume changes in one chamber necessitate equal and opposite volume changes in another chamber (i.e., *interventricular dependence*). Thus, venous return and atrial filling largely occur during ventricular systole. Similarly, the normal respiratory effects on hemodynamics are exaggerated such that inspiratory increases in right-sided filling impair left-sided filling. This may lead to the classic finding of pulsus paradoxus, a drop in systolic blood pressure by more than 10 mm Hg on inspiration.

Epidemiology

Given the variety of conditions that can lead to a pericardial effusion and subsequent tamponade physiology, it is difficult to estimate the true incidence of tamponade. Tamponade is more likely to occur in patients whose pericardial effusion is malignant, bacterial, mycobacterial, or fungal in origin, and in patients with underlying human immunodeficiency virus (HIV).

Etiology

Any condition that can lead to acute pericarditis can ultimately lead to a pericardial effusion and subsequent tamponade physiology (see Table 10-1).

ACUTE MANAGEMENT AND WORKUP

Tamponade should be considered in any patient who presents with hypotension and an elevated jugular venous pressure.

The First 15 Minutes

Cardiac tamponade is a cardiovascular emergency, so you need to move quickly to establish the diagnosis and initiate treatment.

Initial Assessment

Cardiac tamponade is a clinical diagnosis made at the bedside. As cardiac output decreases, patients become tachypneic and tachycardic with low-volume pulses. Beck's triad of muffled heart sounds, hypotension, and jugular venous distention is suggestive of tamponade physiology. While often difficult to see without invasive hemodynamic monitoring, loss of the Y descent on jugular venous pulse examination is also suggestive. As previously described, the exaggerated increase in right heart filling with inspiration is reflected by pulsus paradoxus. To measure the pulsus paradoxus, inflate the blood pressure cuff above the systolic pressure. Very slowly deflate the cuff until Korotkoff sounds are heard only during expiration. Further deflate the cuff until Korotkoff sounds are heard throughout the respiratory cycle. The difference between the two points is the pulsus paradoxus. A difference >10 mm Hg is considered abnormal. Pulsus paradoxus may also be palpable whereby the peripheral arterial pulse disappears during inspiration. If your initial assessment suggests possible cardiac tamponade, urgent cardiology consultation is indicated.

Admission Criteria and Level of Care Criteria

All patients with cardiac tamponade should be stabilized in a coronary care unit with close monitoring of hemodynamics and cardiac rhythm.

The First Few Hours

Once you have recognized the likelihood of tamponade, urgent management to ensure hemodynamic stability should be the focus of your efforts.

History

Patients with large pericardial effusions may be asymptomatic if the effusion has accumulated over a long period of time. However, patients with tamponade are usually uncomfortable and describe symptoms consistent with a low cardiac output state, such as dyspnea, light-headedness, and diaphoresis. Many patients with tamponade will also complain of pericarditislike pain that is relieved with sitting forward. In addition to exploring the nature and duration of your patient's symptoms, it is helpful to search for underlying conditions such as malignancy, HIV, recent trauma, or surgery that may predispose to tamponade.

Physical Examination

The physical examination is the most important aspect of the evaluation because it will lead you to the diagnosis and suggest the urgency of pericardiocentesis. In addition to the cardiac findings described previously, patients may have associated left lower lobe atelectasis and bronchial breath sounds. You should look for signs of end-organ hypoperfusion and search for associated

conditions that can predispose to pericardial effusions, such as rheumatologic disease or malignancy.

Labs and Tests to Consider

While tamponade is a diagnosis made at the bedside, there are a number of
ancillary tests that may prove useful.

Imaging

An ECG might reveal acute pericarditis or reduced voltage consistent with
a pericardial effusion. Electrical alternans, if present, also suggests the presence of a large pericardial effusion, as the heart swings from side to side with
each contraction. Chest radiography may show a characteristic "flasklike"
appearance of the heart with an enlarged cardiac silhouette. Likewise, computed tomography or magnetic resonance imaging may reveal an effusion
and may help to characterize the pericardium itself. Echocardiography will
reveal the presence of a pericardial effusion and may also provide clues about
its hemodynamic significance. Early diastolic collapse of the right ventricle
is strongly suggestive of increased pericardial pressures. Increased right-
sided and decreased left-sided Doppler velocities across the atrioventricular
valves on inspiration are also suggestive. However, remember that the diagnosis of tamponade is made most reliably at the bedside.

Treatment

Pericardiocentesis should be performed when tamponade is present. Because
tamponade effectively limits preload, patients can be temporized with aggressive intravenous fluids, but there will be a limit to the hemodynamic benefits
of such an intervention. Emergent drainage via a subxiphoid approach may
be indicated in unstable patients. If the clinical scenario allows, it is preferable to perform pericardial drainage in a controlled setting using echocardiography or fluoroscopy for guidance. Surgical drainage with the creation of a
pericardial window may be required for recurrent and/or malignant effusions, or in cases in which the effusion cannot be effectively drained with a
small catheter (i.e., hemorrhagic effusions with adherent clot).

In patients with moderate to large effusions and no clinical evidence of tamponade, pericardiocentesis is occasionally performed for diagnosis but is usually of little yield. The diagnosis in these cases is often evident from the history and diagnostic testing or remains elusive despite extensive investigation.

EXTENDED IN-HOSPITAL MANAGEMENT

The hospital course of a patient with cardiac tamponade will be dictated by
his or her hemodynamics and, to a lesser extent, his or her diagnostic
workup. If an underlying etiology for the pericardial effusion is discovered
(i.e., occult malignancy, rheumatologic condition, etc.), patients should be
further evaluated and managed accordingly.

DISPOSITION

Discharge Goals

Patients are ready for discharge once hemodynamic stability has been assured and a plan has been made regarding follow-up. If a pericardiocentesis was performed, patients should undergo repeat echocardiography to evaluate for recurrence of the effusion and to help plan the duration of interval follow-up.

Outpatient Care

Patients with a history of cardiac tamponade should follow up with an outpatient cardiologist to monitor for disease recurrence and to continue the evaluation for the root cause.

 WHAT YOU NEED TO REMEMBER

- Prompt diagnosis of pericarditis and tamponade requires a careful history and physical exam.
- Many patients with acute pericarditis can be managed in the outpatient arena. Patients with known malignancy, large effusions, tamponade physiology, heart failure myocarditis or an anticoagulation should be admitted.
- Most cases of acute pericarditis are "idiopathic" and are likely caused by viral syndromes.
- Cardiac tamponade is a clinical diagnosis. An echocardiogram cannot make or break the diagnosis.

REFERENCES

1. Imazio M, Bobbio M, Cecchi E, et al. Colchicine in addition to conventional therapy for acute pericarditis: results of the COlchicine for acute PEricarditis (COPE) trial. *Circulation.* 2005;112:2012–2016.

SUGGESTED READINGS

Lange R, Hillis LD. Acute pericarditis. *N Engl J Med.* 2004;351:2195–2202.

Reddy PS, Curtiss EI, Uretesky BF. Spectrum of hemodynamic changes in cardiac tamponade. *Am J Cardiol.* 1990;66:1487–1491.

Roy C, Minor M, Brookhart M, et al. Does this patient with a pericardial effusion have tamponade? Rational clinical exam. *JAMA.* 2007;297:1810–1181.

Shabetai R. Pericardial disease: etiology, pathophysiology, clinical recognition, and treatment. In: Willerson J, Cohn J, Wellens H, et al., eds. *Cardiovascular Medicine.* 3rd ed. London: Springer; 2007:1483–1508.

Zayas R, Anguita M, Torres F, et al. Incidence of specific etiology and role of methods for specific etiologic diagnosis of primary acute pericarditis. *Am J Cardiol.* 1995;75:378–382.

Bradyarrhythmia

OVERVIEW

Definition

The term *bradyarrhythmia* refers to an abnormality in the initiation or propagation of cardiac electrical impulses that results in a heart rate <60 bpm.

Pathophysiology

Bradyarrhythmias result from either failures of automaticity or propagation. Failure of automaticity in the form of sinoatrial node dysfunction is the most common cause of bradycardia. Failure of the propagation of electrical impulses generated in the atrium to travel normally to the ventricles is termed either *heart block* or *atrioventricular (AV) block*. It is the result of disease within the AV node or lower down within the His-Purkinje conduction system.

Epidemiology

Bradycardia occurs commonly in both healthy and ill patients; therefore, its presence does not necessarily indicate a disease state. Idiopathic degeneration is the most common cause of sinus node dysfunction, and its incidence increases with age. Endurance athletes are the most common patients to have nonpathologic bradycardia.

Etiology

Table 11-1 lists the most common causes of bradyarrhythmias.

ACUTE MANAGEMENT AND WORKUP

The initial management of a patient with clinically significant bradycardia is similar to other encounters in advanced cardiac life support (ACLS) scenarios. The initial focus should be placed on the patient's ability to protect his or

TABLE 11-1
The Etiology of Bradyarrhythmias

Sinus Node Dysfunction	Atrioventricular Block
Idiopathic degenerative disease	Drugs
Coronary artery disease	Coronary artery disease
Cardiomyopathy	Acute myocardial infarction
Hypertension	Idiopathic fibrosis of conduction system
Infiltrative disorders	Congenital heart disease
Collagen vascular disease	Calcific valvular disease
Myocarditis/pericarditis	Cardiomyopathy
Surgical trauma (valve surgery, transplant)	Infiltrative diseases
Congenital heart disease	Endocarditis
Drugs	Myocarditis
Excessive vagal tone	Collagen vascular diseases
Carotid sinus syndrome	Malignancies including metastatic disease
Excessive vagal tone	Electrolyte abnormalities
Endurance-trained athletes	Cardiac surgery
Hyperkalemia	Iatrogenic (radiation, catheter ablation, or trauma)
Hypercarbia	Addison disease
Hypothyroidism	Carotid sinus syndrome
Increased intracranial pressure	Vasovagal syncope
Hypothermia	Neuromyopathic disorders
Sepsis	

her airway followed by attention to whether the patient has a pulse and is adequately perfusing vital organs.

The First 15 Minutes
How a patient tolerates an abnormal rhythm is highly dependent on his or her underlying cardiovascular status. The patient in the encounter is

experiencing episodes of intermittent lightheadedness, suggesting that his bradycardia may be hemodynamically significant. Cardiac output is the product of heart rate and stroke volume, and when a patient develops brady-cardia, he or she must be able to increase his or her stroke volume to main-tain a sufficient cardiac output. Heart failure in the form of inability to pump (systolic dysfunction) or inability to relax (diastolic dysfunction) can lead to symptoms from insufficient cardiac output during bradycardia. Hemody-namic compromise will require that the patient be immediately assessed for temporary pacing. Available pacing methods include immediate external pacing and the more reliable intravenous temporary pacing.

Initial Assessment

When evaluating a bradyarrhythmia, you should focus on the presence of nonconducted P waves, the occurrence of symptoms, and the rate. Are there nonconducted P waves? If not, evaluate the PR interval. If it is <200 ms, the tracing likely represents sinus bradycardia, whereas a PR interval >200 ms represents first-degree AV block. If there are nonconducted P waves, the rhythm may be characteristic of second-degree Mobitz I, which shows an increasing prolongation of the PR interval, or Mobitz II, which displays intermittently dropped P waves without PR prolongation. Third-degree heart block displays complete dissociation of P waves and QRS complexes (Fig. 11-1). If the rate of atrial depolarization decreases below the intrinsic rate of depolarization of either the AV node (approximately 40 bpm) or the ventricular myocardium (approximately 30 bpm), a junctional or ventricular escape rhythm may occur, respectively.

Now that you have identified the type of bradycardia, you need to deter-mine whether the patient experienced symptoms due to the bradycardia. Older patients and those with comorbid cardiovascular disease are more likely to be intolerant of a low heart rate as the compensatory mechanisms to increase stroke volume, and thus cardiac output, are not effective. As a result, these are the patients who tend to be symptomatic as a result of bradycardia.

CLINICAL PEARL

To facilitate determination of Mobitz I, compare the PR interval of the last conducted P wave prior to the dropped beat to that of the PR interval of the first conducted P wave following the dropped beat (see Fig. 11-1A). Due to properties of the AV node, this comparison provides the largest difference in PR intervals.

Admission Criteria and Level of Care Criteria

Patients with symptomatic bradycardia and asymptomatic Mobitz II should be admitted to a unit with cardiac monitoring. Patients with third-degree heart block or those who are hemodynamically unstable require coronary care unit–level care.

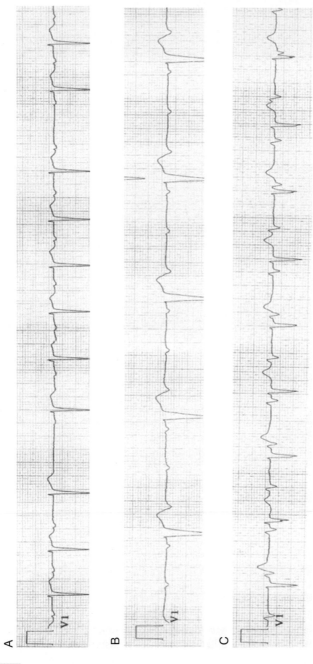

FIGURE 11-1: **A:** Second-degree Mobitz I atrioventricular (AV) block. **B:** Second-degree Mobitz II AV block. **C:** Third-degree (complete) AV block. (Modified from Rimmerman CM, Jain AK *Interactive Electrocardiography.* Philadelphia: Lippincott Williams & Wilkins, 2003:7, 348, 432.)

The First Few Hours

As with the evaluation of tachyarrhythmias discussed in Chapter 12, obtain old electrocardiogram (ECG) tracings, and continue to pursue clues to the etiology of the bradycardia.

History

Similar to tachyarrhythmias, the most important information to determine from the history is whether the patient was symptomatic from the bradyarrhythmia and whether there are clues in the history to the underlying etiology. Symptoms are varied and include fatigue, angina, falls, nausea/vomiting, and shortness of breath. Remember to inquire about how often the patient has symptoms, as well as the duration, the time of first occurrence, and precipitating factors.

Medication use is a common cause of bradyarrhythmias, and a thorough history to elicit new medications or dose changes is necessary. Beta-blockers, calcium channel blockers such as verapamil and diltiazem, and digoxin can all cause bradycardias.

Physical Examination

The physical examination is oftentimes nonspecific in cases of bradyarrhythmias. A thorough cardiovascular examination is critical to assess for signs of heart failure and/or end-organ hypoperfusion. The remainder of the physical examination should search for clues that might reveal the etiology of the bradyarrhythmia.

Labs and Tests to Consider

Arrhythmias have a vast list of potential etiologies, and there are no diagnostic laboratory tests that can definitively uncover the cause of a bradycardia. Electrolyte abnormalities, including hypokalemia and hyperkalemia, are potential causes of bradyarrhythmias, so an analysis of a metabolic profile is indicated. Other laboratory tests should include a complete blood count to look for anemia and thyroid function tests to assess for hypothyroidism. Cardiac enzymes can be used to assess for evidence of ischemia, although it is not unusual to see mild elevations in the setting of bradycardia without significant coronary artery disease. Remember that medications, including beta-blockers, calcium channel blockers, clonidine, and digoxin, are a major cause of bradyarrhythmias. When possible, patients should be tested for the levels of suspected medications, such as digoxin.

Key Diagnostic Labs and Tests

The ECG is the most important diagnostic test in the evaluation of bradyarrhythmias and, in the majority of cases, the specific type of bradyarrhythmia can be identified. Try to obtain an ECG during the arrhythmia and measure the PR interval. If the patient has an implantable cardioverter-defibrillator or pacemaker, it can be interrogated for helpful information about the bradyarrhythmia. A cardiology consultation by a specialist in arrhythmias may be appropriate to help with assessing the underlying rhythm and to determine if an electrophysiology study or intervention is indicated.

Imaging

Echocardiograms should be ordered in patients with findings suggestive of congestive heart failure or valvular disease.

Treatment

Acute treatment of hemodynamically significant bradycardia is usually accomplished with atropine in the case of sinus node dysfunction and in AV block when the level of the heart block is at the AV node. In situations with third-degree (complete) heart block and a resulting ventricular escape rhythm, atropine will not be effective. In these cases patients will require temporary cardiac pacing. Cardiac pacing can be performed on an emergent basis transcutaneously using the defibrillator pad. However, this should only be used as a temporizing measure. Stabilizing the patient will require placement of a temporary pacing wire in the right ventricle via a central venous catheter. Depending on whether the heart block is temporary (as from a medication overdose) or permanent, a permanent pacemaker may be required. Many bradycardias are medication induced, and all potential culprits should be discontinued. In the patient encounter, the dose of metoprolol should be reduced or the medication discontinued entirely pending further evaluation. Sinus bradycardia and AV block may be caused by ischemia, and reperfusion therapy should be pursued rapidly. The decision about whether to implant a permanent pacemaker (PPM) in many cases depends on whether a patient is symptomatic. The American College of Cardiology (ACC) and the American Heart Association (AHA) have specific guidelines that determine pacemaker indications. In general, almost any sinus node dysfunction and AV block that is symptomatic and due to irreversible causes, along with asymptomatic second-degree Mobitz II and third-degree heart block, warrant PPM placement.

EXTENDED IN-HOSPITAL MANAGEMENT

In most cases of bradyarrhythmias due to reversible causes, the patient should remain on a cardiac monitor until the underlying condition has resolved. In patients requiring PPM placement, these procedures are ideally performed when the patient has resolved most other medical issues that require hospitalization and is nearing discharge. Postprocedure recovery from noncomplicated PPM placement is 1 hospital day.

DISPOSITION

Discharge Goals

A patient is ready for discharge when the cause of the bradyarrhythmia has been identified and reversed, or when medical or device therapy has been successfully implemented.

Outpatient Care

Patients should follow up with their primary care physician in 1 to 2 weeks, as well as with a cardiologist within 1 to 2 weeks. Patients who underwent PPM placement should follow up with their electrophysiologist as directed.

WHAT YOU NEED TO REMEMBER

- Bradyarrhythmias range from asymptomatic to fatal.
- Bradycardias commonly occur in healthy and ill patients, and their presence does not necessarily indicate a disease state.
- Medications are a common cause of bradyarrhythmias.
- Structural heart disease and coronary artery disease are risk factors for bradyarrhythmias.
- Patients who experience hypotension, unresponsiveness, altered mental status, respiratory distress, and chest pain due to a bradyarrhythmia may require pacing.
- In order to make treatment decisions, it is important to determine whether a patient was symptomatic from a bradyarrhythmia.
- The evaluation of a bradyarrhythmia should include identification of the etiology.

SUGGESTED READINGS

Gregoratos G, Abrams J, Epstein AE, et al. ACC/AHA/NAPSE 2002 guideline update for implantation of cardiac pacemakers and antiarrhythmia devices. *Circulation.* 2002;106:2145–2161.

Kaushik V, Leon AR, Forrester JS Jr, et al. Bradyarrhythmias, temporary and permanent pacing. *Crit Care Med.* 2000;28(10 Suppl):N121–128.

Mangrum JM, DiMarco JP. The Evaluation and management of bradycardia. *N Engl J Med.* 2000;342:703.

Ufberg JW, Clark JS. Bradydysrhythmias and atrioventricular conduction blocks. *Emerg Med Clin North Am.* 2006;24(1):1–9.

Wazni O, Cole C. Bradyarrhythmias and pulseless electrical activity. In: Griffin BP, Topol EJ, eds. *Manual of Cardiovascular Medicine.* 2nd ed. Philadelphia: Lippincott Williams & Wilkins; 2004.

12 Tachyarrhythmia

A 52-year-old woman without significant past medical history is brought to the emergency department by her husband with palpitations of 4 hours' duration. She reports lightheadedness, but denies chest pain or shortness of breath. She has had three similar episodes over the past 2 months, but they were self-limited and <15 minutes in duration. In the emergency department, her blood pressure is 95/60 mm Hg with a heart rate of 150 bpm. Electrocardiogram reveals a regular, narrow QRS-complex tachycardia.

OVERVIEW

Definition

The term *tachyarrhythmia* refers to an abnormality in cardiac electrical conduction that results in ventricular rhythms that are >100 bpm.

Pathophysiology

An important distinction to understand is where in the conduction system the rhythm originates. Supraventricular tachyarrhythmias occur when the depolarization is initiated above or within the atrioventricular (AV) node as usually characterized by a narrow QRS complex. This is in contrast to a ventricular tachyarrhythmia that displays a wide QRS complex and originates from within the ventricle. Remember that cardiac output is equal to the product of stroke volume and heart rate. In tachyarrhythmias, the heart rate is increased; a reduction in cardiac output must occur due to a decrease in stroke volume. Stroke volume is reduced by either impairment of left ventricular (LV) contraction or reduction of LV preload and therefore filling. Impairment of LV contraction occurs in the case of ventricular fibrillation due to the presence of multiple electrical impulses that result in failure to achieve a coordinated depolarization of the left ventricle. All other tachyarrhythmias result in decreased cardiac output from reduction in LV preload due to loss of LV filling from the atrium or in decreased diastolic filling time.

Epidemiology

Tachycardia may occur in patients with and without structural heart disease. Acquired conditions such as valvular heart disease and coronary artery disease (CAD) tend to present later in life as compared to congenital abnormalities that may present even in early childhood.

Etiology

Table 12-1 describes the most common types and etiologies of tachyarrhythmias.

ACUTE MANAGEMENT AND WORKUP

Arrhythmias vary greatly in severity from immediately fatal to asymptomatic. Your initial evaluation needs to focus on identifying the abnormal rhythm and the clinical stability of the patient.

The First 15 Minutes

How a patient tolerates an abnormal rhythm is highly dependent on his or her underlying cardiovascular status. A younger patient with a structurally normal heart may tolerate a fast rhythm without difficulty, whereas another patient with underlying heart failure may be clinically unstable from the same rhythm. Hemodynamic instability and symptoms such as unresponsiveness, altered mental status, respiratory distress, and chest pain should prompt consideration of immediate direct current cardioversion.

Initial Assessment

First, determine whether the QRS complex is narrow (as in our patient encounter) or wide (i.e., is it >120 ms?). The presence of a wide complex is more concerning than a narrow complex because of the high mortality associated with ventricular tachycardia and fibrillation.

When evaluating wide-complex tachycardias that are presumably ventricular in origin, it is important to observe the pattern of QRS morphology, ventricular rate, and the duration of the arrhythmia. An important pattern to recognize is that ventricular fibrillation has a low amplitude, has a chaotic pattern without discernable QRS complexes (Fig. 12-1A), and requires ACLS resuscitation. Ventricular tachycardia (VT) (Fig. 12-1B), another important wide-complex tachycardia, can have an appearance of QRS complexes that are nearly identical in amplitude and morphology to each other, known as *monomorphic VT*, or that are different in width and amplitude, known as *polymorphic VT*. A special type of polymorphic VT that displays an undulating amplitude is known as *torsades de pointes* (Fig. 12-1C). VT is defined as three or more ventricular QRS complexes at a rate of >100 bpm, and runs of VT <30 seconds are referred to as *nonsustained VT*.

To evaluate a narrow-complex tachycardia or supraventricular tachycardia (SVT), you need to first determine whether the rhythm is regular or irregular.

TABLE 12-1
The Etiology of Tachyarrhythmias

Tachyarrhythmia	Etiologies
Ventricular Tachyarrhythmias (VTs)	
Ventricular fibrillation	Myocardial infarction, idiopathic, progression from VT
Monomorphic VT	Dilated or hypertrophic cardiomyopathy, drug induced (i.e., class I antiarrhythmics, digoxin), right ventricle/left ventricular outflow tract (structural), muscular dystrophy, mitral valve prolapse, repaired tetralogy of Fallot, arrhythmogenic right ventricular dysplasia, Wolff-Parkinson-White (WPW) syndrome, myocarditis
Polymorphic VT	Ischemia, idiopathic, Brugada syndrome, commotio cordis, drug induced
Torsades de pointes	Congenital long QT syndrome, drug induced (i.e., antipsychotics, tricyclic antidepressants, macrolides, fluoroquinolones), subarachnoid hemorrhage, bradycardia, myocarditis, hypokalemia, hypomagnesemia, hypocalcemia
Supraventricular Tachycardias	
Atrial fibrillation/ atrial flutter	Discussed separately in Chapter 13
Sinus tachycardia	Fever/infection, hypovolemia, hypoxemia, congestive heart failure (CHF), anxiety, pulmonary embolism, anemia, thyrotoxicosis, caffeine, nicotine, atropine, catecholamines, alcohol withdrawal
Multifocal atrial tachycardia (MAT)	Pulmonary disease (chronic obstructive pulmonary disease), CHF
Atrioventricular nodal re-entrant tachycardia (AVNRT)	Idiopathic, presence of slow/fast pathways surrounding atrioventricular node
Atrioventricular re-entrant tachycardia (AVRT)	Atrioventricular accessory pathway, WPW, idiopathic, congenital, Ebstein anomaly

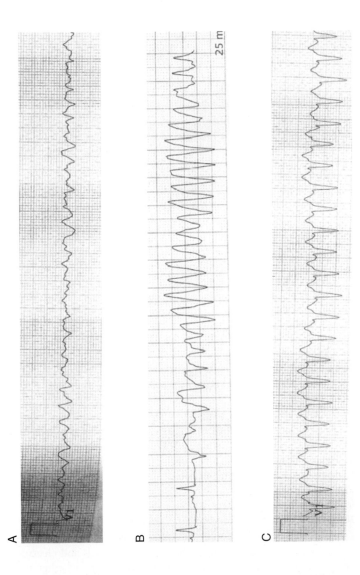

FIGURE 12-1: A: Ventricular fibrillation. **B:** Torsades de pointes. **C:** Monomorphic ventricular tachycardia. (A,C: Modified from Rimmerman CM, Jain AK. *Interactive Electrocardiography.* Philadelphia: Lippincott Williams & Wilkins; 2003:211, 458. B: Courtesy of William Fischer II, MD, Division of Pulmonary and Critical Care, The Johns Hopkins Hospital, with permission.)

25 m

Atrial fibrillation, which is an irregular tachycardia, and atrial flutter are encountered commonly and are discussed in Chapter 13. The other irregular supraventricular tachycardia is multifocal atrial tachycardia (MAT). It requires the presence of three or more P waves in one lead with different morphologies (P waves are best seen in leads II, III, and V1) and variation in the PR interval.

> ## CLINICAL PEARL
>
> *MAT occurs most commonly in patients with pulmonary disease such as chronic obstructive pulmonary disease.*

Included in the narrow-complex tachycardias with a regular rhythm are sinus tachycardia and the group that comprises the atrioventricular re-entrant tachycardias: atrioventricular nodal re-entry tachycardias (AVNRTs) and atrioventricular re-entry tachycardias (AVRTs). Sinus tachycardia is a narrow-complex tachycardia with a conducted P wave that precedes each QRS; it can reach rates as high as 200 bpm in younger patients. It is critical to look for the primary cause of sinus tachycardia. Life threatening conditions such as sepsis, pulmonary embolism, or congestive heart failure may present with sinus tachycardia as the first sign. Other common causes of sinus tachycardia include fever and pain.

AVNRT and AVRT (i.e., Wolff-Parkinson-White syndrome) may both cause narrow-complex SVTs. They may occur in younger patients and those without known cardiovascular disease. Clinical features are very similar between the two. Heart rates may range between 150 and 250 bpm.

Admission Criteria and Level of Care Criteria

All patients being admitted because of an arrhythmia need to be kept on a cardiac monitor. Episodes of sustained VT and ventricular fibrillation universally require coronary care unit–level care. Sinus tachycardia that can be attributed to an underlying etiology should be triaged based on that etiology.

The First Few Hours

Once the patient is stable and on a cardiac monitor, you can return to the underlying etiology of the arrhythmia. Obtaining old records and electrocardiograms (ECGs) from other hospitals can help determine whether the arrhythmia is a new finding. This is especially important if you are considering ischemia among the differential diagnoses.

> ## CLINICAL PEARL
>
> *Always look at several rhythm strips and 12-lead ECGs when assessing a patient with a tachycardia. When possible, try to find old ECGs for comparison.*

History

Points to focus on are the symptoms, frequency, and severity, including any episodes of syncope or injury. A patient may notice precipitating factors and whether there is anything he or she can do to alleviate the symptoms. Many patients with AVNRT or AVRT have discovered how to utilize vagal maneuvers, such as coughing or holding their breath to terminate the arrhythmia.

Information from the history is useful in helping to determine an etiology. Symptoms and risk factors for ischemia due to acute coronary syndrome should be elicited because it is responsible for many arrhythmias. In such cases, reperfusion therapy will be required.

The most common conditions associated with various arrhythmias are ischemic heart disease, valvular disease, and heart failure. A history of dilated cardiomyopathy is a common risk factor for VT, atrial fibrillation/atrial flutter, and MAT. A myocardial scar from a prior myocardial infarction is a common cause of monomorphic VT. A family history of sudden cardiac death, especially in young relatives, might suggest an undiagnosed congenital disorder.

It is necessary to secure a thorough history to elicit any new medications or herbal therapies, or dose changes. Torsades de pointes is caused by a wide variety of medications that prolong the QT interval. Medications that cause electrolyte derangements, such as diuretics, should also be considered.

Physical Examination

The physical examination is oftentimes nonspecific in cases of tachyarrhythmias. A thorough cardiovascular examination is critical to assess for signs of heart failure and/or end-organ hypoperfusion. Such signs may either be the cause of the tachycardia or the result of the hemodynamic consequences of such a fast heart rate. The remainder of the physical examination should search for clues that might reveal the etiology of the tachyarrhythmia.

Labs and Tests to Consider

Electrolyte abnormalities, including potassium, calcium, and magnesium, are among the most common causes of tachyarrhythmias; a metabolic profile and a magnesium level should be ordered. Other laboratory tests should include a complete blood count to look for anemia or infection and thyroid function tests to assess for hyperthyroidism. Cardiac enzymes can be used to assess for evidence of ischemia, although it is not unusual to see mild elevations in the setting of tachycardia without significant coronary artery disease.

Key Diagnostic Labs and Tests

The ECG is the most important diagnostic test in the evaluation of arrhythmias and, in the majority of cases, the specific type of tachyarrhythmia can be identified. Try to obtain an ECG during the arrhythmia. If the patient has an implantable cardioverter-defibrillator (ICD) or pacemaker, it can be interrogated for helpful information about the tachyarrhythmia. A cardiology consultation by a specialist in arrhythmias may be appropriate to help with assessing the underlying rhythm and for assessment of electrophysiologic studies and specific interventions such as ablation and cardioversion.

Imaging

On first presentation of an arrhythmia, a transthoracic echocardiogram (TTE) should be performed to look for structural heart disease. A cardiac magnetic resonance image can give insight into true myocardial structural and tissue disease in circumstances, such as right ventricular dysplasia, that may not be seen on the TTE.

Treatment

Ventricular tachycardias should be acutely managed in the emergency department or intensive care unit (ICU). Electrical cardioversion is the treatment of choice in the setting of hemodynamic compromise; antiarrhythmics such as amiodarone may be considered if the patient is stable. Correction of reversible causes should proceed rapidly, with reperfusion in the case of ischemia, and correction of electrolyte disturbances. For a patient with torsades de pointes, acute management with intravenous magnesium can be used, and any medications that prolong the QT interval should be removed. During the hospitalization, ICD implantation for secondary prevention should be considered in all patients after a sustained ventricular tachyarrhythmia, especially if the underlying cause was not clearly reversible. Consultation with an electrophysiologist should be obtained for recommendations about preventing sudden death with ICD placement and for cases that may require ablation.

The most commonly encountered SVT is atrial fibrillation and flutter, and its treatment is discussed separately in Chapter 13. The SVTs, especially when occurring at rapid rates, can be difficult to differentiate from each other. A diagnostic challenge with intravenous adenosine, which temporarily blocks AV conduction, can be very helpful in distinguishing between these rhythms (make sure you record a continuous ECG during the adenosine administration). Sinus tachycardia may represent an appropriate physiologic response to increased drive or demand, and therefore treatment should be aimed at the cause. AVNRT and AVRT are often minimally symptomatic, but in certain patients, they may cause hemodynamic compromise. Acute termination can often be accomplished with carotid massage, patient-induced Valsalva maneuvers, or adenosine challenge; these maneuvers should be considered for the patient from our encounter. Those cases resulting in hemodynamic instability should be addressed with cardioversion. MAT is acutely managed with rate control with calcium channel blockers or beta-blockers, and long-term treatment is aimed at the underlying disorder.

EXTENDED IN-HOSPITAL MANAGEMENT

The hospital course for a patient admitted with a tachyarrhythmia depends largely on the underlying cause. A patient who had a ventricular tachyarrhythmia due to a large myocardial infarction (MI) may have a prolonged complicated ICU stay related to post-MI care, whereas a patient admitted with VT may undergo prompt ICD placement or ablation and be ready for discharge the next day. In most cases of arrhythmias due to reversible causes, the patient should remain on a cardiac monitor until the underlying condition has resolved.

DISPOSITION

Discharge Goals

A patient is ready for discharge when the cause of the arrhythmia has been identified and reversed, or when medical therapy, treatment with a device, or ablative therapy has been successfully implemented.

Outpatient Care

Patients should follow up with their primary care physician in 1 to 2 weeks, as well as with a cardiologist within 1 to 2 weeks. Patients who underwent ICD placement or ablation or who are being considered for future ablation should follow up with their electrophysiologist as directed.

 WHAT YOU NEED TO REMEMBER

- Tachyarrhythmias range from asymptomatic to fatal.
- Structural heart disease and coronary artery disease are risk factors for tachyarrhythmias.
- How a patient tolerates a tachyarrhythmia is highly dependent on his or her underlying cardiovascular status.
- Patients who experience hypotension, unresponsiveness, altered mental status, respiratory distress, and chest pain due to a tachyarrhythmia may require cardioversion.

- In order to make treatment decisions, it is important to determine whether a patient was symptomatic from a tachyarrhythmia.
- The evaluation of a tachyarrhythmia should include identification of the etiology.
- Wide-complex tachyarrhythmias are associated with a high degree of mortality.

SUGGESTED READINGS

Ellis K, Dresing T. Tachyarrhythmias. In: Griffin BP, Topol EJ, eds. *Manual of Cardiovascular Medicine*. 2nd ed. Philadelphia: Lippincott Williams & Wilkins; 2004.

Gregoratos G, Abrams J, Epstein AE, et al. ACC/AHA/NAPSE 2002 guideline update for implantation of cardiac pacemakers and antiarrhythmia devices. *Circulation*. 2002;106:2145–2161.

O'Keefe JH, Hammill SC, Freed M. *The Complete Guide to ECGs*. Brimingham, MI: Physicians Press; 1997.

Zipes DP, Camm AJ, Borggrefe M, et al. ACC/AHA 2006 guidelines for management of patients with ventricular arrhythmias and the prevention of sudden cardiac death. *J Am Coll Cardiol*. 2006;48:246–346.

Atrial Fibrillation and Atrial Flutter

THE PATIENT ENCOUNTER

A 57-year-old woman comes to the emergency department complaining of shortness of breath and chest palpitations. Her heart rate is 135 bpm, her blood pressure is 140/95 mm Hg, and her initial electrocardiogram is notable for a narrow-complex, irregularly irregular rhythm.

OVERVIEW

Definition

Atrial fibrillation and atrial flutter are the two most common supraventricular tachycardias that you will encounter. Atrial fibrillation is characterized by an irregularly irregular rhythm in the absence of clear P waves on electrocardiography (ECG). Atrial flutter can be regular or irregular, and classically has characteristic flutter waves on ECG.

Pathophysiology

Atrial fibrillation can occur in a healthy or diseased heart, although it is far more common to see atrial fibrillation in patients with structural heart disease. Left atrial dilation from pressure or volume overload, valvular heart disease, or even atrial infiltration or inflammation may predispose to the development of atrial fibrillation. Atrial fibrillation may be (a) paradoxical (self-terminating), (b) persistent (lasting >7 days), (c) permanent (lasting >1 year) or (d) lone (occurring in the absence of structural heart disease). Regardless of the underlying cause, the end result is a series of dysregulated fibrillatory waves (F waves) in the range of 300 to 600 bpm that gives the atria a characteristic "bag of worms" appearance. Only a handful of these waves is conducted through the atrioventricular (AV) node, leading to irregularly irregular ventricular contractions usually in the range of 90 to 170 bpm.

Atrial fibrillation may have several hemodynamic consequences. F waves do not result in effective atrial contractions. As a result, ventricular filling is entirely passive and will depend on diastolic filling time. The loss of this atrial kick is poorly tolerated in patients with stiff, noncompliant, or poorly contracting ventricles and may lead to a dramatic reduction in cardiac output and subsequent heart failure. This effect will be even greater at faster heart rates because diastolic filling time will be further reduced. In patients with underlying coronary artery disease, the increase in myocardial oxygen demand from tachycardia may also lead to myocardial ischemia, which will further contribute to hemodynamic compromise.

In the long term, the absence of normal atrial contractions can lead to stasis and the formation of thrombi, especially in the left atrial appendage. Arterial embolization can occur in virtually any vascular distribution and may lead to stroke, bowel ischemia, or limb ischemia.

Atrial flutter occurs in many of the same situations as atrial fibrillation, although it is far less common. In some cases, atrial flutter may even promote the development of atrial fibrillation. Atrial flutter is classically divided into two types: (a) type 1 (typical, counterclockwise) flutter and (b) type II (atypical) flutter. Type I flutter is characterized by a macro re-entry circuit within the right atrium that follows a predictable counterclockwise path in the isthmus between the inferior vena cava and the tricuspid valve. Atrial contractions usually occur at about 300 bpm as a consequence of the circuit length and are most often conducted in a rate of 2:1, although variable conduction may occur. Atrial contractions do result in ventricular filling, so the hemodynamic effects of atrial flutter are not as severe as atrial fibrillation and are mostly related to tachycardia. Atrial fibrillation produces much higher atrial rates than flutter. However, many of these impulses are not transmitted due to concealed conduction. It is often difficult to control the ventricular rate in atrial flutter due to the ability of the AV node to conduct one out of every two impulses it receives. Even following cardioversion, a single premature atrial contraction close to the circuit can reinitiate the tachycardia.

Prolonged tachycardia in either case can predispose to the development of a tachycardia-related cardiomyopathy.

Epidemiology

The prevalence of atrial fibrillation increases with age, in part because of the increased likelihood of heart disease in older patients, and may be as high as 1%. The lifetime risk of developing atrial fibrillation may be as high as 25%, depending on the population studied. Atrial flutter is less common than atrial fibrillation but, again, is seen more frequently in patients with underlying structural heart disease.

Etiology

There are a number of reasons why a patient may present with atrial fibrillation or atrial flutter. Hyperthyroidism, infection, or any hyperadrenergic state may initiate and propagate atrial fibrillation or atrial flutter. Structural heart disease, as may be seen in valvular disorders, left ventricular dysfunction, or even poorly controlled hypertension, may promote the development of atrial arrhythmias, especially when the left atrium is dilated from chronic pressure or volume overload. Ischemia, while part of the differential diagnosis, is a rare cause of atrial fibrillation or atrial flutter, but could be the inciting event, especially if the patient is in heart failure from ischemia. Lung disease, including chronic obstructive pulmonary disorder and acute pulmonary embolism, may present with atrial arrhythmias as well.

ACUTE MANAGEMENT AND WORKUP

In order to manage atrial fibrillation or atrial flutter, you first need to recognize the presence of an arrhythmia.

The First 15 Minutes

Atrial fibrillation is fairly easy to recognize as an irregularly irregular rhythm with absent P waves. F waves may occasionally be seen but do not have to be present to make the diagnosis (Fig. 13-1A). Atrial flutter can be more difficult to recognize in a patient with a fast heart rate, especially if the flutter waves are hidden in the QRS complex and T waves. In general, a narrow complex tachycardia at a rate of 150 bpm with no apparent P waves should raise your suspicion for atrial flutter. If flutter waves are not definitively seen, adenosine can be administered to transiently block the AV node to reveal the presence of the flutter waves (Fig. 13-1B).

Initial Assessment

Once you recognize the presence of atrial fibrillation or atrial flutter, the first question you need to consider is whether or not acute cardioversion is indicated. Any patient with a rapid ventricular response (RVR) (pulse >110 bpm) and profound hypotension should be immediately electrically cardioverted. In the absence of hypotension or shock, you need to decide whether or not to attempt to slow down the heart rate immediately. This decision will be largely determined by two issues: (a) whether or not the patient is at risk for coronary ischemia from the increased oxygen demand produced by his or her tachycardia, and (b) whether or not the patient has signs and symptoms of heart failure. Evidence of ongoing ischemia either by symptoms or ECG should prompt immediate intervention. Heart failure can be the cause of atrial fibrillation or flutter from high left atrial pressures and atrial stretch, or may be a result of the arrhythmia. In either case, it may be necessary to slow the heart rate down to promote diastolic filling time and to reduce left atrial pressures. The patient in our encounter has atrial fibrillation with RVR. While her relatively normal blood pressure is reassuring in that she does not need immediate cardioversion, her dyspnea may reflect evolving heart failure that may require aggressive rate control.

Once you have performed your initial hemodynamic assessment, it is important to discern the cause of the patient's acute presentation. A focused history and physical should search for underlying cardiovascular and pulmonary disease, thyroid disease, and acute infectious or metabolic processes that may contribute to the arrhythmia.

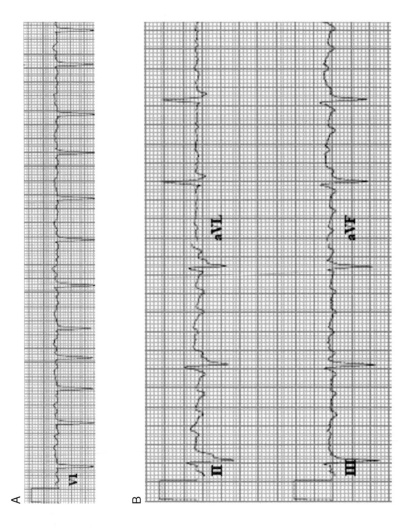

FIGURE 13-1: **A:** Rhythm strip demonstrating an irregularly irregular tachyarrhythmia consistent with atrial fibrillation with rapid ventricular response. **B:** Inferior leads of a 12-lead electrocardiogram demonstrating the downward sawtooth flutter waves of type I (typical) atrial flutter. (Courtesy of Brian T. Garibaldi, MD, Division of Pulmonary and Critical Care Medicine, The Johns Hopkins Hospital.)

Admission Criteria and Level of Care Criteria

Patients with new-onset atrial fibrillation or flutter, or patients with a rapid ventricular response, should be admitted to a cardiac telemetry bed for close observation. Patients with ongoing ischemia, either as the cause or as the end result of their arrhythmia, should be managed in a coronary care unit (CCU). Patients in heart failure or with evidence of end-organ perfusion should also likely be managed initially in the CCU, even if emergent cardioversion is successful.

The First Few Hours

The first few hours should be spent on identifying the cause of the underlying arrhythmia and ensuring continued hemodynamic stability.

History

Patients with atrial fibrillation or atrial flutter may present with noticeable palpitations, lightheadedness, dizziness, or even syncope. It is important to get a sense of the duration of symptoms because they may provide a clue to the onset of the arrhythmia. Be sure to ask patients about prior cardiovascular and pulmonary disease that may predispose to arrhythmias or place the patient at a higher risk of cardiopulmonary compromise. Because myocardial ischemia and pulmonary embolism are potentially life-threatening causes of atrial arrhythmias, it is important to screen patients carefully for symptoms and risk factors of those conditions. A good review of systems should search for any symptoms of infection or metabolic derangements that could be causative. Remember to screen for drug use such as cocaine and methamphetamines that might contribute to a hyperadrenergic state. If patients are unsure of their past medical history, it may also be helpful to review their medications to see if they are on a nodal blocking agent or thyroid medication. If you are considering anticoagulation, it is helpful to ask your patient about recent bleeding as well as to identify risk factors for anticoagulation.

Physical Examination

The jugular venous pulsation may help to differentiate atrial fibrillation from flutter and also provides information about volume status. Remember that the F waves of atrial fibrillation do not correspond to effective atrial contractions. As a result, you will not see true A waves in your exam. This can sometimes make it difficult to use the jugular venous pressure to estimate right atrial pressure. In atrial flutter, you may occasionally see flutter waves in the venous pulsations. Likewise, you would not expect to hear a true S_4 in atrial fibrillation because an S_4 is thought to result from atrial contraction and subsequent filling of a stiff ventricle. A neurologic exam should search for focal deficits that could be caused by arterial thrombi. The remainder of your examination should focus on identifying underlying cardiovascular and pulmonary disease that may contribute to atrial arrhythmias, as well as searching for other comorbid conditions that may alter a patient's risk or response to atrial fibrillation or atrial flutter.

Labs and Tests to Consider

Laboratory studies should be guided by the patient's clinical presentation.

Key Diagnostic Labs and Tests

All patients with new-onset atrial fibrillation or atrial flutter should have thyroid function testing performed because hyperthyroidism has been implicated in up to 20% of new cases. Serial cardiac enzymes should be measured to assess for ischemia, either as the causal event or as the result of tachycardia.

Imaging

Most patients with newly diagnosed atrial fibrillation or atrial flutter should undergo echocardiography to evaluate for valvular disease, reduced ejection fraction, diastolic dysfunction, and atrial size. This will provide useful information about underlying cardiac function and may provide prognostic information regarding the likelihood of successful cardioversion. A chest radiograph may also be helpful in evaluating for heart size, heart failure, and underlying pulmonary disease.

Treatment

There are three keys issues to consider when caring for a patient with atrial fibrillation or atrial flutter: (a) rate control, (b) rhythm control, and (c) anticoagulation.

Rate Control

There are a number of potential medications that can be used to achieve rate control. The choice of medication will be determined by how quickly you need to achieve rate control and whether or not the patient's blood pressure can tolerate certain medications. In cases in which rapid rate control is needed (i.e., active demand ischemia from tachycardia), an intravenous formulation of a beta-blocker such as metoprolol is probably the most effective choice. The calcium channel blocker diltiazem may also be used, with the chief advantage being its ability to be used as a continuous intravenous infusion. If the patient's blood pressure is borderline, he or she may not be able to tolerate these medications. Intravenous amiodarone may be more appropriate in this setting. Digoxin is also a potential choice. All of these medications can be used in their oral formulations for the management of chronic atrial fibrillation and atrial flutter.

Rhythm Control

The restoration of normal sinus rhythm leads to a rapid increase in left ventricular function and cardiac output, especially in the case of atrial fibrillation.

In theory, the maintenance of normal sinus rhythm should also decrease the risk of thromboembolic events. However, despite these potentially attractive advantages, at the present time it does not appear that achieving and maintaining sinus rhythm over rate control in atrial fibrillation confers a long-term benefit in the majority of patients, even in those with underling congestive heart failure. That being said, it is important to consider the circumstances of your particular patient when making treatment decisions. Ventricular rates in atrial flutter are oftentimes more difficult to control and atrial flutter may degenerate into atrial fibrillation. As a result, the restoration of normal sinus rhythm is more frequently attempted in atrial flutter.

Electrical Cardioversion. Patients with hemodynamic instability should undergo an emergent attempt at synchronized direct current (DC) electrical cardioversion. Stable patients should be considered for cardioversion if the acute cause of the atrial fibrillation or atrial flutter is likely to be reversible. The rate of success is inversely proportional to the length of time the patient has been in the arrhythmia and the size of the left atrium.

Chemical Cardioversion. Electrical cardioversion is favored over chemical cardioversion because of its greater success rate and less proarrhythmic side effects. Ibutilide, flecainide, dofetilide, propafenone, and, to a lesser degree, amiodarone have all been used as chemical agents and are useful if anesthesia is not available for safe DC cardioversion. The use of these medications to maintain normal sinus rhythm following successful cardioversion is not indicated except in patients who have shown that they cannot tolerate episodes of atrial fibrillation or atrial flutter without significant ischemia or hemodynamic compromise.

Ablation. Patients with chronic atrial fibrillation or atrial flutter may be candidates for ablation if they fail to achieve or maintain normal sinus rhythm after attempts at electrical cardioversion. Because of the predictable site of the macro re-entry circuit, in about 95% of cases, patients with typical atrial flutter can undergo successful catheter-directed radiofrequency ablation. Atypical flutter and atrial fibrillation are more difficult to isolate and ablate, although in recent years, pulmonary vein isolation and left atrial ablation techniques have been increasingly successful.

Anticoagulation

Patients with atrial fibrillation and atrial flutter are at increased risk of arterial thromboembolic events after as little as 48 hours of atrial arrhythmia. In atrial fibrillation the per-year risk of stroke is probably on the order of 3%, although this increases with increasing age. Atrial flutter in isolation may convey a slightly reduced risk of stroke, but many patients with atrial flutter also have intermittent atrial fibrillation, which raises the incidence of stroke to that of atrial fibrillation. This yearly risk of stroke translates into a very low per-day risk of events. As a result, anticoagulation in a patient with chronic atrial fibrillation or atrial flutter is not an emergent issue but one that needs to be addressed before discharge.

There are some factors that predict a higher likelihood of stroke and can be remembered using the acronym *CHADS2*: **C**ongestive heart failure, **H**ypertension, **A**ge older than 75, **D**iabetes, and **S**econdary prevention of stroke or transient ischemic attack (1). In the absence of these risk factors (i.e., "lone" atrial fibrillation or atrial flutter), a patient may benefit from full-dose aspirin alone. Most other patients with chronic atrial fibrillation or atrial flutter should be strongly considered for full-dose anticoagulation with warfarin therapy.

At the time of attempted cardioversion or ablation, there is an increased risk of embolizing a previously formed clot. As a result, patients who have been in atrial fibrillation or atrial flutter for more than 48 hours should be anticoagulated several weeks before attempted return to sinus rhythm, or they should have a transesophageal echocardiogram to confirm the absence of a thrombus.

CLINICAL PEARL

In the case of hemodynamic instability, emergent cardioversion should be attempted without waiting to confirm the absence of thrombus. Following cardioversion, there is also a well-known phenomenon called atrial stunning in which the atria do not contract efficiently for as long as 3 weeks after the return of sinus rhythm. As a result, patients should be anticoagulated for up to 4 weeks after successful cardioversion if there are no obvious contraindications.

EXTENDED IN-HOSPITAL MANAGEMENT

The extended in-hospital management should focus on identifying potentially reversible causes of atrial fibrillation and atrial flutter.

DISPOSITION

Discharge Goals

Patients are ready for discharge once hemodynamic stability has been assured and a plan has been made regarding the three phases of treatment (i.e., rate control, rhythm control, and anticoagulation).

Outpatient Care

Patients should follow up with their primary care doctor within 2 weeks of discharge for atrial fibrillation or atrial flutter. Depending on their underlying risk factors, they may benefit from continued outpatient cardiology follow-up. Patients discharged on anticoagulation therapy should have regular follow-up arranged with an appropriate anticoagulation clinic before discharge.

 WHAT YOU NEED TO REMEMBER

- Atrial fibrillation and atrial flutter are most common in patients with underlying heart disease.
- Unstable patients should undergo immediate attempts at electrical cardioversion.
- In most cases, typical atrial flutter can be successfully ablated.
- Despite potential advantages, there is no clear benefit to rhythm control versus rate control in patients with chronic atrial fibrillation.
- The CHADS2 score can help to identify patients who are most likely to benefit from full-dose anticoagulation.

REFERENCE

1. Gage BF, Waterman AD, Shannon W. Validation of clinical classification schemes for predicting stroke: results from the National Registry of Atrial Fibrillation. *JAMA*. 2001;285:2864.

SUGGESTED READINGS

Aronow WS. Treatment of atrial fibrillation and atrial flutter: part II. *Cardiol Rev.* 2008;16(5):230–239.

Roy D, Talajic M, Nattel S, et al. Rhythm control versus rate control for atrial fibrillation and heart failure. *N Engl J Med.* 2008;358(25):2667–2677.

Van Gelder IC, Hagens VE, Bosker HA, et al. A comparison of rate control and rhythm control in patients with recurrent persistent atrial fibrillation. *N Engl J Med.* 2002;347(23):1834–1840.

Wyse DG, Waldo AL, DiMarco JP, et al. A comparison of rate control and rhythm control in patients with atrial fibrillation. *N Engl J Med.* 2002;347(23):1825–1833.

Valvular Heart Disease

THE PATIENT ENCOUNTER

A 70-year-old man is brought to the emergency department complaining of shortness of breath. On examination, he is found to have a late-peaking III/VI systolic crescendo-decrescendo murmur at the right upper sternal border. Carotid upstrokes are noted to be weak and delayed. He has bibasilar rales and an elevated jugular venous pressure.

OVERVIEW

Definition

This chapter will focus on two valvular heart diseases that are commonly seen on the wards, aortic stenosis (AS) and mitral regurgitation (MR), to provide a basis for the assessment of valvular disease.

Aortic stenosis is defined as the reduction in diameter or narrowing at the site of the aortic valve that causes obstruction of blood flow from the left ventricle (LV) to the aorta during systole. Mitral regurgitation is the flow of blood from the LV back into the left atrium (LA) during systole as a result of an incompetent or leaking valve.

Pathophysiology

The aortic valve must be reduced to one-fourth its normal size before hemodynamic consequences occur. Aortic stenosis is thought to progress at a rate of 0.1 cm^2 reduction in aortic valve area per year. There are several factors that can affect this rate of progression, including smoking, age, and chronic kidney disease.

As the valve area gets smaller, the LV must generate more pressure in order to overcome the obstruction to flow. Hypertrophy of the LV occurs and the stroke volume is preserved at a cost of greater work and oxygen consumption as defined by the area of the loop in Figure 14-1. As the AS progresses, the LV initially hypertrophies and ultimately dilates. The result is an increase in the end-systolic volume at a rate greater than the end-diastolic volume. This results in a reduced stroke volume as defined by the width of the pressure–volume loop (see Fig. 14-1).

The mitral valve is a complex structure that includes leaflets, chordae tendineae, papillary muscles, and the annulus. Mitral regurgitation can occur with dysfunction in any part of the mitral apparatus or changes in LV

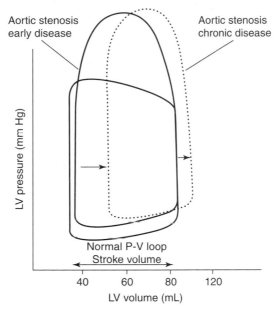

Aortic stenosis
early disease

Aortic stenosis
chronic disease

LV pressure (mm Hg)

Normal P-V loop
Stroke volume

40   60   80   120

LV volume (mL)

FIGURE 14-1: Pressure–volume loop in aortic stenosis. In order to over-come the obstruction to flow, the pressure in the left ventricle (LV) has to increase, leading to increased work. As the disease progresses, the LV end-diastolic volume increases but not at the same rate as the end-systolic volume. Stroke volume therefore decreases despite the increased work done by the left ventricle.

geometry. The LV responds to chronic MR by dilating to accommodate both the forward flow into the aorta and the backward flow into the LA. The resulting pressure from the regurgitated volume is transmitted to the LA and consequently to the pulmonary veins and lungs. In response to this increased pressure, the LA dilates to reduce the pressure; over time, this results in an increased incidence of atrial fibrillation. The resulting pressure–volume loop from MR is seen in Figure 14-2. There is a marked increase in the end-diastolic volume and an increase in the end-diastolic pressure. There is no true isovolumetric contraction during systole because blood will flow back through the mitral valve into the LA via the path of least resistance. Stroke volume is greater with a reduced end-systolic volume in an attempt to preserve output from the LV into the aorta. As you can see, ejection fraction, as measured by the percentage of volume ejected from the LV, can be greater than normal as a significant portion of blood is flowing back into the LA. Again, work and oxygen consumption as shown by the area of the loop are increased in this disease.

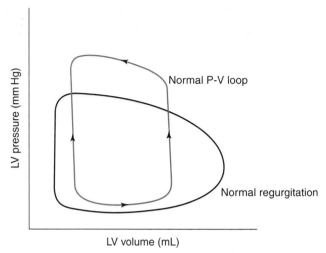

FIGURE 14-2: Pressure–volume loop in mitral regurgitation. In mitral regurgitation, end-diastolic volume and work increase. However, the resulting stroke volume is an overestimation of forward flow because a significant amount of that volume is ejected along the path of least resistance back into the left atrium.

Epidemiology

Aortic stenosis is present in 2% to 4% of the U.S. population over the age of 65 (1). Mitral regurgitation has been estimated to affect more than 3 million people in the United States.

Etiology

Worldwide, the most common cause of AS is rheumatic heart disease. In the United States, AS is caused primarily by calcific degeneration of tricuspid aortic valves or congenital bicuspid aortic valves.

Mitral regurgitation can be divided into two categories: acute and chronic MR. Acute MR is caused by a flail leaflet, chordae tendineae rupture, or papillary muscle dysfunction. The mechanisms for these three etiologies can be found in Table 14-1.

Chronic MR is caused by dysfunction in the mitral valve apparatus or changes in LV geometry. The most common causes of chronic MR in the developed world are mitral valve prolapse and ischemic heart disease. Mitral valve prolapse with or without MR is found in 2% to 3% of the population. In underdeveloped countries, rheumatic heart disease is still the predominant cause of chronic MR.

TABLE 14-1
Etiologies of Acute Mitral Regurgitation

Flail Leaflet	Chordae Tendineae Rupture	Papillary Muscle Dysfunction
• Mitral valve prolapse • Trauma • Infective endocarditis	• Trauma • Acute rheumatic fever • Infective endocarditis • Idiopathic rupture	• Acute myocardial infarction • Active ischemia • Trauma

ACUTE MANAGEMENT AND WORKUP

When evaluating a patient with decompensated valvular function, return to the basic premise of evaluating and stabilizing the airway and circulation if needed. Patients with acute decompensation will require immediate attention to identify the affected valve.

The First 15 Minutes

You will encounter many patients with valvular disease who present to the hospital with a variety of chief complaints. Once you recognize that they have valvular disease, it is important to carefully evaluate their hemodynamic status and determine if they are able to maintain adequate perfusion to their organs.

Initial Assessment

Your initial assessment should focus on the patient's symptoms and clinical state. A thorough cardiopulmonary examination is essential. Tachycardia and a narrow pulse pressure may indicate that the patient's stroke volume is reduced and his or her heart rate has increased to compensate. Shortness of breath or a new oxygen requirement, as seen in the patient from our encounter, might be signs of pulmonary edema. Tachyarrhythmia may reflect congestive heart failure or may be a marker of a dilated left atrium. Lightheadedness or delirium suggests poor cerebral perfusion. Cool extremities could indicate an increased afterload in the setting of decompensated heart failure.

Next, your attention should turn to the chronicity of the illness because this will have implications for the patient's ability to compensate and also give clues to the etiology of the valvular disease.

Remember that patients with valvular disease often present to the hospital for other reasons. Be sure to carefully evaluate and address their chief complaint in addition to focusing on their valve process.

Admission Criteria and Level of Care Criteria

There are no formal admission criteria for patients with valvular heart disease. In general, all patients with symptomatic heart failure, arrhythmias, syncope, chest pain, and hypoxia should be admitted. All patients will require cardiac monitoring. Any patient with a significant oxygen requirement and/or hemodynamic instability should be cared for in an intensive care unit or intermediate care unit.

The First Few Hours

The initial hours should be spent gaining a detailed history of the patient's symptoms and their time course.

History

The patient with AS may be asymptomatic for quite a long time. Symptoms of AS vary a great deal depending on the patient's activity level. The classic triad of symptoms is angina pectoris, syncope, and dyspnea. As many as 50% of patients with AS have coronary artery disease (CAD) that leads to angina. Even patients without significant CAD can have angina due to LV hypertrophy and increased oxygen demand. Patients may describe dyspnea or orthopnea, which may indicate heart failure and more advanced AS. Dyspnea initially occurs with exertion and is a result of the inability to increase cardiac output with exercise. Exercise induces peripheral vasodilation and the normal response to this is to augment cardiac output. If there is a fixed obstruction (aortic stenosis), the increase in cardiac output is minimal, which may lead to hypotension and syncope. Diastolic dysfunction from long-standing LV pressure overload likely also plays a role (see Chapter 7).

The history that you take from a patient with acute MR versus chronic MR might be very different. In acute MR, patients may be quite sick with a significant amount of pulmonary edema and hemodynamic instability due to the noncompliant LA and previously normal LV. The most common presenting symptoms of chronic MR are dyspnea and fatigue. In chronic MR, the LV and LA have had time to compensate by dilating. Therefore, patients may have had mild to moderate MR for an extended period before developing symptoms. MR can also lead to supraventricular arrhythmias, such as atrial fibrillation, due to the dilated LA. Patients may describe a history of palpitations or an irregular heart rate. Your history should also focus on other constitutional symptoms, which may indicate infective endocarditis. Be sure to ask if the patient had rheumatic fever or ever lived in an underdeveloped country.

It is important to determine the chronicity of symptoms, because this can give important clues to the etiology of the valvular heart disease. Patients with congenital AS or mitral valve prolapse may give a history of a murmur since childhood.

Physical Examination

A detailed cardiovascular examination is informative in valvular heart disease because it provides clues to the affected valve as well as to the degree of heart failure present.

Aortic Stenosis

In aortic stenosis, the pulses are classically described as *pulsus parvus et tardus* (small and delayed) and should be palpated at the carotid artery. Examination of the precordium in the early stages may reveal an LV heave due to the resulting LV hypertrophy. A displaced, sustained apex beat would indicate a failing and dilated LV and a more severe clinical scenario. The murmur of AS is classically described as a systolic crescendo-decrescendo sound that starts just after the first heart sound (S_1) and ends before the second heart sound (S_2). The murmur is usually harsh and is heard best at the right upper border of the sternum, radiating to the carotid arteries. The loudness of the murmur does not always correlate with the severity of the stenosis. However, the timing of the murmur does correlate with the severity of the stenosis. Mild to moderate AS peaks early in systole, whereas severe AS is late peaking. The second heart sound (A_2) that represents closure of the aortic valve is soft and can be absent in severe AS.

CLINICAL PEARL

The quality of the pulse can be one of the best bedside indicators of the severity of the aortic stenosis.

Mitral Regurgitation

Atrial fibrillation as a result of LA enlargement is a common finding in MR and suggests chronicity. The apex beat as a marker of LV dilatation will become laterally and inferiorly displaced. As the systolic function declines, the apex beat will also become sustained and enlarged. The murmur of mitral regurgitation is classically described as holosystolic, located at the apex and radiating to the axilla. A thrill may be palpated at the apex. The murmur begins just after S_1 and continues into and over S_2. S_1 is usually diminished, reflecting the inability of the mitral valve to close properly. It should be noted that the intensity of the murmur does not vary with the respiratory cycle, unlike tricuspid regurgitation. In mitral valve prolapse, a midsystolic click may be heard followed by a murmur later in systole. Acute MR may not be audible in cases of acute ischemia. The murmur may not even be holosystolic due to the inability of the noncompliant LA to accommodate the regurgitant blood throughout systole.

The remainder of your exam should focus on other signs of heart failure, such as rales, elevated jugular venous pressure, lower extremity edema, and a third heart sound (S_3). You should also do a careful skin exam, looking for embolic or immunologic phenomenon of infective endocarditis, as this can be an important cause of mitral regurgitation.

Labs and Tests to Consider

Important imaging and laboratory studies include a 12-lead electrocardiogram (ECG), a comprehensive metabolic panel, chest radiography, echocardiography, and possibly cardiac catheterization.

Key Diagnostic Labs and Tests

All patients admitted with suspected valvular heart disease should have a 12-lead ECG performed. An acute posterior myocardial infarction leading to ischemic MR, atrial fibrillation, and atrial chamber enlargement are some findings that may be seen. Comparison to prior ECGs, when possible, is essential. A comprehensive metabolic panel should be drawn to evaluate renal function, liver function, and electrolytes. Significant heart failure from valvular disease may lead to renal dysfunction from poor renal perfusion secondary to low cardiac output.

Imaging

All patients admitted with suspected valvular heart disease should have a chest radiograph. This is helpful for ruling out other causes of dyspnea and can show pulmonary edema, cardiomegaly, and vascular and sometimes even valvular calcification.

The most useful diagnostic tool for assessing valvular heart disease is Doppler echocardiography. Doppler echocardiography can evaluate the severity of AS by measuring velocities below and through the aortic valve. By measuring the corresponding outflow tract diameter, a calculation of the LV-to-aorta pressure gradient can be made and therefore an aortic valve area can be estimated. Both of these quantifications are used in assessing severity and planning treatment in AS. Table 14-2 classifies the severity of AS based

TABLE 14-2

Classification of the Severity of Aortic Valve Stenosis in Adults

	Mild	Moderate	Severe
Mean gradient (mm Hg)	<25	25–40	>40
Valve area (cm²)	>1.5	1.0–1.5	<1.0

on mean gradients and aortic valve area. Echocardiography can also assess for a bicuspid aortic valve, and will also give a very accurate assessment of LV function (or ejection fraction) and cardiac dimensions.

Doppler echocardiography is also essential in evaluating the severity and etiology of mitral regurgitation. Vegetations, leaflet prolapse, chordae rupture, and rheumatic valves can all be seen with two-dimensional echocardiography. An estimation of severity can be made, taking into account the size of the LA, the volume and flow of the regurgitation jet, the width of the jet at the neck, and the extent that it flows into the pulmonary veins.

Cardiac catheterization can be used to assess the severity of AS by measuring a simultaneous LV and aortic peak-to-peak gradient across the aortic valve in cases of equivocal echocardiographic measurements. Right heart catheterization can be invaluable for measuring elevated right heart pressures, pulmonary pressures, and LA pressure as complications of valvular disease.

Treatment

The treatment of valvular heart disease falls into two main categories: medical management and surgical management. Options for medical management are limited.

Aortic Stenosis

Unfortunately, there is no medical management that has been shown to slow the progression of aortic stenosis. Medical management focuses on improving symptoms, such as heart failure, with diuretics and blood pressure control.

CLINICAL PEARL

Remember to be careful when giving diuretics, nitrates, or vasodilators to patients with severe aortic stenosis as this can decrease preload. These patients are very preload dependent and this can result in significant hypotension. In general, nitrates and vasodilators should be avoided in all patients with severe AS.

Surgical replacement of the aortic valve is the only effective treatment for symptomatic AS at this time, and is most likely indicated in the patient from our encounter. The timing of when to recommend a patient for aortic valve replacement (AVR) should focus on symptoms. AVR is recommended for all symptomatic patients with AS because there is a close correlation between the development of symptoms and mortality. Patients who are asymptomatic yet have echocardiographic evidence of severe AS should also undergo AVR because survival is decreased when valve replacement is delayed.

Coronary angiography is routinely performed in all patients at risk of coronary artery disease before AVR in order to perform concomitant coronary artery bypass grafting at the time of valve replacement if indicated.

Mitral Regurgitation

The management of acute, symptomatic mitral regurgitation is almost always surgical. The medical management of acute MR should focus on hemodynamic stabilization prior to surgery. Mitral regurgitation is an afterload-dependent disease, so vasodilator therapy with angiotensin-converting enzyme inhibitors, hydralazine, and nitroprusside should be the mainstay of medical treatment to slow progression in chronic symptomatic MR prior to surgery. When technically possible, mitral valve repair as opposed to replacement is the surgery of choice in patients with severe MR as it preserves the unique apparatus and architecture of the valve. Even if replacement is required, the surgeon will take great lengths to maintain the apparatus as destruction of this leads to a change in LV dimension and function, even when the replaced valve is functioning well.

The choice of valve replacement with a mechanical versus a bioprosthetic valve is largely dependent on age and other comorbid conditions. Mechanical valves last longer but require lifelong anticoagulation with warfarin due to the increased risk of thromboembolism. Bioprosthetic valves need to be replaced sooner, but do not require anticoagulation. Generally, mechanical valves are used in patients younger than 65 years of age, assuming there are no contraindications to anticoagulation.

EXTENDED IN-HOSPITAL MANAGEMENT

Most patients with severe, symptomatic valvular heart disease will eventually require surgical intervention. Patients with other significant comorbidities, such as chronic obstructive pulmonary disease, LV dysfunction, and chronic kidney disease, encounter a significantly higher operative mortality. Particular attention should be paid to identifying appropriate surgical candidates and optimizing their condition before surgery.

DISPOSITION

Discharge Goals

A significant number of patients will need to remain in the hospital until they have valve surgery; their postoperative course will need to be largely managed by the surgical team. If it is determined that your patient will not need surgery, then you will want to make sure that his or her volume status and other hemodynamic parameters have been stabilized before discharge.

Outpatient Care

Patients with valvular heart disease will need to be followed closely for the development of symptoms and/or imaging criteria that might trigger the need for valve surgery. Patients should be educated about the signs or symptoms of progression in the severity of their disease.

WHAT YOU NEED TO REMEMBER

- There are three common types of aortic stenosis: congenital bicuspid valve AS, degenerative AS, and rheumatic AS.
- Mitral regurgitation can be caused by changes in the mitral valve apparatus itself or by changes in LV geometry.
- Aortic stenosis produces a harsh systolic murmur at the right upper sternal border that radiates to the carotids.
- Mitral regurgitation produces a holosystolic murmur, best heard at the apex, which radiates to the axilla.
- Valvular surgery is the only truly effective treatment for severe valve disease.
- Patients who do not require surgery during their admission should be followed closely both clinically and with echocardiography to determine the timing of any needed valve surgery.

REFERENCE

1. Freeman RV, Otto CM. Spectrum of calcific aortic valve disease: pathogenesis, disease progression, and treatment strategies. *Circulation*. 2005;111(24):3316–3326.

SUGGESTED READINGS

Bonow RO, Carabello BA, et al. ACC/AHA 2006 guidelines for the management of patients with valvular heart disease. *Circulation*. 2006;114(5):e84–231.

Boon NA, Bloomfield P, Kanu C, et al. The medical management of valvular heart disease. *Heart*. 2002;87(4):395–400.

Otto CM. Timing of surgery in mitral regurgitation. *Heart*. 2003;89(1):100–105.

Otto CM. Valve disease: timing of aortic valve surgery. *Heart*. 2000;84(2):211–218.

Syncope

A 60-year-old man is brought to the emergency department by his family after he passed out at home. They were eating dinner when he complained that his "heart was racing." He then lost consciousness for <1 minute. There was no limb shaking. When he awoke, he was lucid but concerned about the event, so his family brought him to the hospital.

OVERVIEW

Definition

Syncope is defined as a sudden and brief loss of consciousness associated with a loss of postural tone followed by spontaneous recovery. Determining the etiology of syncope can oftentimes be challenging. Equally challenging is distinguishing syncope from other similar conditions. This chapter will focus on the approach, diagnosis, and treatment of syncope.

Pathophysiology

Syncope results from a sudden decrease in cerebral blood flow, which leads to loss of consciousness and postural tone. Although this is the final common pathway, the mechanism by which blood flow is reduced depends on the underlying etiology.

Epidemiology

Between 20% and 50% of adults will experience one or more episodes of syncope in their lifetime. The prevalence increases with age—more than 75% of adults over the age of 70 will experience at least one episode of syncope. Syncope is very common, accounting for 1% to 3% of all emergency visits annually, and 6% of all medical admissions (1). Syncope can also result in injuries ranging from falls to motor vehicle accidents, so these numbers may underestimate the true incidence of syncope.

Etiology

Syncope can be frustrating because the etiology of up to 30% of cases remains unidentified. It is important not to misdiagnose similar conditions as syncope. For example, vertigo or dizziness is not syncope as there is no loss of consciousness.

One of the most challenging distinctions to make is that of syncope or seizure. The events just prior to the episode can help distinguish between these conditions. A loss of consciousness preceded by chest pain, palpitations, exercise, defecation, or stress is more likely syncope than a seizure. Seizures are more typically preceded by an aura, and seizure patients recover more slowly with prolonged confusion (i.e., a postictal state). Loss of bowel or bladder control is also much more likely with seizures.

CLINICAL PEARL

Seizurelike movements can occur in up to 12% of patients presenting with true syncope.

Once a diagnosis of syncope is made, it is helpful to use four categories to determine the etiology: (a) reflex mediated, (b) cardiac, (c) orthostatic hypotension, and (d) neurologic (Table 15-1).

TABLE 15-1
Categories of Syncope

Reflex mediated (30%–60%)
  Vasovagal
  Carotid hypersensitivity
  Situational (micturition, defecation, coughing, etc.)

Cardiac (10%–30%)
  Myocardial ischemia
  Malignant arrhythmias
  Heart block (second-degree Mobitz II, third-degree)
  Long QT syndrome
  Brugada syndrome
  Pulmonary embolism
  Aortic stenosis
  Hypertrophic cardiomyopathy

Orthostatic hypotension (2%–24%)

Neurologic (1%)
  Vertebrobasilar insufficiency
  Stroke

Reflex-mediated syncope has three common causes: vasovagal, carotid hypersensitivity, and situational (micturition, defecation, coughing, etc.). In normal, healthy individuals, cerebral perfusion is maintained by complex neurohormonal autoregulation. With decreased venous return, there is increased sympathetic tone and hypercontractility of the left ventricle. In patients with reflex-mediated syncope, the body misinterprets the increased left ventricular contractions as increased volume, and falsely inhibits the sympathetic system while activating the parasympathetic drive. This leads to hypotension, bradycardia, and, ultimately, syncope.

Syncope due to cardiac causes has the greatest risk for significant adverse outcomes. All-cause mortality is nearly doubled in patients with cardiac syncope. Myocardial ischemia and malignant arrhythmias, particularly ventricular arrhythmias, have the greatest immediate mortality risk. Other serious causes of cardiac syncope include heart block, especially Mobitz type II (second-degree) and third-degree heart block, aortic stenosis, hypertrophic cardiomyopathy, long QT syndrome, and pulmonary embolism.

Orthostatic hypotension may be related to volume depletion usually from dehydration. It can also occur from medications such as antihypertensives or from autonomic failure from a comorbid condition such as diabetes.

Syncope from cerebrovascular disease is very rare. Transient ischemia from vertebrobasilar insufficiency can lead to syncope; however, other neurologic symptoms are often present. Finally, syncope can occur in psychiatric conditions such as conversion disorder. However, this is a diagnosis of exclusion once organic causes have been completely ruled out.

ACUTE MANAGEMENT AND WORKUP

The acute management of a patient with syncope should first focus on hemodynamic stability but quickly moves toward identifying the underlying etiology.

The First 15 Minutes

After an episode of syncope, the initial assessment is critical to rule out potentially life-threatening causes.

Initial Assessment

First, assess the mental status of the patient. If the patient appears confused or is difficult to arouse, he or she may have a more serious neurologic problem, such as a stroke or a seizure, rather than simple syncope. It is also important to determine if the patient had any symptoms of myocardial ischemia or arrhythmias prior to the event. Simply asking the patient if he or she experienced any chest pain, shortness of breath, or palpitations prior to the event is sufficient in the initial assessment.

Next, observe the patient and make sure there is no facial asymmetry that would suggest a stroke. Vital signs should also be reviewed, with particular attention paid to the patient's blood pressure. Blood pressure must be checked in both arms and orthostatic measurements must be obtained. A brief cardiac exam should also be completed, listening for murmurs, particularly of aortic stenosis or hypertrophic cardiomyopathy.

Finally, an electrocardiogram (ECG) should be obtained immediately. Although an etiology for syncope is established in <5% of cases based on the ECG, it is an inexpensive and easy tool that helps to rule out serious conditions, including myocardial infarctions and ongoing arrhythmias. In the case of the patient from our encounter, his prodromal symptom of palpitations suggests a possible underlying arrhythmia or cardiac condition that might be picked up early by ECG.

Admission Criteria and Level of Care Criteria

It is often a difficult task to determine who needs to be admitted to the hospital after a syncopal event. In general, patients with advanced age or those with suspected serious cardiovascular or neurologic conditions should be admitted. Patients with frequently occurring symptoms but no diagnosis may also warrant admission. Patients with likely vasovagal syncope but no heart disease or abnormal ECG findings can typically be evaluated as an outpatient.

Because the decision to admit a patient after a syncopal event is often unclear, the San Francisco Syncope Rule was established to aid in this process. If a patient has one of the following five abnormalities—shortness of breath, an abnormal ECG, a hematocrit <30, systolic blood pressure <90 mm Hg, or a history of congestive heart failure—he or she should be admitted. This validated set of criteria has 96% sensitivity and 62% specificity for predicting adverse events in 7 days. If used properly, it can also reduce the number of syncope admissions by 10% (2,3). If the history, physical exam, and electrocardiogram suggest underlying structural heart disease or arrhythmia, a patient must be admitted to a floor with 24-hour cardiac monitoring capability.

The First Few Hours

Once you have made sure that the patient does not have an immediate life-threatening condition, you can begin to collect more information that will aid in establishing a potential diagnosis.

History

It is helpful to begin asking the patient about symptoms and circumstances preceding the syncopal event. Using the four syncope categories can help you to remember the necessary questions. For patients with possible reflex-mediated syncope, it is important to ask about the precipitating event or situation. Prolonged standing, emotional stress, trauma, pain, or postural changes can all lead to vasovagal syncope. Ask if the patient experienced any light-headedness, dizziness, or sweating prior to the event. If the patient fainted after turning his or her head or was wearing a shirt with a tight collar, this might suggest carotid hypersensitivity. Patients can also have a syncopal event during defecation, micturition (urination), or coughing, so patients should be specifically asked if they were recently engaging in these activities.

For patients with possible cardiac syncope, questions should focus on recent chest pain, shortness of breath, or palpitations. It should be determined if the event was related to exercise. They should also be questioned about their past medical history, specifically about heart conditions and medications. A family history of sudden death is also important to ascertain, as this may point to an underlying cardiac condition such as long QT syndrome, Brugada syndrome, or hypertrophic cardiomyopathy.

The patient should be asked about symptoms with postural changes and about fluid intake as dehydration can lead to orthostatic hypotension. It is also important to obtain a detailed past medical history and medication list when considering orthostatic hypotension as the etiology.

Finally, the patient should be asked about neurologic symptoms such as weakness, headaches, or blurry vision as these could suggest an underlying neurologic disorder. The patient should also be asked about a loss of bowel or bladder control, prolonged confusion, or an aura preceding the event as this suggests seizure activity. Finally, the patient should be questioned about recent alcohol or drug use as well as possible psychiatric disorders as these can also contribute to syncope.

Physical Examination

After evaluating the vital signs and doing a quick cardiac exam, a more detailed examination should be conducted with particular attention paid to the cardiovascular and neurologic systems. Initially inspect the patient and look for signs of volume depletion, such as poor skin turgor and dry mucous membranes. Assess the jugular venous pulse as this can aid in your evaluation of the patient's volume status. Evaluate for any irregularity in the pulse as this could point toward an arrhythmia. Also palpate the chest for the heart's point of maximal impulse. Next, you should auscultate the carotids, listening for any bruits. Finally, listen to the heart, paying close attention to any murmurs that might suggest valvular disease.

Next, a thorough neurologic exam should be performed, including assessing mental status, as well as performing cranial nerve, motor, and sensory exams. Focal neurologic deficits could point to an underlying neurologic condition and should prompt consultation with a specialist.

Labs and Tests to Consider

An electrocardiogram and basic laboratory tests (including renal function, glucose, and hemoglobin) should be ordered on every patient with syncope. Further testing should be ordered based on the data obtained from the history and physical exam.

Key Diagnostic Labs and Tests

If the initial ECG or the history suggests an underlying arrhythmia, the patient should be monitored for at least 24 hours to evaluate for recurrence of the arrhythmia. If this does not occur, other options include outpatient Holter monitoring; however, the diagnostic yield is rather low (only 4% of patients have an event in conjunction with a documented arrhythmia). Implantable continuous-loop event monitors, which can be used for weeks to months, can also be considered. Electrophysiologic testing is reserved for patients with recurrent syncope in which the diagnosis has not yet been identified but in whom arrhythmia is still the prime suspect. Echocardiography should be performed in any patient in whom you suspect structural or valvular heart disease. Stress testing for underlying ischemia may also be warranted.

Head-up tilt-table (HUTT) testing can be considered in patients with a likely diagnosis of reflex-mediated vasovagal syncope. HUTT testing uses changes in position to reproduce a syncopal event. The use of provocative agents such as isoproterenol can improve the yield of HUTT testing, with the sensitivity approaching 90% in patients with unexplained recurrent syncope. This should only be considered when other causes have been clearly eliminated and the patient continues to experience syncope.

Carotid sinus massage can be performed on patients with a probable history of carotid sinus hypersensitivity. This should be performed only after listening for carotid bruits, and only in patients without recent myocardial infarction or stroke.

CLINICAL PEARL

Never massage both carotid arteries at the same time because this can lead to decreased perfusion to the brain and can precipitate syncope or even a watershed infarct.

Imaging

Few patients require advanced neurologic testing. Head computerized tomography (CT) provides new diagnostic information in <4% of cases, and should only be used if focal neurologic deficits are seen on examination, or if the patient had head trauma as a result of the syncopal episode. An electroencephalogram should only be ordered if the patient likely suffered a seizure—it should not be used as a tool to distinguish syncope from seizure. Carotid Doppler ultrasound also has low yield in the workup of syncope unless the history or physical exam suggests some abnormality.

Treatment

Treatment depends on the underlying cause of the syncope. In patients with orthostatic hypotension secondary to dehydration, they will require aggressive fluid resuscitation. If their issues are related to medication side effects, the offending medicine should be stopped and an alternative medication chosen. Unfortunately, for most patients with recurrent reflex-mediated syncope, there are few proven treatment options. Some patients with neurocardiogenic syncope derive benefit from midodrine, fludrocortisone, and compressive stockings, but definitive data are lacking. Permanent cardiac pacing should not be used to treat syncope unless the patient has high-grade conduction system disease. For the patient in the clinical encounter, treatment would likely be dictated by the results of his cardiovascular workup since from his presentation, a cardiovascular cause is suspected.

EXTENDED IN-HOSPITAL MANAGEMENT

Most patients do not require more than 24 hours of hospitalization. They are typically placed on a cardiac monitor, and if the workup reveals no cardiac disease, they can be safely discharged home with outpatient follow-up.

DISPOSITION

Discharge Goals

Patients can be discharged once life-threatening causes of syncope have been ruled out by history, examination, and appropriate diagnostic testing. HUTT testing is not required in the inpatient setting unless the patient has recurrent admissions for syncope without a diagnosis. Some patients are set up with Holter monitoring or loop recorders prior to discharge if an arrhythmia is still high on the differential.

Outpatient Care

All patients should follow up with their primary care physician within 1 to 2 weeks of discharge from the hospital. Their primary care doctor can consider further testing as medically appropriate.

WHAT YOU NEED TO REMEMBER

- Syncope is a common problem that affects many people as they age.
- The etiology of a syncopal event can be difficult to determine and often remains undiagnosed.
- Seizure and syncope are two different entities.
- Syncope due to neurologic causes is uncommon.
- Syncope related to cardiac conditions has the greatest morbidity and mortality.

- The history and physical exam are essential in the workup of syncope and often lead to a diagnosis.
- Admission to the hospital is not required for every patient with syncope.
- The syncope workup often continues for an extended period of time in the outpatient arena.

REFERENCES

1. Calkins H. Syncope. In Zipes D, Jalife J, eds. *Cardiac Electrophysiology*. 4th ed. Philadelphia: Saunders; 2004.
2. McKeon A, Vaughan C, Delanty N. Seizure versus syncope. *Lancet Neurol.* 2006;5: 171–180.
3. Miller TH, Kruse JE. Evaluation of syncope. *Am Fam Physician.* 2005;72: 1492–1500.

SUGGESTED READINGS

Kapoor WN. Syncope. *N Engl J Med.* 2000;343:1856–1862.
Kaufmann H, Wieling W. Syncope: a clinically guided diagnostic algorithm. *Clin Auton Res.* 2004;14(Suppl 1):I/87–I/90.
Quinn JV, Stiell IG, McDermott DA, et al. Derivation of the San Francisco rule to predict patients with short-term serious outcomes. *Ann Emerg Med.* 2004;43: 224–232.
Sun BC, Edmond JA, Camargo CA Jr. Characteristics and admission patterns of patients presenting with syncope to U.S. emergency departments, 1992–2000. *Acad Emerg Med.* 2004;11:1029–1034.

16

Approach to the Pulmonary Evaluation

It is important to remember that the cardiovascular and pulmonary systems serve the same ultimate goal: delivering oxygen to the tissues of the body. This chapter will help you develop a framework in which to think about patients with pulmonary problems, but it is critical to remember that the cardiovascular and pulmonary systems are inextricably linked.

Pulmonary Physiology

The primary function of the respiratory system is gas exchange. Oxygen enters blood through the alveoli and carbon dioxide moves out. The lung plays a role in the metabolism of certain substances as well as in host defense, but these are by and large secondary functions.

Lung Mechanics

In order to initiate a breath, the diaphragm contracts and moves downward, causing a more negative intrathoracic pressure relative to the atmosphere. This allows air to flow along a pressure gradient. The volume of air that enters the chest depends on the pressure difference generated and the compliance of the respiratory system. Exhalation is passive during tidal breathing as the lung and chest wall move toward their equilibrium positions. During forceful breathing or hyperventilation, the abdominal muscles provide additional force for moving air out of the lungs.

Compliance

Compliance is the change in volume for a given change in pressure of a system. It is not possible to separate lung compliance from chest wall compliance at the bedside because the lung is essentially a balloon sitting inside another container. As a result, we often speak of respiratory system compliance. Certain disease states, such as chronic obstructive pulmonary disease (COPD), make the lung more compliant, while other diseases make the lung stiffer, such as idiopathic pulmonary fibrosis. Chest wall diseases can also affect respiratory system compliance by making the chest wall stiffer. For example, severe kyphoscoliosis can make the system stiffer and limit the volume that enters the chest with the same inspiratory effort.

The compliance of the lung changes with changing lung volume. As lung volume increases, lung compliance decreases since elastic forces tend to collapse the lung. This relationship also changes with inspiration and expiration (called hysteresis) because surfactant in the alveoli acts to decrease surface tension.

Resistance

Airway resistance is an important determinant of airflow and, when increased, can cause significant problems. It is helpful to remember that total airway resistance is in part a function of lung volume. At lower volumes, small airways tend to collapse and total resistance is higher. At higher lung volumes, these airways are pulled open. This helps to explain why patients with significant airflow obstruction breathe at higher lung volumes—the total airway resistance is lower. However, breathing at higher lung volumes takes a lot of additional energy and patients may fatigue more rapidly.

Ventilation

Not all the gas that passes into our mouth on inspiration reaches the alveoli. Some remains in the oropharynx and the larger conducting airways of the respiratory system. This is referred to as *anatomic dead space*. A normal person has about 1 mL of dead space per pound of ideal body weight. For an average tidal breath of 500 mL, about 150 mL of that air never reaches the alveoli to participate in gas exchange.

> ### CLINICAL PEARL
>
> *Because anatomic dead space is essentially fixed, rapid shallow breathing results in less alveolar ventilation because a greater proportion of each breath is relegated to dead space.*

Gas Exchange

Once the gas reaches the alveoli, two important events happen: Carbon dioxide is unloaded and oxygen is taken up. Oxygen is normally diffusion limited—most hemoglobin is fully saturated in about a third of the time it takes a red cell to traverse the pulmonary capillary bed—but in disease states it may become perfusion limited. Carbon dioxide is about 20 times more soluble than oxygen and is almost always diffusion limited.

Ventilation–Perfusion Relationships

The balance between ventilation (V) and perfusion (Q) in the lung is critical in determining the final oxygen content of the blood that returns to the left side of the heart from the lungs. Areas with ventilation but no blood flow will not participate in gas exchange. The trachea and larger airways are part of this "dead space," as we have already seen. An area of lung that gets no blood flow after a pulmonary embolism will also contribute to the overall dead space. Areas with blood flow but no ventilation will not participate in gas exchange and will make the final O_2 content of the blood lower. These areas of "shunt" are an important cause of hypoxia. Areas of V/Q mismatch also contribute to hypoxemia (see Chapter 17).

Pulmonary Blood Flow

The mechanics of pulmonary blood flow are beyond the scope of this chapter, but it is critical to remember one key fact about the pulmonary vasculature: It tends to constrict in areas of low oxygen tension. As a result, less blood flow is sent to areas that have little or no ventilation, which works to improve overall V/Q matching. Disease states or even medications that impair this hypoxic pulmonary vasoconstriction can lead to greater than expected degrees of hypoxemia for a given reduction in ventilation.

Control of Ventilation

Ventilation is tightly regulated by respiratory control centers in the pons and medulla. These centers receive information about changes in PCO_2 from both central and peripheral chemoreceptors, and adjust ventilation accordingly to maintain a relatively stable pH in the surrounding cerebrospinal fluid. There are also peripheral chemoreceptors for sensing changes in PaO_2 as well as stretch receptors in the lung that play a role in ventilation. The control of ventilation is beyond the scope of this chapter, but it is important to remember that disorders of ventilation are not always caused by primary lung pathology (see Chapter 18).

PATIENT EVALUATION

Now that we've reviewed some basic pulmonary physiology, we can begin to develop an approach to a patient with an apparent pulmonary disorder.

History

A thorough exploration of the timing and character of dyspnea, cough, and chest pain is critical to understanding a patient's underlying pulmonary process. It is important to ask about both environmental and occupational exposures because these may help to frame the risk for specific disease processes. Likewise, a thorough travel and social history may also help to uncover important clues. A good smoking history is also important to ascertain. Remember to ask about pets and other animal exposures because they can be vectors for certain diseases or the antigen responsible for a hypersensitivity reaction. A good medication history is helpful to elicit because certain medications predispose to infectious, vascular, or parenchymal abnormalities. Remember to take a sleep history, especially in obese patients, because obstructive sleep apnea is often suggested by a careful history and physical examination. Be sure to observe your patient carefully while taking your history because confusion, anxiety, or an inability to speak in full sentences may provide insight into the severity of his or her respiratory complaints.

Physical Examination

Observation is one of the most important parts of a thorough pulmonary evaluation.

Pulmonary Examination

First, observe the patient breathing at rest. *Is he or she tachypneic or breathing fast?* A normal respiratory rate is usually 10 to 12 breaths per minute, not the ubiquitous "20" recorded in every patient's bedside chart. Bradypnea, or a slow respiratory rate, is not as common as tachypnea but suggests central nervous system depression from either medications/ingestions or possibly an intracranial process.

Note the patient's pattern of breathing. *Is he or she taking deeper breaths than normal?* This may be Kussmaul's sign and is oftentimes seen in patients with metabolic acidosis as they try to increase their minute ventilation to blow off more carbon dioxide. *Is he or she having episodes of rapid, shallow breathing followed by slower, deeper breaths?* Such Cheyne-Stokes respirations may be a sign of decompensated heart failure or an evolving intracranial process. *Is his or her breathing labored or is he or she using accessory muscles?* If you see contractions of the sternocleidomastoids, nasal flaring, or intercostal retractions, the patient is working hard to breathe and is likely in distress.

Is he or she demonstrating paradoxical respirations? When you take in a breath, your diaphragm pushes down on your intra-abdominal contents. This raises intra-abdominal pressure and pushes your abdominal wall outward. If the diaphragm is paralyzed or too weak from excessive use, it will not move or will actually be pulled up into the chest as the accessory muscles drop intrathoracic pressure. As a result, intra-abdominal pressure will not change or will actually fall, and the abdominal wall will not move or will be drawn inward with inspiration. You can sometimes observe this, but putting one hand on the chest and the other on the patient's belly will confirm this dyssynchronous or paradoxical motion.

Is the patient pursing his or her lips or contracting his or her abdominal muscles on exhalation? Remember that exhalation is usually a passive process, as the elastic recoil of the normal lung will provide the force to exhale. If a patient has an obstruction to airflow, he or she may need to purse his or her lips and contract his or her intra-abdominal muscles to help stent open his or her airways and provide additional force for exhalation. In someone with severe obstructive lung disease, you may also notice *tripoding*—sitting upright with extended arms resting on the knees. This helps to stabilize the shoulders and maximize intrathoracic volume.

After careful observation, you should palpate the patient's posterior chest wall to see if he or she has normal chest wall movement. Asymmetry could be secondary to muscular weakness or to local changes in chest wall compliance, such as from a pleural effusion. Next, percuss the lungs from top to bottom, again looking for asymmetry and lung size. Dullness to percussion can be from a local mass, consolidation, or pleural effusion. If you can appreciate the lower edge of the diaphragm, you can have the patient take a deep breath and measure the diaphragmatic excursion. A normal excursion is about 1 cm with tidal breathing but can be as high as 10 cm with deep breathing.

You should then feel for tactile fremitus. Place the base of your hand along the patient's back and ask him or her to say "toy truck" or "ninety-nine." If you cannot feel the vibrations in your hand, there may be either a mass or pleural effusion that is limiting sound transmission. If you feel increased vibrations, there is likely a consolidation in that area.

Finally, you can take your stethoscope and listen to the patient's breath sounds.

Rales, or crackles, are generated by alveoli opening with inspiration. They usually imply consolidation or fibrosis in that area. Bronchial breath sounds are generated by air moving through a larger tube, implying that the alveoli and small airways around that tube are filled with fluid (i.e., consolidation). Egophony, or "E" sounding like "A," occurs in areas of consolidated lung. Decreased breath sounds can be from atelectasis or possibly a pleural effusion. You would expect increased fremitus in the former and decreased in the latter. Wheezes are generated by turbulent airflow. They can be monophonic if only one airway is obstructed (as in a foreign body aspiration), or more commonly polyphonic if multiple airways are obstructed (as in asthma or COPD). Remember to listen above the trachea to exclude stridor as the cause of respiratory distress.

Cardiovascular Examination

In addition to a careful pulmonary examination, a good cardiovascular examination is crucial to exclude cardiac disease as the underlying cause of the patient's symptoms or to see if his or her underlying lung disease has caused undue strain on the heart. For example, a loud P_2 can be a sign of pulmonary hypertension. You may notice large expiratory swings in jugular venous pulsations in a patient who is obstructed and is generating high pleural pressures to exhale. Pulsus paradoxus, an inspiratory drop in systolic blood pressure by >10 mm Hg, can also be caused by such wide swings in pleural pressure.

Other Examination Findings

Lip color or skin color may tell you if a patient is cyanotic or frankly hypoxemic. Nail changes, such as clubbing, can be a clue to either chronic hypoxia or systemic diseases, such as an occult malignancy. Palpation of the trachea should also be performed because shift of the trachea to one side might indicate volume loss on that side from atelectasis or increased volume of the contralateral side from a pleural effusion or pneumothorax.

Key Diagnostic Evaluations

Chest radiography is a critical component of the pulmonary evaluation. In addition to confirming findings from the history and physical examination, patterns on both chest radiograph and computed tomography are essential to refining differential diagnoses and directing further testing. It is important to look at all of your patient's radiographic studies with an experienced clinician or radiologist as this is by far the best way to learn how to interpret key findings.

We will review radiography and other diagnostic tests as they relate to specific disease processes in the chapters within this section.

 WHAT YOU NEED TO REMEMBER

- The pulmonary and cardiovascular systems are intimately connected—it is oftentimes not easy to separate one from the other when examining a patient at the bedside.
- Observation is a critical component of the pulmonary examination.
- Auscultation should always be the last part of the pulmonary physical examination.
- Always look at your patient's chest radiographs yourself. When possible, review the films with an experienced clinician or radiologist.

SUGGESTED READINGS

Bickley LS, ed. *Bates' Guide to Physical Examination and History Taking*. 9th ed. Philadelphia: Lippincott Williams & Wilkins; 2007.

Mann H, Bragg D. *Chest Radiology*. Chicago: Year Book Medical Publishers; 1989.

West JB. *Respiratory Physiology. The Essentials*. 7th ed. Philadelphia: Lippincott Williams & Wilkins; 2005.

Hypoxemic
Respiratory Failure

THE PATIENT ENCOUNTER

A 33-year-old woman with a history of asthma presents with worsening shortness of breath for the past week after a viral upper respiratory infection. In the emergency department, vital signs reveal tachycardia, a respiratory rate of 40 breaths per minute, and an oxygen saturation of 85% on room air. A chest radiograph reveals hyperinflated lungs, and an arterial blood gas is notable for a pH of 7.44, a $PaCO_2$ of 35 mm Hg, and a PaO_2 of 55 mm Hg.

OVERVIEW

Definition

Respiratory failure is defined as the inability of the respiratory system to provide adequate gas exchange to meet the requirements of the individual patient. Hypoxemic respiratory failure is said to occur when arterial PaO_2 is low (i.e., <60 mm Hg) despite normal or increased ventilation. The inability to remove sufficient carbon dioxide from blood defines hypercapnic respiratory failure ($PaCO_2$ >45 mm Hg with respiratory acidosis and a normal alveolar-arterial gradient). Both processes can occur in the same patient.

This chapter will focus on the approach and early management of patients with hypoxemic and mixed respiratory failure. Hypercapnic respiratory failure will be discussed in the following chapter.

Pathophysiology

The respiratory system is composed of three major components: a controller (the central nervous system), a pump (the peripheral nervous system, the rib cage, and its musculature), and the lungs. Dysfunction in any of these components may lead to hypoxemia.

Hypoxemia is the sine qua non for respiratory failure. The five general mechanisms of hypoxemia are as follows: (a) decreased barometric pressure, (b) hypoventilation, (c) shunt, (d) ventilation–perfusion (V/Q) mismatch, and (e) impaired diffusion.

1. *Decreased barometric pressure* is seen at high altitudes (i.e., mountain sickness and air travel). It is important to remember that the inspired concentration of FiO_2 is the same regardless of elevation. The lower alveolar

oxygen concentration is a function of the reduced atmospheric pressure as demonstrated in the alveolar gas equation:

$$PAO_2 = PiO_2 - PaCO_2/R,$$

in which R is the respiratory quotient (R = 0.8) and PiO_2 is the oxygen concentration in inhaled air. $PiO_2 = FiO_2 \times$ (atmospheric pressure [760 at sea level] – vapor pressure of water [47]).

2. *Hypoventilation* refers to diminished alveolar ventilation (V_A), and occurs in diseases that affect the controller and/or pump components of the respiratory system. When it occurs, a new steady state in alveolar gas concentrations (PAO_2 and $PACO_2$) is reached with a decrease in both CO_2 clearance and O_2 delivery. The end result is an increased $PACO_2$ and a decreased PAO_2. When hypoventilation occurs in the presence of normal lungs, the alveolar-arterial oxygen gradient (A-a gradient), which is the driving force for O_2 diffusion into blood, is unchanged from baseline. The combination of hypercapnia, hypoxemia, and a normal A-a gradient is referred to as hypercapnic respiratory failure in an effort to differentiate it from the other three clinically relevant mechanisms of hypoxia. Hypoventilation will be discussed in more detail in Chapter 18.

3. *Shunt* occurs when venous blood reaches the arterial system without passing through ventilated regions of the lung. Shunt can be extrapulmonary, such as right-to-left intracardiac shunt, or intrapulmonary, such as pulmonary arteriovenous malformations (i.e., hepatopulmonary syndrome), or alveoli filled with pus (pneumonia), fluid (pulmonary edema, acute respiratory distress syndrome [ARDS]), or blood. As the shunted blood is not exposed to alveolar oxygen, increasing FiO_2 and, therefore, PAO_2 will not raise the PaO_2 level substantially. This feature can be used diagnostically at the bedside: If a patient's PaO_2 level does not increase substantially on 100% oxygen, then shunt is likely playing a large role in his or her hypoxia.

4. In normal lungs, ventilation and perfusion are tightly matched in order to allow for efficient gas transfer. Whenever an area of the lung has *ventilation–perfusion (V/Q) mismatch*, abnormalities in gas transfer ensue. Areas with low V/Q, such as those distal to an airway obstruction, will be relatively hypoventilated, will have a lower PaO_2 level, and therefore will have hypoxemic blood leaving these units. Clinically, areas with low V/Q have a strong depressive effect on arterial oxygen concentration. It is sometimes helpful to think of shunt as an extreme form of V/Q mismatch (i.e., an area of blood flow with no ventilation; V/Q = 0). Areas with high V/Q, such as alveolar units distal to a pulmonary embolism, will increase overall dead space, thus increasing $PACO_2$ steady-state concentration at any given alveolar ventilation, and finally decreasing PaO_2. Excluding the other three mechanisms of hypoxemia generally identifies V/Q mismatch. Disease entities with underlying V/Q mismatch include asthma and chronic obstructive pulmonary disease (COPD).

5. *Diffusion impairment* means that equilibration does not occur between PAO_2 and PaO_2. Under normal resting conditions, the capillary PO_2 reaches PaO_2 in one-third the total contact time with the alveolar-capillary membrane. Even with exercise, when the increased cardiac output reduces contact time, equilibration occurs in the normal lung. In conditions in which the blood–gas barrier is thickened, the diffusion of oxygen can be slowed enough so that equilibration does not happen. In fact, any hypoxemia that occurs at rest will be exaggerated in situations of increased cardiac output (e.g., exercise, sepsis). Diffuse parenchymal lung diseases, connective tissue diseases affecting the lungs, and alveolar cell carcinoma are examples of conditions with hypoxemia resulting from diffusion impairment.

Shunting, diffusion impairment, and V/Q mismatch have variable effects on CO_2 transfer; however, in most cases, ventilation is increased through stimulation of the controller component. This will increase alveolar minute ventilation, resulting in a decreased $PaCO_2$, and therefore an increased A-a gradient. Hypoxemia in the presence of an elevated A-a gradient is referred to as hypoxemic respiratory failure.

Low venous oxygen saturation, as can be seen in low cardiac output states or in states with increased oxygen consumption, is considered a separate cause of hypoxemia by some. It will accentuate the effects of the other mechanisms, rather than independently cause hypoxemia.

Epidemiology

There is a multitude of causes of hypoxemic respiratory failure. As a result, it is difficult to estimate the incidence and prevalence of hypoxia in hospitalized patients.

Etiology

As shown in Table 17-1, identifying the mechanisms of hypoxemia in individual patients will help narrow the differential diagnosis of hypoxemic respiratory failure.

ACUTE MANAGEMENT AND WORKUP

Few encounters in internal medicine are as time sensitive as respiratory failure. The main objectives of the initial evaluation of the hypoxic patient are identifying the most likely cause of respiratory failure, assessing the likelihood of respiratory arrest, and ensuring appropriate ventilatory support if needed.

The First 15 Minutes

The first step in evaluating a patient in respiratory distress is to determine if he or she is hypoxic.

TABLE 17-1
Mechanisms of Hypoxia

Mechanism of Hypoxia	Disease
Ventilation–perfusion mismatch	• Airway diseases (asthma, COPD, pneumonia) • Interstitial lung diseases • Pulmonary vascular diseases (pulmonary embolism, pulmonary hypertension) • Pneumothorax
Shunt	• Intrapulmonary shunts (AVMs, hepatopulmonary syndrome) • Alveolar filling (pneumonia, atelectasis, ARDS, pulmonary edema, alveolar hemorrhage) • Intracardiac (septal defects, PFO)
Diffusion impairment	• Diffuse parenchymal lung diseases (idiopathic, collagen vascular diseases, drug related)
Hypoventilation	• Narcotics or other sedating medications • Hypothyroidism • Congenital hypoventilation syndromes • Obesity hypoventilation syndrome
Decreased barometric pressure	• High altitude • Air travel

ARDS, acute respiratory distress syndrome; AVM, arteriovenous malformation; COPD, chronic obstructive pulmonary disease; PFO, patent foramen ovale.

Initial Assessment

Pulse oximetry can allow a rapid bedside assessment of hemoglobin saturation and, if <90%, strongly implies hypoxia. However, pulse oximetry may not be reliable in certain instances and does not provide any information regarding ventilation or $PaCO_2$. Arterial blood gas (ABG) analysis should be performed in patients to confirm hypoxemia and evaluate ventilatory status.

> ## CLINICAL PEARL
>
> *The pulse oximeter is unreliable in the presence of abnormal hemo-globins, such as carboxyhemoglobin from CO poisoning (normal PaO_2 and O_2 saturation reading on oximeter but low measured oxygen saturation) and methemoglobinemia (erratic reading and normal PaO_2 with low measured oxygen saturation). Always confirm abnormal oxygen saturation on pulse oximetry with a measured saturation level on ABG.*

Once it is determined that a patient is hypoxic, assess him or her using the ABC (airway, breathing, circulation) approach. A safe airway requires a preserved mental status. Delirium, drowsiness, and lethargy are all manifestations of progressive hypoxemia and hypercapnia, which blunt the sensation of dyspnea. If the patient is unresponsive, lethargic, or incoherent, then his or her airway is unprotected in the case of vomiting or abnormal head posture. Furthermore, a blunted sensation of dyspnea will precipitate a cycle of hypoventilation, acidemia, more hypoventilation, and ultimately cardiorespiratory arrest. For those reasons, the safest course of action in such a patient includes endotracheal intubation and mechanical ventilation.

After performing an airway assessment, follow it with a quick evaluation of the patient's breathing and circulatory status. An inability to speak in full sentences (if at all), the use of accessory muscles (sternocleidomastoid muscles in the neck, abdominal muscles, and intercostal muscles), paradoxical respirations, and severe tachypnea (respiratory rate >40 breaths per minute) all indicate severe respiratory distress. However, a seemingly normal breathing pattern often precedes respiratory fatigue and ultimately arrest. A focused exam must include skin palpation (warm and bounding pulses versus cool, clammy, and thready pulses), assessment of the jugular venous pressure (JVP), tracheal palpation, a lung exam, and a cardiac exam.

The cornerstone of the evaluation of respiratory failure lies in the interpretation of the arterial blood gas, which will narrow the differential diagnosis and direct treatment. In addition to identifying underlying acid–base disorders, the ABG will help obtain accurate PaO_2 and $PaCO_2$ measures, which then can be used to calculate the A-a O_2 gradient:

$$\text{A-a gradient} = PAO_2 - PaO_2 = [(760 - 47) \times FiO_2 - PaCO_2/0.8] - PaO_2$$

The age-appropriate A-a gradient in the normal lung is the result of baseline V/Q mismatch and can be estimated by the formula (age/4) + 4. As seen in Figure 17-1, an elevated A-a gradient suggests V/Q mismatch, shunt, or diffusion defect as mechanisms for hypoxemia, while a normal A-a gradient suggests pure hypercapnic respiratory failure (if elevated $PaCO_2$) or a low barometric pressure (if normal $PaCO_2$).

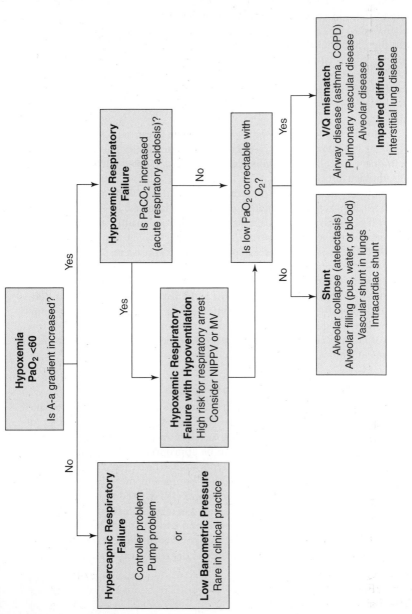

FIGURE 17-1: Approach to determining the mechanism of hypoxic respiratory failure.

In addition, the ABG will help reveal respiratory fatigue by detecting elevated $PaCO_2$ in a patient in respiratory distress. This is of considerable value when looked at serially; rising $PaCO_2$ suggests worsening respiratory fatigue and therefore the need for ventilatory support. For example, the patient in our encounter has an elevated A-a gradient of 51 mm Hg, and a low-normal $PaCO_2$. If a repeat ABG 15 minutes later were to show a pH of 7.36 and a $PaCO_2$ of 45 mm Hg with persistent hypoxemia and respiratory distress, this would suggest worsening respiratory fatigue and the need for ventilatory support.

As soon as hypoxia is recognized, a portable chest radiograph should be obtained and interpreted. A radiograph can help identify pulmonary edema, pulmonary vascular congestion, pneumothorax, consolidations, and other intrathoracic processes.

By the end of the first 15 minutes, you should be able to identify a mechanism for hypoxemia, formulate a differential diagnosis, secure the patient's airway as necessary, and initiate attempts at hemodynamic stabilization and ventilatory support (ranging from supplemental oxygen to mechanical ventilation). The goal is to correct hypoxemia and decrease respiratory drive to avoid respiratory muscle fatigue.

You should increase inhaled oxygen to maintain an oxygen saturation >90%. This should be done as soon as hypoxemia is suspected or confirmed. In the absence of improvement in either oxygen saturation or respiratory distress, quickly initiate positive pressure ventilation (PPV) in the form of noninvasive positive-pressure ventilation (NIPPV) or endotracheal intubation and mechanical ventilation.

Admission Criteria and Level of Care Criteria

Hypoxemic respiratory failure requires admission for close monitoring and further treatment. The level of care required depends on the etiology of hypoxemia and the level of stability reached in the emergency room. In general, quickly reversible causes can be appropriately managed on a regular floor. This is often seen in patients with a heart failure exacerbation who receive diuretics in the emergency room. On the other side of the spectrum, intubated patients and those on NIPPV need to be admitted to an intensive care unit (ICU). In general, when the course of the disease is uncertain (such as in refractory asthma) and when patients have decreased cardiopulmonary reserve (e.g., elderly patients or those with congestive heart failure, COPD, or end-stage renal disease), you should admit the patients to the ICU.

The First Few Hours

Once the patient has been stabilized, a thorough history and physical examination will help to pinpoint the cause of the patient's decline.

History

Determining the onset and character of symptoms provides clues about the possible etiology of hypoxemia. Other chapters will provide more information on common causes of hypoxia, such as pneumonia, COPD, asthma, and pulmonary embolism. One scenario that tends to be under-appreciated is the rapid development of acute lung injury (ALI)/ARDS in patients with sepsis or systemic inflammatory response syndrome from both pulmonary and nonpulmonary etiologies (e.g., burns, pancreatitis, and urosepsis). A thorough history will help you identify such risk factors. This will allow appropriate discussions with the patient, early intervention, and endotracheal intubation in a more controlled setting if necessary.

Physical Examination

A patient in respiratory failure is often unable to provide a history; a detailed physical exam is therefore essential. The key components of the pulmonary examination are reviewed in Chapter 16. A volume status examination is helpful. An elevated JVP with bilateral diffuse crackles and an S_3 on cardiac exam suggest cardiogenic pulmonary edema. A low JVP, with a hyperdynamic heart exam and warm extremities, suggests low systemic vascular resistance and possible shock, the most common cause of which is sepsis. In this case, hypoxemic failure can be secondary to ALI/ARDS or pneumonia. A bedridden patient with sacral pressure ulcers and a percutaneous endoscopic gastrostomy tube makes aspiration pneumonitis high on the list of differential diagnoses. Tracheal deviation, asymmetric chest expansion, and absent air movement in a lung field suggests either pneumothorax or pleural effusion (the trachea is deviated away from the field of absent air movement) or lung collapse (the trachea is deviated toward the field of absent air movement).

Labs and Tests to Consider

Laboratory and radiologic testing should be directed toward the pathophysiologic process causing the hypoxemic respiratory failure.

Key Diagnostic Labs and Tests

As mentioned previously, the most crucial and emergent lab to obtain is an ABG. Another important blood test to obtain is a serum lactic acid. When elevated, it is a good marker for tissue hypoxia, the end result of hypoxemia. Measured serially, it may help determine the efficacy of the therapy in reversing anaerobic metabolism.

The differential diagnosis will help guide other diagnostic testing (i.e., cardiac enzymes and brain natriuretic peptide in a patient with suspected heart failure). Obtaining a urine toxicology screen is oftentimes useful. Many illicit drugs such as cocaine and heroin may directly cause and/or worsen preexisting hypoxemic respiratory failure. A basic metabolic profile should be obtained to assess renal function, as well as obtaining a complete blood count to look for markers of infection and anemia. Blood and sputum cultures should be obtained as appropriate.

Imaging

The chest radiograph is essential to the diagnosis and management of hypoxemic respiratory failure. The initial radiograph will be informative about any gross intrathoracic process. Things to look for include localized infiltrates (pneumonia), bilateral infiltrates (pulmonary edema, ARDS, alveolar hemorrhage), pleural effusions, pneumothorax, a widened vascular pedicle, cardiomegaly, diaphragmatic flattening, and hyperinflation. Serial radiographs can be useful in the case of rapidly progressive pulmonary processes. For example, prompt resolution of infiltrates that correlates with clinical improvement will favor cardiogenic pulmonary edema over ARDS as an underlying etiology of hypoxia.

Further imaging will depend on the differential diagnosis. For example, a thoracic computed tomography (CT) scan with intravenous contrast can identify pulmonary embolism, a noncontrast CT can assess for parenchymal lung disease, and an echocardiogram can help to assess cardiac function.

Treatment

Therapy is directed at correcting hypoxemia and addressing the underlying etiology of hypoxia. Figure 17-2 schematizes the management of hypoxemia. The first step is to administer enough supplemental oxygen to increase oxygen saturation to >90% while relieving dyspnea. A safe approach would be to start with maximal oxygen through a nonrebreather facemask (close to 90% FiO_2) and then titrate the FiO_2 downward based on response. If the hypoxemia and clinical status do not correct within minutes, PPV should be initiated. NIPPV has been proven to be beneficial in cardiogenic pulmonary edema, acute COPD exacerbations, and certain instances of hypoxemic respiratory failure with superimposed hypercapnia, such as community-acquired pneumonia in patients with COPD. It is likely safe to attempt NIPPV in these situations in the absence of contraindications (intolerance to the mask, altered mental status, active vomiting, inability to handle secretions) and in the presence of trained personnel. If there is no improvement or stabilization in the patient's clinical status within 1 hour, endotracheal intubation is indicated. In all other cases of refractory hypoxemia, endotracheal intubation must not be delayed.

Ultimately, therapy should be focused on the underlying etiology: diuresis for cardiogenic pulmonary edema; bronchodilators and corticosteroids for COPD and asthma, as in the case of our patient encounter; antibiotics for pneumonia, etc.

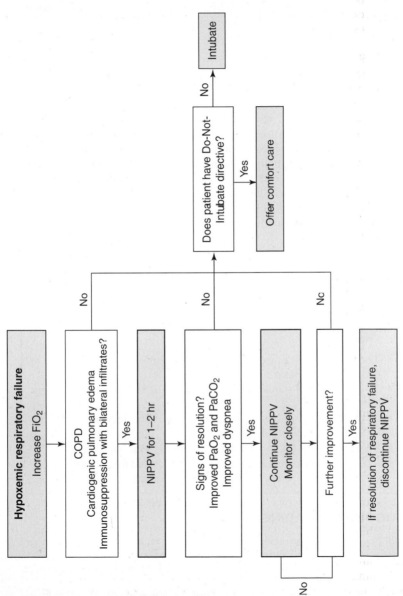

FIGURE 17-2: Approach to the management of hypoxic respiratory failure.

EXTENDED IN-HOSPITAL MANAGEMENT

The hospital course of patients with hypoxemic respiratory failure depends on the underlying etiology. The length of stay varies from a few days in the case of an uncomplicated asthma exacerbation to possibly months in the case of ARDS.

DISPOSITION

Discharge Goals

Patients are ready for discharge once the etiologies of hypoxemia have been identified and addressed. Some patients will have a complete return to baseline, while others might need extended rehabilitation as outpatients. In the case of progressive lung diseases such as pulmonary fibrosis and COPD, it is important to check for home oxygen requirements on discharge. Patients with oxygen saturation <88% at rest or with ambulation need to be discharged on home oxygen. Finally, appropriate immunizations need to be administered prior to discharge, and patients need to be educated about potential triggers of hypoxemic respiratory failure.

Outpatient Care

Appropriate outpatient follow-up will be largely determined by the underlying cause of hypoxemia.

WHAT YOU NEED TO REMEMBER

- The first 15 minutes are critical in the evaluation and management of patients with hypoxia.
- Assessing mental status is key in determining the need for emergent intubation.
- At the first sign of hypoxemia, obtain an ABG, increase FiO_2, and order a chest radiograph.
- Always calculate the A-a gradient in patients with hypoxemia.
- If there is no improvement in oxygen saturation and dyspnea within minutes of initiating therapy, consider endotracheal intubation or NIPPV.

SUGGESTED READINGS

Hill NS, Brennan J, Garpestad E, et al. Noninvasive ventilation in acute respiratory failure. *Crit Care Med.* 2007;35(10):2402–2407.

Isakow W, Kollef M. *Respiratory Failure* [eBook]. ACP Medicine; 2007. Available at: www.acpmedicine.com/acpmedicine/.

Lee W, Slutsky A. Hypoxic respiratory failure. In Mason RJ, ed. *Murray & Nadel's Textbook of Respiratory Medicine.* 4th ed. Philadelphia: Elsevier; 2005.

Truwi JD, Bernard GR. Noninvasive ventilation—don't push too hard. *N Engl J Med.* 2004;350(24):2451–2460.

Hypercapnic Respiratory Failure

THE PATIENT ENCOUNTER

A 45-year-old previously healthy man presents with worsening shortness of breath for the past few hours. He also reports ascending weakness that started 48 hours ago. In the emergency department, vital signs reveal a respiratory rate of 30 and a room air oxygen saturation of 88%. Physical examination reveals symmetrically limited chest expansion and decreased air entry but normal auscultation and percussion. On neurologic examination he has severe, symmetric lower extremity weakness. A chest radiograph is normal, and an arterial blood gas reveals a pH of 7.24, a $PaCO_2$ of 62, and a PaO_2 of 55.

OVERVIEW

Definition

Hypercapnic respiratory failure is defined as hypoxemia (PaO_2 <60) *and* acute respiratory acidosis (pH <7.34 and $PaCO_2$ >45) in the absence of an acute disruption in the mechanisms of oxygen delivery.

Pathophysiology

Hypoventilation refers to diminished alveolar ventilation (V_A), and occurs in diseases affecting the controller and/or pump components of the respiratory system. When it occurs, a new steady state in alveolar gas concentrations (lower PAO_2 and higher $PACO_2$) is reached. The relationship between arterial $PaCO_2$ and alveolar ventilation is the following:

$$PaCO_2 = k \times (CO_2 \text{ production})/V_A,$$

in which k is a constant. **Arterial CO_2 levels are inversely proportional to alveolar ventilation and will therefore always rise in the face of hypoventilation.** This leads to a decrease in PAO_2 according to the alveolar gas equation:

$$PAO_2 = PiO_2 - PaCO_2/R,$$

in which *R* is the respiratory quotient (R = 0.8) and PiO_2 is the oxygen concentration in inhaled air [$PiO_2 = FiO_2 \times (760 - 47)$]. **$PAO_2$ must decrease when $PaCO_2$ increases.** Furthermore, when hypoventilation occurs in the absence of parenchymal or vascular disease, the alveolar-arterial oxygen gradient (A-a gradient), which is the driving force for O_2 diffusion into blood, is unchanged from baseline. The combination of hypercapnia, hypoxemia, and a normal A-a gradient is referred to as hypercapnic respiratory failure in an effort to differentiate it from the other mechanisms of hypoxia in which increasing ventilation is not the only therapeutic intervention needed to correct the low PaO_2.

It is important to remember that hypercapnia can also occur in situations of increased CO_2 production in the face of limited ventilatory reserve. Such conditions (exercise, overfeeding, hyperthyroidism, burns, fever, and sepsis) will worsen or even cause hypercapnic respiratory failure and therefore need to be identified and corrected.

Hypercapnic respiratory failure entails the absence of an acute disruption in oxygen delivery, such as ventilation–perfusion (V/Q) mismatch or shunting. Normally, hypercapnia does not occur in these circumstances because a normal individual can augment his or her alveolar ventilation in response to this insult. This may not correct hypoxemia but usually results in a normal or even a low $PaCO_2$. However, patients with chronic lung disease, such as chronic obstructive pulmonary disease (COPD) or interstitial lung disease, are unable to augment their alveolar ventilation in response to an acute insult and are at high risk of developing acute hypoventilation and subsequent hypercapnic respiratory failure.

Epidemiology

Because there are so many potential causes of hypercapnic respiratory failure, it is difficult to estimate the incidence and prevalence of this disorder in patients who present to the hospital.

Etiology

As shown in Table 18-1, the causes of hypercapnic respiratory failure are diseases that affect the controller and/or the pump components of the respiratory system. Remember that conditions that increase CO_2 production can cause or contribute to preexisting hypercapnia as well.

The most common cause of hypercapnic respiratory failure is probably hypoxemic respiratory failure. The increased respiratory drive and impaired pulmonary mechanics related to the underlying etiology will tremendously increase the workload on the respiratory system. The combination of muscular fatigue, decreased chest wall compliance, and central nervous system (CNS) depression from hypoxia will disrupt all elements of the controller and pump components and ultimately lead to hypoventilation and therefore superimposed hypercapnic respiratory failure. This is often referred to as *mixed respiratory failure*; the ultimate reason for ventilatory support is hypoventilation, but the primary pathophysiologic mechanism is impaired oxygen exchange. This distinction is important because it represents the group of patients who are at highest risk of respiratory arrest (see Fig. 17-1).

TABLE 18-1
Etiologies of Hypercapnic Respiratory Failure

Mechanism of Hypercapnia	Possible Causes
Decreased ventilatory drive	• CNS disease (stroke, tumor, encephalitis) • Narcotic or benzodiazepine overdose • Sleep apnea/obesity hypoventilation • Multiple sclerosis • Myxedema • Congenital hypoventilation
Neuromuscular disorders	• Anterior horn cell (poliomyelitis, amyotrophic lateral sclerosis, tetanus, trauma) • Peripheral nerve (Guillain-Barré syndrome, diphtheria, phrenic nerve palsy) • Myopathy (muscular dystrophy, polymyositis/dermatomyositis) • Neuromuscular junction (myasthenia gravis, Lambert-Eaton syndrome, botulism) • Metabolic (hypercalcemia, hypophosphatemia)
Decreased chest wall compliance	• Obesity • Ascites • Kyphoscoliosis • Pneumothorax or pleural effusion
Primary lung pathology	• COPD • Asthma • Cystic fibrosis • Interstitial lung disease • Pulmonary embolism • Pneumonia • Pulmonary edema • Pneumothorax
Increased CO_2 production	• Burns • Trauma • Sepsis • Infection • Hyperthyroidism • Hyperalimentation

CNS, central nervous system; COPD, chronic obstructive pulmonary disease.

ACUTE MANAGEMENT AND WORKUP

The initial encounter with patients in hypercapnic respiratory failure is essentially the same as patients in hypoxemic failure, because both will present with hypoxemia (see Chapter 17).

The First 15 Minutes

The main objectives are identifying hypercapnic respiratory failure, assessing the likelihood of respiratory arrest, and ensuring appropriate ventilatory support.

Initial Assessment

From the onset, there are important clues that suggest hypercapnic respiratory failure and its etiology. Contrary to patients with hypoxemic respiratory failure, who often appear in distress, patients with respiratory acidosis present predominantly with symptoms of CNS depression, such as somnolence, lethargy, dysarthria, and altered mental status. As a result, a good history is often difficult to obtain. A very common and crucial piece of information is drug history (i.e., narcotic or benzodiazepine overdose). On physical examination, severe acidemia can cause cardiovascular dysfunction and, subsequently, hypotension. Certain findings can suggest specific etiologies. A large body habitus will decrease respiratory compliance, while an emaciated patient could lack the musculature needed for appropriate ventilation. Evidence of stroke on examination suggests CNS pathology as the cause of hypoventilation.

The arterial blood gas will provide quick and crucial information. The presence of hypoxemia, acute respiratory acidosis, and a normal A-a gradient (or one unchanged from baseline) is diagnostic of hypercapnic respiratory failure. The presence of an underlying chronic respiratory acidosis suggests disorders of ventilation like many listed in Table 18-1; exacerbations of those diseases will often manifest as hypercapnic respiratory failure. The degree of acidemia will also dictate certain interventions, such as mechanical ventilation. A portable chest radiograph can show small lung fields, elevated hemidiaphragms (phrenic nerve pathology), pleural effusion, parenchymal lung disease, or pneumothorax.

As in hypoxemic respiratory failure, patients are frequently very unstable, necessitating immediate interventions prior to further data gathering. In patients with pure hypercapnic failure, **increasing FiO_2 should be done cautiously** as it can worsen hypercapnia through several mechanisms (see Chapter 21). The most important intervention is to increase ventilation. Naloxone and flumazenil should be administered if narcotic or benzodiazepine overdose is a possibility. In almost all other situations, ventilation should be increased by using positive-pressure ventilation in the form of intubation and mechanical ventilation (MV) or noninvasive ventilation (NIV). In the absence of contraindications, NIV should be attempted first

TABLE 18-2
Contraindications to Noninvasive Positive-pressure Ventilation

- Coma or confusion
- Inability to protect airway
- Severe acidosis at presentation (pH <7.2)
- Vomiting
- Inability to handle secretions
- Obstructed bowel
- Hemodynamic instability
- Orofacial abnormalities that interfere with the mask

and is often enough to correct the physiologic disturbance. In the presence of contraindications or lack of clinical improvement after approximately 1 hour of NIV, then MV should be instituted (Table 18-2). However, if the clinician has the slightest inclination that the patient will fare better with MV (i.e., the patient appears "very sick"), then intubation should not be delayed.

Admission Criteria and Level of Care Criteria

Patients with respiratory failure should be admitted for evaluation and further management. The level of care depends on the initial response to treatment and the underlying etiology. Intubated patients should be admitted to the intensive care unit. Patients who require NIV for a prolonged period of time and who are stable and tolerating the mask should be admitted to an intermediate level of care because of the close monitoring required for NIV. Finally, patients whose hypercapnia is stable on NIV but whose underlying etiology has yet to be reversed should be monitored in the intensive care unit.

The First Few Hours

Once hypercapnia has been recognized and initially managed, you can begin to explore the potential etiologies of the patient's respiratory failure.

History

Ascending paralysis in an otherwise healthy individual, such as the patient described in the clinical vignette, should suggest Guillain-Barré syndrome. Difficulty rising from a chair or combing one's hair suggests proximal muscle weakness from a possible inflammatory myopathy. Dysarthria, diplopia, and repetitional fatigue may be signs of myasthenia gravis. Somnolence and hypercapnia in a patient with lymphoma should raise suspicion for hypercalcemia, while a similar presentation in an alcoholic patient can be a manifestation of hypophosphatemia. A history of COPD, asthma, or other obstructive lung disease might suggest a flare of that underlying disorder. A careful sleep history should be obtained because patients with obstructive sleep apnea may have worsening hypoventilation at night or may have an overlap syndrome with features of obesity hypoventilation. Orthopnea is often thought of as a sign of heart failure but may also be caused by diaphragmatic weakness or paralysis, or poor chest wall compliance. An acute infection in a patient with poor ventilatory reserve might increase CO_2 production to the point in which acute respiratory acidosis occurs. Finally, lung pathology, such as severe pneumonia, ARDS, pulmonary embolism, or even pulmonary edema from heart failure, may worsen V/Q mismatch or dead space enough to cause hypercapnia, especially in a patient with chronic lung disease.

CLINICAL PEARL

Patients with diaphragmatic dysfunction feel more short of breath when their abdomen is under water because the surrounding water pressure makes it more difficult to push the abdominal contents down to allow lung expansion.

Physical Examination

You should evaluate a patient's work of breathing by looking for tachypnea, accessory muscle use, and paradoxical motion of the diaphragm. You should also look for signs of severe airflow obstruction as described in Chapter 16. Examination of the chest can also reveal decreased chest expansion, kyphoscoliosis, or findings suggestive of a pneumothorax or pleural effusion.

It is important to calculate a patient's body mass index and look for features suggestive of sleep apnea (i.e., macroglossia, retrognathia, pharyngeal soft tissue hypertrophy, etc.). Cachectic patients could have underlying neuromuscular disease, such as amyotrophic lateral sclerosis or muscular dystrophies, malignancies with secondary pleural effusions, or hypercalcemia. Abdominal examination may reveal evidence of ascites, which can impair respiratory system compliance.

A complete neurologic exam should be conducted. Mental status should be frequently assessed because it can be a reliable indicator of the severity of the respiratory failure. A neuromuscular exam can help identify weakness in specific groups, such as proximal muscle weakness in proximal dystrophies and inflammatory myopathies, and ascending paralysis with absent reflexes and a normal sensory exam in demyelinating polyneuropathies. Focal neurologic defects suggest cerebrovascular disease or inflammatory processes such as multiple sclerosis.

Labs and Test to Consider

An arterial blood gas and serum bicarbonate are the most important lab tests to obtain in patients with hypercapnic respiratory failure.

Key Diagnostic Labs and Tests

Serial arterial blood gases are very helpful in determining whether or not a patient needs ventilatory support as well as in following the effectiveness of such support. An elevated bicarbonate level, especially if known to be old, is suggestive of a metabolic alkalosis in response to a chronic respiratory acidosis and may help to frame the clinical context of the patient's current presentation. Other lab tests should be ordered according to the differential diagnosis.

Imaging

Chest imaging should be ordered if intrathoracic pathologies are suspected. Specific neurologic imaging can be useful if CNS diseases are diagnostic possibilities.

Treatment

The ultimate goal of therapy is to increase alveolar ventilation. At the time of presentation, the latter is achieved through either NIV or MV. The effectiveness of the ventilatory support in correcting the acute respiratory acidosis is assessed by serial arterial blood gases. Once an acceptable degree of stability is achieved, further treatment is aimed at the underlying etiology. For example, an exacerbation of myasthenia gravis will likely be treated with acetylcholinesterase inhibitors and steroids, while treatment for Guillain-Barré syndrome, as in the case of the patient from our encounter, involves plasma exchange and intravenous immune globulin (IVIG).

EXTENDED IN-HOSPITAL MANAGEMENT

The hospital course of patients with hypercapnic respiratory failure depends on the underlying etiology. The length of stay varies from a few days in the case of CNS depressant intoxication to possibly weeks in the case of refractory myopathies.

DISPOSITION

Discharge Goal

Patients are ready for discharge once the etiologies of hypercapnia have been controlled. Some patients will have a complete return to baseline, while others might need extended rehabilitation as outpatients. In the case of progressive diseases such as many neuromuscular diseases, home NIV for nocturnal support is occasionally necessary.

Outpatient Care

Most patients can follow up with their primary care physician in 1 to 2 weeks after discharge from the hospital. Patients with chronic ventilatory problems should be referred to a pulmonologist.

WHAT YOU NEED TO REMEMBER

- Acute respiratory acidosis and a normal A-a gradient are the hallmark of hypercapnic respiratory failure.
- Hypercapnia can be the result of decreased alveolar ventilation, increased carbon dioxide production, or a combination of the two.
- The presence of an elevated A-a gradient suggests hypoxemic respiratory failure as the primary disorder.
- The initial treatment is aimed at increasing alveolar ventilation through MV or NIV.
- Remember that NIV is not appropriate for every patient.

SUGGESTED READINGS

Isakow W, Kollef M. Respiratory failure [eBook]. ACP Medicine; 2007. Available at: www.acpmedicine.com/acpmedicine/.

Pierson DJ, Hill NS. Acute ventilatory failure. In: Mason RJ, ed. *Murray & Nadel's Textbook of Respiratory Medicine.* 4th ed. Philadelphia: Elsevier Saunders; 2005.

Truwi JD, Bernard GR. Noninvasive ventilation—don't push too hard. *N Engl J Med.* 2004;350(24):2451–2460.

Pulmonary Embolism

A 60-year-old man presents to the emergency department with a sudden onset of chest pain and shortness of breath. On examination, he is hypotensive and hypoxemic. His lungs are clear, his jugular venous pressure is elevated, and he exhibits unilateral lower extremity edema. A computed tomography scan confirms the presence of pulmonary embolism.

OVERVIEW

Definition

Deep venous thrombosis (DVT) is the formation of a blood clot in the deep venous system. A pulmonary embolism (PE) is a clot that dislodges and travels to the pulmonary arterial bed. This chapter will focus on the identification and management of pulmonary embolism.

Pathophysiology

Stasis, hypercoagulability, and trauma (Virchow's classic triad) are conditions that predispose to clot formation. A fresh blood clot is rich in enzymatic activity. Clot formation begins with platelet activation and is followed by thrombin generation. Although they may develop in any vascular location, clots frequently form in the venous system of the lower extremities below the knee. When such clots extend above the knee, they may dislodge and travel to the pulmonary arterial vasculature, where they block perfusion to an area of ventilated lung. This can increase dead space and can lead to hypercapnia. Local effects cause alveolar collapse in the surrounding lung tissue through which blood may shunt, leading to hypoxia. If the clot burden is high, the increased resistance in the pulmonary vascular bed can lead to pulmonary hypertension, right heart failure, and even death.

Epidemiology

The incidence of pulmonary embolism has been reported to be from 23 to 69 per 100,000 people per year (1). The rate in populations at increased risk, such as hospitalized patients, is much higher and is thought to be considerably underdiagnosed.

Etiology

The causes of venous thromboembolism are directly related to the patho-physiology—hypercoagulability, trauma, and stasis. Hypercoagulable states are associated with surgery, malignancy, hormones such as oral contraceptives, pregnancy, heritable abnormalities such as factor V Leiden, acquired abnormalities such as antiphospholipid antibody syndrome, and obesity. Trauma may be surgical, nonsurgical, or central-line related. Hematologic stasis may result from local compression or a general lack of flow due to inactivity. For example, the right iliac artery may compress the left iliac vein as it passes over it, resulting in a propensity for left-sided DVTs (i.e., May-Thurner syndrome). Generalized stasis can explain the occurrence of clots during periods of immobility, such as a long airplane trip or a prolonged hospitalization.

It may be most clinically useful to consider the etiology in terms of categories that predict recurrence. From the lowest to the highest risk of recurrence, categories of risk factors include (a) postsurgical, (b) identifiable nonsurgical, and (c) idiopathic.

ACUTE MANAGEMENT AND WORKUP

Pulmonary embolism can present in many ways. The most important part of the initial management is to stabilize the patient and to make the diagnosis.

The First 15 Minutes

A quick history as well as a focused cardiopulmonary examination can go a long way in helping to determine a patient's likelihood of having a pulmonary embolism.

Initial Assessment

PE may cause chest pain, cough, hemoptysis, syncope, and dyspnea. Symptoms are classically acute in onset but insidious progression does not rule out PE. The sudden onset of symptoms may be more helpful in ruling out alternative diagnoses such as heart failure. If pulmonary infarction occurs, patients may complain of pleuritic chest pain that is worse with deep breathing and cough. Because infarction often takes several hours to develop, these symptoms may be absent at the time of initial presentation. A more gradual onset of dyspnea may be the result of right heart failure from either an acute PE or chronic PEs. Fever is not atypical for PE, but high fever (>38.9°C [102°F]) is unusual and should prompt consideration of alternate or complicating etiologies. In patients presenting with what would appear to be otherwise unexplained exacerbations of chronic obstructive pulmonary disease (COPD), the prevalence of PE may be as high as 25%.

TABLE 19-1
Modified Wells Score for Predicting Pulmonary Embolism (PE)

Risk Factor	Score
Clinical signs or symptoms of deep venous thrombosis (DVT)	3 points
Alternative diagnosis less likely	3 points
Heart rate >100	1.5 points
Immobilization or surgery in past 30 days	1.5 points
Previous DVT or PE	1.5 points
Hemoptysis	1 point
Known malignancy	1 point

Adapted from Wells PS, Anderson DR, Rodger M, et al. Derivation of a Simple Clinical Model to categorize patients probability of pulmonary embolism: increasing the models utility with the SimpliRED D-dimer. *Thromb Haemost.* 2008;83(3):416–420.

A number of clinical prediction rules have been established to help make the diagnosis of PE. Probably the best known is the Well's score, which includes a point system to help define a pretest probability for PE (Table 19-1). A score <2 predicts a low likelihood of PE, while a score >6 gives a high probability of PE.

It is important to recognize massive pulmonary embolism in the initial evaluation because these patients have a high mortality and will require intensive care unit (ICU)–level care for consideration of thrombolytic therapy and close hemodynamic monitoring. A massive pulmonary embolism is defined as one that causes a systolic blood pressure of <90 mm Hg, or a sustained drop in blood pressure >40 mm Hg. Massive PE, as well as cardiogenic shock and tamponade, should be considered in any patient who is hypotensive and has elevated neck veins, as is the case in the patient from the encounter. Patients with tachycardia, high oxygen requirements, and evidence of right ventricular strain may not meet the strict definition of massive PE but warrant very close monitoring.

Any patient with a moderate pretest probability for PE should undergo diagnostic testing such as computed tomography (CT) angiogram and lower extremity compression ultrasonography (often referred to as "Dopplers") as soon as possible to help guide further management. If the pretest probability is high, it may be reasonable to start anticoagulation therapy before confirming the diagnosis.

Admission Criteria and Level of Care Criteria

PE generally warrants hospital admission because the risks attributable to the clot as well as to anticoagulation therapy are highest during the first few hours and days. PE patients are most often sent to an ICU setting when there is hemodynamic compromise that requires close observation and/or invasive monitoring. Patients who require vasoactive medications or ventilatory support or who are being considered for thrombolytic therapy should be triaged to the ICU as well.

The First Few Hours

Once the diagnosis of PE is made, it is useful to revisit the history and physical for therapeutic and prognostic implications.

History

A thorough history should aim to identify any potential risk factor that may have contributed to thrombosis. Be sure to ask about recent surgery, trauma, immobilization, prolonged travel, symptoms attributable to malignancy, the status of age-appropriate cancer screening, the use of oral contraceptives, and pregnancy. It is important to ask your patients about known cancer diagnoses. Cancer predisposes to DVT/PE, but also imparts an increased risk of recurrent events that may impact the duration and type of anticoagulation. It is also important to ask your patients about a family history of clotting or bleeding disorders to help frame your suspicion for a hereditary hypercoagulable state. Rheumatologic conditions and chronic infections such as syphilis, hepatitis, and human immunodeficiency virus may also predispose to the antiphospholipid antibody syndrome, so a thorough review of systems with this in mind is warranted.

Physical Examination

Although PE may cause a focal wheeze, generally, the lung exam is unremarkable. The relative clarity of the lungs helps differentiate PE from alternative diagnoses such as heart failure or pneumonia. Pulmonary hypertension associated with PE leads to a loud P_2, a holosystolic murmur of tricuspid regurgitation, and a right ventricular heave. If tricuspid regurgitation is severe, the liver may be pulsatile as well. Lower extremities should be evaluated for the presence of edema, which could represent right heart failure or the presence of DVT.

Labs and Tests to Consider

In pulmonary embolism, a number of tests have diagnostic, therapeutic, and prognostic implications.

Key Diagnostic Labs and Tests

An arterial blood gas (ABG) can provide interesting information but is rarely of significant diagnostic utility. PE can cause hypoxemia, with a resulting compensatory respiratory alkalosis, or PE can cause hypercarbia via increased dead space. The former is the most common blood gas finding, and the latter would be unlikely in a patient with normal lungs prior to PE. A normal ABG does not rule out PE but would be unusual in a large PE.

Cardiac enzymes are often checked in patients presenting with chest pain and may cause diagnostic confusion when they are abnormal. Elevated troponins have been associated with a worse prognosis in PE and are likely the result of right ventricular subendocardial ischemia from increasing right heart pressures.

Brain natriuretic peptide (BNP) elevation is generally considered evidence of heart failure and is often ordered in patients presenting with dyspnea. Patients who die from PE in actuality die from right heart failure, and it has been found that BNP elevation is a negative prognostic indicator in this setting.

Rarely useful in ruling in the diagnosis, a negative D-dimer in a patient with a low pretest likelihood of venous thromboembolism may help rule out the diagnosis and can help focus diagnostic attention elsewhere.

Markers of renal function play an important role in the evaluation and management of pulmonary embolism. Impaired renal function complicates diagnosis, as nephrotoxic dye is necessary for a PE-protocol CT scan, and therapeutic options are more limited because low-molecular-weight heparins such as enoxaparin require relatively normal renal function for metabolic processing and elimination.

In the right clinical context, it may be useful to test for the presence of an antiphospholipid antibody. In addition to increasing the risk for DVT or PE, these antibodies have the ability to spuriously affect the tests used to monitor the efficacy of anticoagulation therapy. If present, the target values for these tests may be higher, or alternative tests may provide better information for monitoring therapy.

Imaging

An electrocardiogram (ECG) can function to screen for alternative diagnoses such as myocardial infarction, as well as to provide information directly pertinent to the diagnosis of PE. Classic findings of PE on ECG include sinus tachycardia with the S1Q3T3 pattern (an S wave in lead I, a Q wave in lead III, and an inverted T wave in lead III); a partial or complete right bundle branch block (RSR' pattern in V1); inverted T waves in leads V1, V2, V3, and sometimes V4; and right axis deviation.

Similarly, chest radiography both evaluates for alternative diagnoses, including pneumothorax and pneumonia, and provides findings more specific to PE. Classic findings include a wedge-shaped infarct (Hampton hump) or a focal area of oligemia (Westermark sign). Atelectasis, a raised hemidiaphragm, or a clear chest radiograph are more common observations.

CLINICAL PEARL

New hypoxemia with a clear chest x-ray is suspicious for PE.

The ventilation/perfusion (V/Q) scan is a well-studied diagnostic modality that is often used in patients with poor renal function in whom the nephrotoxic contrast dye needed for CT angiography should be avoided. The hallmark of pulmonary embolism on V/Q is an area of lung that is well ventilated but not perfused, a so-called mismatched defect. The V/Q scan plays an important role in the detection of chronic thromboembolic disease, which tends to create small peripheral lesions that are usually less apparent on CT than on V/Q (see Chapter 8).

CT angiogram has become the test of choice for the diagnosis of pulmonary embolism, largely obviating the need for invasive pulmonary artery angiography. In addition to providing a view of the pulmonary vascular bed, it allows simultaneous evaluation of other structures in the thorax pertinent to alternative diagnostic considerations, such as aortic dissection, a condition with a very different management strategy than pulmonary embolism (Fig. 19-1).

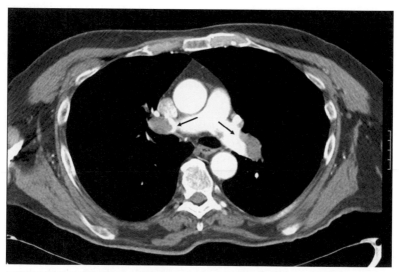

FIGURE 19-1: Bilateral proximal pulmonary emboli (*arrows*) as seen on computed tomography angiography. (*Courtesy of Brian T. Garibaldi, MD, Division of Pulmonary and Critical Care Medicine, The Johns Hopkins Hospital.*)

CLINICAL PEARL

It is a common misconception that people allergic to seafood have an increased risk of reaction to iodinated contrast because seafood contains high quantities of iodine. In fact, seafood allergy is mediated by allergy to a protein called tropomyosin. Severe allergic reactions of any kind convey a slightly increased risk of other allergies, but beyond this general allergic propensity, there is no greater risk from seafood allergy than from a severe peanut allergy, for example.

Echocardiography is the test of choice in the unstable patient. When a PE is large, it may present similarly to other conditions that can be identified by echocardiogram. For example, echocardiogram can reveal segmental wall motion abnormalities from a myocardial infarction, a large pericardial effusion that causes cardiac tamponade, or perhaps even evidence of aortic dissection. Furthermore, echocardiography provides prognostic information for PE because it allows some quantification of right heart function. In this way, the echo gives the practitioner a sense of the patient's cardiopulmonary reserve. For example, a patient with severe right heart strain and a significant clot burden remaining in the deep veins would likely be considered for an inferior vena caval (IVC) filter or for thrombolytic therapy, even if the patient's vitals signs were "normal." Echocardiography may also identify a right ventricular thrombus or a patent foramen ovale, either of which might prompt consideration of thrombolytic therapy even in the absence of hemodynamic compromise.

Treatment

As in any case, the first step in treatment is to stabilize the patient. If the patient's blood pressure is low, fluids, vasopressors, and ICU-level care should be administered. Anticoagulation with heparin or low-molecular-weight heparin should be started as soon as possible. A patient with significant hemodynamic compromise or cardiogenic shock has a "massive" pulmonary embolism and should be considered for clot lysis with intravenous alteplase. The patient in our encounter is hypotensive and would be a candidate for thrombolytic therapy. In patients who are unstable but who have absolute contraindications to thrombolytic therapy, catheter-directed thrombectomy or even surgical thrombectomy have been performed. Patients with evidence of right heart strain on echocardiography or who have positive biomarkers of cardiac injury have evidence of "submassive" PE. There is continuing debate about the role of thrombolytics in these patients, and such decisions should be made on a case-by-case basis in consultation with either a cardiologist or pulmonologist.

In a stable patient in whom it is unlikely that alteplase will be used, enoxaparin is preferred over unfractionated heparin by some clinicians, assuming the patient has relatively normal renal function. An additional benefit to enoxaparin is that, unlike unfractionated heparin, it can be self-administered by the patient at home while warfarin is being titrated to therapeutic levels.

IVC filters should not routinely be placed in patients with DVT or PE, and should be reserved for only those patients who have proven significant clot burden remaining in the lower extremities as well as poor cardiopulmonary reserve such that they would be at high risk for death from embolization of the clot. Alternatively, an IVC filter could be placed in the setting of a lower extremity clot with a strict contraindication to anticoagulation. In either situation, a removable filter is generally preferred over a permanent filter and anticoagulation should be initiated as soon as it is safe to do so. Plans to remove a filter should be made at the time of placement.

EXTENDED IN-HOSPITAL MANAGEMENT

It is important to monitor patients closely for evidence of clinical deterioration despite the use of anticoagulation. If patients did not initially require thrombolytic therapy but subsequently develop signs of shock or worsening hypoxemia, thrombolytic therapy should be considered.

DISPOSITION

Discharge Goals

Patients who are hemodynamically stable from their PE can be quickly transitioned to oral warfarin therapy, and even discharged on enoxaparin while they await a therapeutic warfarin level. Patients with "massive" or "submassive" PE or those with extensive clot burden should be observed in the hospital for at least 3 to 4 days before discharge is considered. Be sure to assess your patient's need for home oxygen early on because this is often forgotten until the time of discharge.

Outpatient Care

Patients should have follow-up with their primary care physician as well as with an anticoagulation clinic at the time of discharge. The optimal duration of anticoagulation is controversial. Thromboembolic events related to surgery (with no other risk factors) are least likely to recur. These patients can be treated for 3 to 6 months and can be reassured of the low risk of recurrence. The presence of any nonsurgical risk factor places the risk of recurrence between that of surgical events (low risk) and idiopathic events (high risk). The standard treatment is 3 to 6 months, after which the likelihood for recurrence is intermediate at a rate of approximately 5% per year.

When a patient has cancer, the likelihood of thromboembolic recurrence is high and the patient should receive a longer course of anticoagulation if clinically feasible. This means at least a year, with most physicians recommending lifelong anticoagulation. In the context of cancer, low-molecular-weight heparins given long term may be preferable to warfarin.

If no risk factor at all is identifiable, the event is termed idiopathic. The risk of recurrence in this context is relatively high—potentially in excess of 10% per year. Current recommendations are to treat these patients for at least 1 year with the option for longer therapy at the discretion of the patient and treating physician.

It is in the setting of these idiopathic events that interest in hypercoagulable studies developed. The goal of such studies is to better identify those patients who would benefit from long-term therapy. Although conceptually elegant, currently available hypercoagulable studies have been clinically disappointing. They fail to predict recurrence and thus lack clinical utility. There is emerging evidence that D-dimer testing 1 month after completion of a recommended course of anticoagulation may help predict a patient's risk of recurrence.

The absolute risk of recurrent, fatal PE is <1% per year. The risk of fatal hemorrhage associated with anticoagulation is also <1% per year. The similar scale of these risks should be appreciated so that clinical factors, such as a propensity to bleed, lifestyle, and patient preferences, can be factored into the anticoagulation decision and discussed with the patient.

If a patient had a known DVT as the cause of his or her PE, the use of TED hose should be encouraged for at least 1 year to help reduce the incidence of the postthrombophlebitic syndrome. Consideration should be given to removing any temporary IVC filters placed during hospitalization.

Venous thromboembolism may be the presenting manifestation of cancer. The best current evidence, however, does not favor an extended search for occult malignancy in this setting. Age-appropriate screening, a thorough history and physical examination, and a symptom-guided approach remain sufficient.

 WHAT YOU NEED TO REMEMBER

- Always include pulmonary embolism in your differential diagnosis for patients presenting with shortness of breath, chest pain, tachycardia, or unexplained hypoxia.
- Massive pulmonary embolism is defined as a systolic blood pressure <90 mm Hg, or a sustained drop of 40 mm Hg. These patients are candidates for thrombolytic therapy and should be admitted to the ICU.

- Hemodynamically stable patients with "submassive" pulmonary embolism do not routinely benefit from thrombolytics but should be carefully monitored in the hospital for several days on anticoagulation therapy before discharge.
- The "hypercoagulable workup" does not predict recurrence and should not be routinely ordered.
- TED hose should be prescribed for at least a year following DVT.
- The duration of anticoagulation therapy depends on the underlying risk factors for DVT/PE.
- The risk of fatal recurrence and the risk of fatal bleeding while on treatment are not dissimilar. Patient-specific factors should be taken into consideration when making treatment decisions.

REFERENCE

1. Konstantinides S. Clinical practice. Acute pulmonary embolism. *N Engl J Med.* 2008;359(26):2804–2813.

SUGGESTED READINGS

Goldhaber SZ. Pulmonary thromboembolism. In: Kasper DL, Braunwald E, Hauser S, et al., eds. *Harrison's Principles of Internal Medicine.* 16th ed. New York: McGraw Hill; 2005.

Kucher N, Goldhaber SZ. Management of massive pulmonary embolism. *Circulation.* 2005;112:e28.

Stein PD, Fowler SE, Goodman LR, et al. Multidetector computed tomography for acute pulmonary embolism. *N Engl J Med.* 2006;354(22):2317–2327.

Tapson VF. Acute pulmonary embolism. *N Engl J Med.* 2008;358(10):1037–1052.

van Belle A, Büller HR, Huisman MV, et al. Effectiveness of managing suspected pulmonary embolism using an algorithm combining clinical probability, D-dimer testing, and computed tomography. *JAMA.* 2006;295(2):172–179.

Wells PS, Anderson DR, Rodger M, et al. Derivation of a simple clinical model to categorize patients probability of pulmonary embolism: increasing the models utility with the SimpliRED D-dimer. *Thromb Haemost.* 2000;83(3):416–420.

Asthma

20

THE PATIENT ENCOUNTER

A 31-year-old woman is brought to the emergency department by paramedics 2 hours after developing shortness of breath, cough, wheezing, and chest tightness. She has been using her inhalers at home with no relief. She is anxious, diaphoretic, and unable to speak in more than two- or three-word sentences.

OVERVIEW

Definition

Asthma is a chronic lung disease caused by continuous airway inflammation and characterized by recurrent episodes of increased airway inflammation and obstruction. These episodes often occur in response to specific triggers and are at least partially reversible, either spontaneously or with treatment.

Pathophysiology

Airflow limitation in asthma results from bronchospasm, airway hyperresponsiveness, airway edema, and mucus hypersecretion. These changes represent the consequences of acute and chronic airway inflammation.

The mechanisms responsible for acute airway hyperresponsiveness and bronchospasm are incompletely understood. Inhaled aeroallergens stimulate the release of inflammatory mediators from mast cells via immunoglobulin E (IgE)–mediated activation. These mediators cause bronchial smooth muscle contraction, increase vascular permeability, and stimulate mucus secretion from goblet cells. Eosinophils and neutrophils are recruited when chemotactic factors are released from mast cells, resident macrophages, and T lymphocytes and augment the inflammatory response by releasing additional mediators that damage the airway epithelium. Epithelial injury may trigger autonomic nerve stimulation, causing reflex increases in smooth muscle contraction and bronchospasm. Chronic airway inflammation results in increased airway wall thickness and remodeling. These changes may be responsible for the component of airflow limitation that is not completely reversible with bronchodilators during acute exacerbations.

Epidemiology

About 11% of the U.S. population suffers from asthma. Worldwide, it is estimated that almost 300 million people are affected (1). While the prevalence of the disease and of attacks has remained fairly stable, asthma-attributed mortality has recently begun to decline.

Etiology

Genetic and environmental factors contribute to the development of asthma. Genetic factors are likely influenced by early environmental exposures and shifts in innate immunity from a T_H1-predominant to a T_H2-predominant (IgE-mediated) response, as suggested by the "hygiene hypothesis."

A variety of "triggers" have been identified as common causes of acute exacerbations. Aeroallergens, including dust mite, pollen, and cockroach antigens, are important triggers of IgE-mediated airway hyperresponsiveness. Non–IgE-mediated triggers include viral infections and a variety of irritants, including tobacco smoke, cold air, perfumes, ozone, and exercise.

ACUTE MANAGEMENT AND WORKUP

During the initial assessment of a patient with an asthma exacerbation, it is critical to confirm the diagnosis, assess the severity of the attack, and evaluate the response to simple therapies like supplemental oxygen and inhaled bronchodilators.

The First 15 Minutes

Remember: All that wheezes is not asthma, and respiratory compromise is a life-threatening emergency. Alternative diagnoses with similar presentations (anaphylaxis, flash pulmonary edema, pulmonary embolism, etc.) can precipitate respiratory failure and require different interventions.

Initial Assessment

Review of the patient's vital signs and a focused physical examination can confirm the diagnosis and allow you to assess the severity of airflow obstruction. Signs of impending respiratory failure include diaphoresis, agitation or obtundation, accessory muscle use, cyanosis, or paradoxical respirations. An inability to speak in more than one- or two-word phrases suggests that the extent of airway obstruction is likely severe, as seen in the patient from our encounter. While tachycardia and hypertension are not uncommon with respiratory distress, bradycardia or hypotension may suggest impending cardiopulmonary collapse. Patients with a severe asthma flare often describe an inability to lie flat. If a patient was in extremis moments earlier and now appears to be lying back and resting comfortably, he or she may have tired out and is now on the verge of respiratory failure.

The extent of bronchoconstriction and airway obstruction can be roughly assessed at the bedside. While diffuse, polyphonic, end-expiratory wheezing is consistent with a mild or moderate exacerbation, loud inspiratory and expiratory wheezes may be heard during a severe exacerbation. Diffusely diminished or absent breath sounds suggest severe airflow obstruction and are of much greater concern. Rales or clear lung fields should prompt consideration of alternative diagnoses. The presence of a localized, monophonic, or strictly inspiratory wheeze may indicate foreign body aspiration or local intrabronchial or extrabronchial obstruction.

An objective measurement of obstruction, either peak expiratory flow rate (PEFR) or forced expiratory volume in 1 second, should also be assessed early to help grade the severity of the acute exacerbation.

CLINICAL PEARL

Diffusely diminished or absent breath sounds indicate a greater degree of airflow obstruction than diffuse wheeze, no matter how loud or extensive.

Admission Criteria and Level of Care Criteria

Guidelines for hospital admission have recently been updated by both the Expert Panel of the National Asthma Education and Prevention Program (2007) and the Global Strategy for Asthma Management and Prevention (2007). All patients should receive inhaled bronchodilators and supplemental oxygen to maintain SaO_2 ≥90%. Systemic corticosteroids should be given early if there is no immediate response to bronchodilators or if the patient was recently on corticosteroids. After 1 to 2 hours, reassessment should include physical examination, spirometry or peak flow evaluation, and pulse oximetry. Patients with a good response to therapy can generally be discharged home safely with a short course of systemic corticosteroids and close follow-up. Patients with an incomplete response to initial therapies will often need hospital admission, but the decision should be individualized based on consideration of several risk factors that predict a poor outcome. These risk factors include a history of previous severe exacerbation (requiring intubation or intensive care unit admission), multiple emergency department visits or hospital admissions for asthma within the preceding month, use of more than two canisters of albuterol within the past month, difficulty perceiving symptom severity, psychiatric illness, low socioeconomic status, illicit drug use, cardiovascular comorbidities, and structural lung disease. Patients who are severely ill or who demonstrate signs of impending respiratory collapse may require intubation and mechanical ventilation and should be evaluated for intensive care unit admission.

The First Few Hours

After a focused, rapid assessment of your patient's respiratory status, the first few hours should focus on monitoring the response to initial therapies and collecting historical information to help guide the development of short- and long-term management plans.

History

A careful review of the presenting symptoms should help rule out alternative diagnoses. Symptoms consistent with asthma exacerbation include chest tightness, cough, wheeze, shortness of breath, and sputum production. You should inquire about the onset of symptoms, any triggers that may have precipitated the current flare, and the frequency of home rescue inhaler use prior to presentation.

It is critical to ask patients about exacerbation and symptom frequency during the initial assessment. Information on the number of emergency room visits, hospitalizations, and prior intubations can help generalize the clinical risk. In addition, a history of recurrent, refractory exacerbations despite good medical management might prompt consideration of an alternative diagnosis (vocal cord dysfunction, allergic bronchopulmonary aspergillosis, Churg-Strauss syndrome). It is also important to make an initial assessment of the frequency of both daytime and nighttime symptoms between acute exacerbations. This information is critical in the classification of disease severity, and will help guide your choice of discharge medications (see Table 20-1).

You should also thoroughly elicit the patient's triggers and the pattern of symptoms as identification and avoidance may be highly effective in reducing symptom frequency and preventing future exacerbations. Smoking cessation and avoidance of secondhand smoke should be strongly encouraged. Be sure to ask (and possibly test for) other drugs that are known to cause bronchospasm and pulmonary pathology, such as heroin, cocaine, and methylphenidate. In urban health centers, such illicit drug use may account for a sizeable percentage of emergency room visits for "asthma" flares. A history of seasonal symptoms or exacerbations around cats or dogs may suggest an IgE-mediated process. A history of recent upper respiratory infection symptoms during the appropriate season might trigger evaluation for influenza. Reflux symptoms may suggest the need for acid-suppressive therapy. A history of worsening symptoms during the workweek, with improvement at home on the weekend, should prompt consideration of a diagnosis of occupational asthma. A careful history of potential environmental exposures should always be pursued. The family history should focus on atopic conditions.

Finally, it is important to assess the patient's understanding of his or her current outpatient medical regimen. Although the medication list may include an inhaled corticosteroid or long-acting bronchodilator, the patient may not be using it appropriately. It is not uncommon for patients to inadvertently use controller medications only when symptomatic.

TABLE 20-1

Asthma Severity Classification Guidelines

Classification	Symptom Frequency	Nocturnal Symptom Frequency	Pulmonary Function	Controller Therapy (All Include PRN Short-acting β_2-Agonist)
Mild intermittent	≤2 days/week	≤2 nights/month	Normal FEV_1 between exacerbations FEV_1/FVC normal	None
Mild persistent	>2 days/week, but not daily	3–4 nights/mo	FEV_1 >80% predicted FEV_1/FVC normal	Low-dose inhaled corticosteroid
Moderate persistent	Daily	>1 night/week, but not nightly	FEV_1 <80% predicted, but >60% predicted FEV_1/FVC reduced 5%	Medium-dose inhaled corticosteroid
Severe persistent	Continuous	Up to nightly	FEV_1 <60% predicted FEV_1/FVC reduced >5%	Medium- or high-dose inhaled corticosteroid ± long-acting β_2-agonist

FEV_1, forced expiratory volume in 1 second; FVC, forced vital capacity.
(Adapted from National Asthma Education and Prevention Program. *Guidelines for the Diagnosis and Management of Asthma.* Available at: www.nhlbi.nih.gov/health/prof/lung.)

Physical Examination

In addition to the pulmonary examination maneuvers described previously, a careful physical exam may provide invaluable clinical information. The cardiovascular examination will frequently identify sinus tachycardia, but you should focus careful attention on evaluating for signs of heart failure or valvular disease as an alternative etiology of symptoms. The cardiovascular examination should also include assessment for *pulsus paradoxus*, a difference of 10 mm Hg in the systolic blood pressure between inspiration and expiration, which may indicate high intrathoracic pressures from airway obstruction and hyperinflation. An augmentation of the jugular venous pulsations with expiration might indicate that a patient is mounting large pleural pressures in an attempt to overcome hyperinflation and air trapping.

> ### CLINICAL PEARL
> *The magnitude of the* pulsus paradoxus *may be helpful in the evaluation of exacerbation severity. However, its absence does not exclude the possibility of a severe flare.*

Conjunctival injection, rhinorrhea, or edematous nasal turbinates may suggest a component of allergic rhinitis. Sinus tenderness or postnasal drip may suggest acute or chronic infection. The presence of nasal polyps may suggest a component of aspirin hypersensitivity and requires careful historical follow-up. Angioedema or stridor suggests the possibility of anaphylaxis. Finally, inspection of the skin may reveal atopic dermatitis, consistent with the integral relationship between asthma and other IgE-mediated pathologies.

Labs and Tests to Consider

Laboratory studies have limited utility in the management of an asthma exacerbation. While not indicated for every patient, arterial blood gas (ABG) assessment may be helpful if there is concern for impending respiratory failure. Respiratory alkalosis and an increased alveolar-arterial gradient are common during an exacerbation. A developing respiratory acidosis (or normalization of the $PaCO_2$ in a patient who had a respiratory alkalosis) suggests respiratory muscle fatigue, and may help predict impending respiratory failure.

Key Diagnostic Labs and Tests

While spirometry is the gold standard, assessment of the PEFR may be the simplest and most readily available measure of airway obstruction. Many asthmatics have been instructed in assessing their own lung function at home with a peak flow meter, and can base the severity of their symptoms (and the need for evaluation) on the percentage of their personal best PEFR reading.

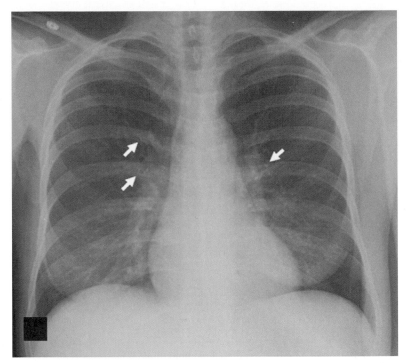

FIGURE 20-1: Arrows identify thickened bronchial walls, characteristic of an asthma exacerbation. (*Courtesy of David Feigin, MD, Department of Radiology, Johns Hopkins Hospital, Baltimore, Maryland.*)

Imaging

Although the diagnosis of asthma exacerbation is generally made based on the history and physical examination, chest radiography may help to exclude alternative diagnoses or uncover complications of asthma, such as pneumothorax or pneumomediastinum. Common radiographic abnormalities during an exacerbation can include hyperinflation, bronchial wall thickening, and peripheral oligemia (Fig. 20-1).

Treatment

Treatment approaches are intended to reverse bronchospastic changes and quiet the inflammatory response. Inhaled bronchodilators and systemic corticosteroids make up the core of the initial management regimen. Both inhaled β_2-adrenergic agonists (such as albuterol) and inhaled anticholinergics (such as ipratropium bromide) can mediate smooth muscle relaxation in the airways and limit bronchospasm. Inhaled anticholinergics may also provide the added benefit of limiting mucus hypersecretion. While the delivery methods are equally efficacious when a spacer chamber is used with a metered-dose inhaler, nebulized bronchodilators may be more effectively delivered in patients who are agitated or in respiratory distress.

Systemic corticosteroids are used to limit and reduce airway inflammation. They are often used in patients with moderate to severe exacerbations, those who do not respond to initial β_2-agonist therapy, or those who have recently been on systemic corticosteroids. Oral and parenteral administration are equally efficacious. Standard therapy includes 40 to 60 mg of prednisone daily for a 5- to 10-day course, and tapering is not necessary.

Other medications have been used in the acute management of asthma exacerbations with limited success. Systemic β-adrenergic agonists (i.e., epinephrine, terbutaline) are no more effective than inhaled β_2-agonists, and their use is complicated by cardiovascular side effects. Intravenous magnesium sulfate may have some benefit in preventing hospitalization in patients with the most severe exacerbations. Phosphodiesterase inhibitors (theophylline, aminophylline) have a narrow therapeutic window and are less effective bronchodilators than inhaled β_2-agonists. Antibiotics generally serve no purpose in the management of an acute exacerbation, unless other comorbidities are functioning to trigger symptoms.

EXTENDED IN-HOSPITAL MANAGEMENT

The primary goals of the hospital stay are symptom alleviation and resolution of airflow obstruction. There are no hard and fast rules for weaning, but bronchodilators are generally tapered to a reasonable outpatient regimen based on improvement in both subjective symptoms and objective measures of airway obstruction.

You should also utilize the inpatient stay to educate the patient about minimizing the chances for recurrent exacerbations. Remember, your goal is to prepare the patient for discharge on an effective regimen that the patient understands in an effort to limit additional exacerbations.

DISPOSITION

Discharge Goals

The decision to discharge is based on similar clinical guidelines as those used for admission. The patient should have good subjective symptom relief, and the physical examination should reveal no signs of respiratory distress. If the patient did not require supplemental oxygen for other reasons prior to admission, he or she should be able to demonstrate an oxygen saturation >90% on room air prior to discharge. A patient should probably not be discharged if he or she requires inhaled bronchodilators more frequently than every 4 to 6 hours.

Outpatient Care

Following hospital discharge, the patient should be advised to follow up with his or her primary physician or an asthma specialist within 3 to 5 days to ensure that the acute exacerbation has completely resolved. Remember, asthma is a chronic disease. Outpatient care should be focused on trigger avoidance and optimization of controller medications in an effort to minimize symptoms and exacerbation frequency. The National Asthma Education and Prevention Program has recently revised guidelines to help guide decision making based on symptom frequency (Table 20-1).

WHAT YOU NEED TO REMEMBER

- Asthma exacerbation can be a life-threatening emergency, so the initial assessment should include a careful evaluation for signs of impending respiratory failure.
- All that wheezes is not asthma, and alternative diagnoses may require urgent interventions.
- Supplemental oxygen, inhaled bronchodilators, and systemic corticosteroids are the foundation of inpatient management of asthma exacerbations.
- Seek out specific triggers and assess symptom frequency in an effort to formulate an effective outpatient regimen.
- The inpatient stay is an ideal time to provide education to your patient regarding his or her disease and medications.

REFERENCE

1. Global Strategy for Asthma Management and Prevention. *Global Initiative for Asthma (GINA)*. 2007. Available at: http://www.ginasthma.org

SUGGESTED READINGS

Cockcroft DW, Davis BE. Mechanisms of airway hyperresponsiveness. *J Allergy Clin Immunol*. 2006;118:551–559.

National Asthma Education and Prevention Program. *Guidelines for the Diagnosis and Management of Asthma*. NIH 08-5846. 2007. Available at: http://www.nhlbi.nih. gov/health/prof/lung

Chronic Obstructive Pulmonary Disease

THE PATIENT ENCOUNTER

A 66-year-old man is brought to the emergency department by ambulance because he cannot catch his breath. He appears to be in distress, is using accessory muscles, and is leaning forward with his forearms resting on his knees. He also complains of 2 days of cough productive of greenish sputum. He had smoked a pack of cigarettes a day for 50 years but quit 2 years ago. Chest radiography reveals hyperinflation, but no focal consolidation.

OVERVIEW

Definition

Chronic obstructive pulmonary disease (COPD) is a progressive disease characterized by airflow obstruction that is not fully reversible. It is caused by an abnormal inflammatory response in the lungs to noxious stimuli, most commonly to cigarette smoking. Classically, COPD has been divided into two diseases: (a) chronic bronchitis, with persistent airway inflammation and mucus production, and (b) emphysema, with enlargement and destruction of distal airspaces and airway walls. In clinical practice, COPD represents a continuum that may involve the central and peripheral airways, as well as the lung parenchyma and vasculature.

Patients with COPD may or may not be symptomatic at rest, but become acutely ill during "exacerbations." Acute exacerbations of COPD are defined clinically by one or more of the following: (a) worsening dyspnea, (b) increased sputum production, and (c) production of purulent sputum.

Pathophysiology

The overwhelming majority of COPD is caused by cigarette smoking, although the exact mechanism of lung injury is not known. Genetic disorders such as a defect in the α_1-antitrypsin gene may lead to early COPD, but smoking usually plays an important causative role in these patients as well. Chronic inflammation leads to mucus oversecretion and problems with ciliary clearance. An imbalance of proteases and antiproteases allows the destruction of lung parenchyma, reducing the elastic forces that help to tether airways open. Both the chronic airway inflammation and this increase in lung compliance lead to airflow obstruction.

Epidemiology

As many as 15% to 20% of smokers develop COPD, but this may be an underestimate, as pulmonary function testing is not done on every smoker. Given the worldwide smoking epidemic and the increasing age of the world's population, it is estimated that COPD will become the third-leading cause of death worldwide by the year 2020 (1). Acute exacerbations are reasonably common, accounting for as many as 500,000 hospitalizations per year. Exacerbations are more likely to occur among patients with more severe airflow obstruction at baseline (2).

Etiology

Exacerbations are caused by an irritant that triggers additional inflammation in an already compromised respiratory system. Chronic inflammatory changes appear to allow pathogens to colonize not merely the upper airway, but also the lower airways; acquiring a new colonizer may incite a flare. Viral infections such as rhinoviruses, influenza, and respiratory syncytial virus may account for up to 50% of exacerbations, but bacterial infections are also likely important triggers. Increased air pollution and even psychological stress have also been implicated.

ACUTE MANAGEMENT AND WORKUP

There are many conditions that can mimic a COPD exacerbation. The initial assessment should focus on ruling out other cardiopulmonary causes of shortness of breath and determining the severity of the acute exacerbation.

The First 15 Minutes

Your initial assessment should focus on the patient's work of breathing and the severity of his or her airflow obstruction.

Initial Assessment

As discussed in Chapter 16, tripoding, as demonstrated by our patient in the encounter; accessory muscle use; intercostal retractions; abdominal contractions; and purse-lipped breathing are all potential signs of severe obstruction. If your patient has abdominal paradox, then respiratory failure may be imminent and an intensive care unit (ICU) consultation is likely warranted.

Wheezing can be a marker of airflow obstruction, but it is important to remember that in patients with a low forced expiratory volume in 1 second (FEV_1), you may not hear any breath sounds at baseline. As with asthma, not hearing anything can be an ominous sign of severe obstruction.

It is important to find out if your patient has ever required noninvasive ventilation or intubation during a COPD flare, because this may give you a sense of the severity of his or her underlying lung disease.

Look for signs of heart failure or pulmonary hypertension, because patients with COPD often have underlying ischemic heart disease or may develop pulmonary hypertension and cor pulmonale from their parenchymal lung disease.

In general, you should have a low threshold to get an arterial blood gas (ABG) in a patient with a COPD flare to evaluate his or her ventilatory status. An ABG can help you determine how far the patient is from his or her baseline and whether or not he or she will need ventilatory support.

Admission Criteria and Level of Care Criteria

It is difficult to create precise guidelines for inpatient versus outpatient therapy. In general, considerations for admission include the patient's other risk factors for a poor outcome. Previous intubations for COPD, pneumonia, diabetes, or the failure of other organs, such as congestive heart failure or renal failure, should lower the threshold to admit a patient to the hospital.

If the patient has an acute respiratory acidosis, he or she will likely require ventilatory assistance in the form of noninvasive positive pressure ventilation (NIPPV) or intubation and mechanical ventilation. Such patients should likely be managed in an intensive care unit because they often worsen quite quickly and need close monitoring.

The First Few Hours

The first few hours are critical for assessing the severity of a patient's exacerbation, but also provide an important window of opportunity to initiate therapies that may prevent further decompensation.

History

Patients often describe a gradual worsening of their shortness of breath, and should describe an increase in sputum production or a change in its nature. Sometimes they describe a recent "cold" and may have sick contacts at home. A sudden onset of acute shortness of breath, with no cough or sputum, is not typical of a COPD flare and may suggest another diagnosis, such as a pulmonary embolism. In fact, up to 20% of COPD "flares" are likely caused by pulmonary embolism, so it is important to screen for thromboembolic risk factors in all patients who present with COPD exacerbations. Remember that in people with very limited reserve, anything that increases the work of breathing can manifest as dyspnea. Even a fever from a simple urinary tract infection can be enough to tip someone over the edge, so be sure to screen for such possibilities.

Many patients with chronic lung disease are told that they have COPD. If possible, try to find records of old pulmonary function testing to confirm the diagnosis. Ask about medications. Pay particular attention to recent steroid use because prolonged or frequent steroid dosing may predispose the patient to opportunistic infections or, if recently tapered, may place the patient at risk for adrenal insufficiency. If the patient uses oxygen at home, find out how long he or she has been on it, and if he or she uses it at rest, with exertion, or when sleeping.

All patients with evidence of obstruction should be screened for active tobacco use and also for other drugs that may cause bronchospasm and lung injury, such as cocaine, heroin, and methylphenidate.

Be sure to ask about known heart disease. Respiratory and cardiac disease are both common in smokers, and it can initially be difficult to distinguish a COPD flare from a heart failure exacerbation.

Physical Examination

In addition to the pulmonary examination features described previously, a careful cardiopulmonary examination should look for signs of heart failure, pulmonary hypertension, and volume overload.

Look for signs of living with a chronic disease; some patients with COPD have been on and off steroids for years, and have developed the associated moon facies and fragile skin. Severe COPD is also associated with anorexia and muscle wasting. Clubbing is very unusual in COPD alone and might suggest another underlying disease, such as bronchogenic carcinoma or pulmonary fibrosis.

Labs and Tests to Consider

There are a number of tests that can both confirm a diagnosis of COPD and help to quantify the severity of a patient's acute presentation.

Key Diagnostic Labs and Tests

An elevated bicarbonate level in a basic metabolic panel may be compensation for a chronic respiratory acidosis from severe obstruction at baseline. If the patient is in respiratory distress, get an ABG and try to find an old one for comparison. A rising $PaCO_2$ in the setting of a COPD exacerbation usually signifies respiratory failure and a need for prompt intervention. In contrast, a fall in $PaCO_2$ >5 mm Hg from a baseline value may suggest the presence of a pulmonary embolism with a relative respiratory alkalosis. An elevated white blood cell count with a neutrophil predominance would support a bacterial infection.

A nasopharyngeal aspirate may provide evidence for a respiratory virus. About 20% to 30% of people with COPD have positive sputum cultures when stable, so the results of cultures have to be considered in the context of the clinical presentation.

Some clinicians advocate measuring levels of brain natriuretic peptide (BNP) to help distinguish a COPD flare (low BNP levels) from congestive heart failure (elevated BNP levels), but results can be nonspecific and must again be interpreted in context.

Imaging

The typical radiographic appearance of a COPD exacerbation is hyperinflation. This is usually best seen on a lateral film (Fig. 21-1). Focal infiltrates

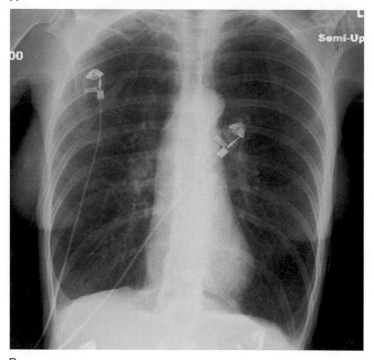

FIGURE 21-1: Radiographic features of chronic obstructive pulmonary disease. **A:** Anteroposterior chest radiograph showing flattened hemidiaphragms and hyperinflation. **B:** Chest computed tomography showing severe emphysematous changes. (*Courtesy of Brian T. Garibaldi, MD, Division of Pulmonary and Critical Care, The Johns Hopkins Hospital.*)

are not typical of a COPD flare and would suggest an acute pneumonia. The chest radiograph may also reveal signs of congestive heart failure. Computed tomography may be indicated in selected patients to rule out pulmonary embolism but may also reveal emphysema or other parenchymal disease.

> ### CLINICAL PEARL
>
> *The degree of emphysematous changes on chest imaging does not necessarily correlate with the severity of airflow obstruction on pulmonary function testing.*

Pulmonary Function Testing. On pulmonary function testing, patients will have evidence of airflow obstruction, usually characterized by a ratio of FEV_1 to forced vital capacity (FVC) of <70%. The severity of their disease is then further classified by the absolute value of their FEV_1 or by comparing their FEV_1 to a predicted value. A normal person has about a 30-mL decline in his or her FEV_1 per year, while a susceptible smoker with COPD loses about 50 to 80 mL per year (Fig. 21-2). In general, patients do not begin to retain CO_2 until their FEV_1 is <1 L. The residual volume also provides valuable information about the severity of airflow obstruction and hyperinflation, but may be artificially low if measured by helium dilution. The diffusing capacity of carbon monoxide may be normal in patients on the chronic bronchitis end of the spectrum but may be markedly reduced in patients with emphysema.

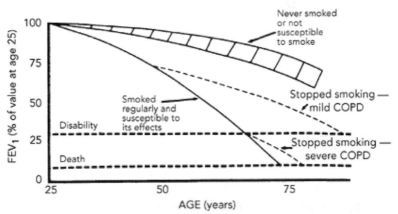

FIGURE 21-2: Decline in forced expiratory volume in 1 second over time in nonsmokers, susceptible smokers, and nonsusceptible smokers.

Electrocardiography and Echocardiography. Electrocardiography may reveal sinus tachycardia in the setting of respiratory distress but may also reveal atrial arrhythmias such as atrial flutter, atrial fibrillation, or multifocal atrial tachycardia. Right atrial enlargement, right access deviation, and right ventricular hypertrophy may suggest pulmonary hypertension. Hyperinflation may result in low voltage. Echocardiography may be helpful to evaluate for evidence of either systolic dysfunction or right-sided disease from pulmonary hypertension.

Treatment

The mainstays of acute COPD management are supplemental oxygen, antibiotics, corticosteroids, bronchodilators, and ventilatory support as needed.

Supplemental Oxygen

In patients who are chronically hypoxemic, supplemental oxygen is the only therapy that has been definitively shown to improve mortality in patients with COPD. However, oxygen in the acute setting is not without some risk and may actually lead to an increase in arterial PCO_2 in certain situations (a topic of much discussion among pulmonary physiologists). Hyperoxia may lead to a decrease in respiratory drive; people with hypoxemia and COPD have been shown to decrease their minute ventilation when oxygen is added. Hyperoxia also likely increases dead space and worsens ventilation/perfusion matching by causing microatelectasis. Patients may also take lower tidal volume breaths on supplemental oxygen, which further increases dead space relative to overall ventilation. There is also the "Haldane effect," whereby oxygenated hemoglobin is less able to unload carbon dioxide in the lungs to be expired, although this effect is probably not clinically relevant. It is important to remember that while hypercarbia is dangerous, a low oxygen level is worse. Do not allow someone to become dangerously hypoxic, with prolonged oxygen saturation <88%, just for fear of increasing his or her CO_2.

Antibiotics

Antibiotics are of demonstrated benefit in COPD flares, especially if the patient has described a change in sputum. Choosing the best antibiotic remains controversial; most clinicians take into account both local bacterial resistance patterns and the patient's risk factors for resistant organisms. That being said, oftentimes a simple 5-day course of Bactrim, doxycycline, or azithromycin is sufficient treatment for a COPD flare.

Corticosteroids

Systemic corticosteroids are of demonstrable benefit in acute COPD exacerbations. Patients treated with steroids are less likely to have treatment failure, and have faster improvements in their FEV_1. There are still not great data on the optimal dose or duration of steroid therapy. In hospitalized patients, typical courses start with methylprednisolone 60 to 125 mg, two to four times a day, and then prednisone 60 mg daily, with a taper lasting 7 to 14 days.

Bronchodilators

Bronchodilators are a cornerstone of therapy and provide rapid improvement in airflow obstruction. Short-acting β-agonists (i.e., albuterol) and anticholinergics (i.e., ipratropium bromide) can be administered via nebulizer or metered-dose inhaler, although the former may be more effective in patients who are markedly short of breath.

Ventilatory Support

Patients who demonstrate signs and symptoms of respiratory failure will likely require ventilatory support until the antibiotics, steroids, and bronchodilators take effect. In patients who are hemodynamically stable, a trial of NIPPV via full facemask (i.e., bilevel positive-pressure ventilation [BiPAP]) may markedly reduce the work of breathing, improve ventilation, and possibly prevent endotracheal intubation. BiPAP is contraindicated if a patient has altered mental status, active vomiting, or hemodynamic instability. In patients with COPD, BiPAP is a bridge to getting better or getting intubated. If a patient does not improve after several hours, he or she should likely be intubated and placed on full ventilatory support in an ICU setting.

EXTENDED IN-HOSPITAL MANAGEMENT

Patients with respiratory failure should be observed for several days to make sure that they have moved beyond the need for ventilatory support. If a patient develops hemodynamic instability or worsening hypoxia, he or she should be evaluated for pneumothorax, pulmonary embolism, or worsening hyperinflation. If airflow obstruction was initially severe, patients may develop a worsening wheeze as their obstruction improves and they move more air. If a patient is still smoking, a multidisciplinary approach to smoking cessation should be implemented while he or she is in the hospital.

DISPOSITION
Discharge Goals

Before you consider discharge, patients should be breathing comfortably without evidence of respiratory distress. Improvement in airflow obstruction can be documented objectively with spirometry, although most patients are able tell when they are approaching their pulmonary baseline. Every patient should be assessed for home oxygen needs. Just because a patient did not have home oxygen prior to his or her hospitalization doesn't mean he or she didn't need it. If a patient is still smoking, it is imperative to warn him or her of the risks of smoking while on oxygen. All patients should receive a pneumonia vaccine as well as an influenza vaccine during the flu season.

Outpatient Care

Having an exacerbation with respiratory failure is a marker for short-term mortality. As a result, good follow-up with either a primary care physician or a pulmonologist is critical in the weeks following an exacerbation. Patients with severe disease should be on a long-acting controller medication, such as salmeterol/fluticasone or tiotropium bromide, to help prevent future exacerbations. Smoking cessation is by far the most important therapeutic intervention and should be a priority in all follow-up visits.

WHAT YOU NEED TO REMEMBER

- COPD is a predominantly smoking-related disease marked by loss of alveolar elasticity (emphysema) and/or persistent airway inflammation (chronic bronchitis).
- Acute exacerbations are defined by increased dyspnea, increased sputum production, and a change in sputum quality.
- Mainstays of therapy are systemic corticosteroids, antibiotics, supplemental oxygen, and positive-pressure ventilation.
- Patients with acute exacerbations of COPD and hypercarbic respiratory failure have a high in-hospital mortality.
- Acute exacerbations are associated with higher long-term mortality.
- Smoking cessation is critical to the patient's long-term outcome.

REFERENCES

1. Global Initiative for Chronic Obstructive Lung Disease. *Am J Respir Crit Care Med.* 2007;176(6):532–555.
2. Anzueto A, Sethi S, Martinez F. Exacerbations of chronic obstructive pulmonary disease. *Proc Am Thorac Soc.* 2007;4:554–556.

SUGGESTED READINGS

Niewoehner DE, Erbland ML, Deupree RH, et al. Effect of systemic glucocorticoids on exacerbations of chronic obstructive pulmonary disease. *N Engl J Med.* 1999;340:1941–1947.
Papi A, Bellettato CM, Braccioni F, et al. Infections and airway inflammation in chronic obstructive pulmonary disease severe exacerbations. *Am J Respir Crit Care Med.* 2006;173(10):1114–1121.

Rabe KF, Hurd S, Anzueto A, et al. Global strategy for the diagnosis, management, and prevention of chronic obstructive pulmonary disease: GOLD executive summary.

Singh JM, Palda VA, Stanbrook MB, et al. Corticosteroid therapy for patients with acute exacerbations of chronic obstructive pulmonary disease: a systematic review. *Arch Intern Med.* 2002;162:2527–2536.

Tillie-Leblond I, Marquette CH, Perez T, et al. Pulmonary embolism in patients with unexplained exacerbation of chronic obstructive pulmonary disease: prevalence and risk factors. *Ann Intern Med.* 2006;144(6):390–396.

Pleural Effusions

THE PATIENT ENCOUNTER

A 60-year-old man presents to the emergency department with fatigue, fevers, cough, and shortness of breath. He notes some right-sided chest discomfort, worse with inspiration, and says that his breathing is worse when he lies on his right side. A chest radiograph reveals a large right pleural effusion.

OVERVIEW

Definition

A pleural effusion is an abnormal collection of fluid in the pleural space. This chapter will focus on the diagnosis and management of pleural effusions.

Pathophysiology

The lungs are surrounded by the visceral pleura, a thin epithelial layer of mesothelial origin. The thoracic cavity is lined by the parietal pleura. A potential space exists between the visceral and parietal pleura; normally, only a miniscule amount of serous fluid exists in this space, serving as a lubricant for normal respiratory motion.

The visceral pleura receives its blood supply from the bronchial circulation and drains via the pulmonary veins. The parietal pleura is supplied by chest wall arteries and drains into the inferior vena cava. Lymphatic drainage of the pleural space itself occurs via stomata (2 to 6 μm in diameter) in the parietal pleura, which leads to a lymphatic system located between the parietal pleura and the chest wall. About 7 to 10 mL of fluid per day "leaks" out of the bronchial and parietal pleural microvasculature, enters the pleural space, and drains via the stomata into the lymphatic system; the volume and protein concentrations of pleural fluid are therefore normally kept constant. However, if either increased pleural fluid production or decreased drainage (or both) occurs, a pleural effusion can develop. There are six mechanisms by which excess pleural fluid can accumulate:

1. *Increased hydrostatic pressure in the circulatory system.* As intravascular pressures rise, more fluid will leak out of the microvasculature at endothelial cell–cell junctions.

2. *Decreased intravascular oncotic pressure.* If serum albumin levels are low, fluid will have a tendency to diffuse out of the vasculature and into the pleural space.
3. *Decreased lymphatic drainage.* If there is obstruction of the lymphatic system from a process such as a malignancy, pleural fluid may accumulate.
4. *Increased vascular permeability.* If the vessels supplying the lung or pleura become damaged or inflamed, fluid will leak more readily across the endothelial barrier.
5. *Transit of peritoneal fluid (i.e., ascites) through diaphragmatic defects.*
6. *Decreased hydrostatic pressure in the pleural space.* If the lung is not allowed to expand because of bronchial obstruction or pleural inflammation, the resulting decrease in hydrostatic pressure may result in the accumulation of pleural fluid.

Epidemiology

Each year in the United States, roughly 1.3 to 1.5 million pleural effusions are diagnosed (1).

Etiology

As a general rule, a pleural effusion due to hydrostatic or oncotic causes is low in protein and is called a transudate. In contrast, an effusion due to lymphatic obstruction or increased vascular permeability has elevated protein levels and is an exudate. Table 22-1 lists several common causes of pleural effusions.

TABLE 22-1
Common Causes of Pleural Effusions

Transudative	Exudative
Congestive heart failure	Infection: parapneumonic/empyema
Pulmonary embolism	Pulmonary embolism
Liver cirrhosis	Tuberculosis
Peritoneal dialysis	Esophageal perforation
Nephrotic syndrome	Pancreatitis
	Chylothorax
	Coronary artery bypass graft surgery
	Malignancy
	Yellow nail syndrome
	Collagen-vascular and rheumatologic Diseases
	Trauma

ACUTE MANAGEMENT AND WORKUP

As with any patient encountered in the clinic, emergency room, or hospital, the first determination that needs to be made is whether the patient is stable.

The First 15 Minutes

The initial assessment should focus on whether the pleural effusion is causing respiratory compromise.

Initial Assessment

Signs of respiratory distress or hypoxia may indicate the need for urgent thoracentesis to improve pulmonary mechanics. However, such signs may be the result of an underlying process such as a pulmonary embolism, pneumonia, or malignancy, and not directly caused by the fluid itself. Signs of infection, as in our patient encounter, are concerning for empyema and also warrant urgent drainage for both diagnosis and source control.

Admission Criteria and Level of Care Criteria

Unlike pneumonia or cardiac ischemia, there are no defined admission criteria or level of care criteria for patients with pleural effusions. You should use common sense to determine a patient's disposition. A stable patient with a pleural effusion can safely be worked up and managed as an outpatient. In contrast, a patient with abnormal vital signs (fever, hypotension, tachycardia, hypoxia) or severe dyspnea needs to be worked up more expeditiously as an inpatient. Profound hypotension or hypoxia or severe arrhythmias warrant admission to an intensive care unit.

The First Few Hours

Once you ensure the stability of the patient, you can give attention to determining the etiology of the pleural effusion.

History

A carefully taken history can elicit possible causes of pleural effusions. Fevers or chills can indicate an infectious cause of pleural effusion. A history of weight loss, poor appetite, or prior malignancy may indicate a malignant pleural effusion. Joint complaints or a history of rheumatic or autoimmune disease may also provide diagnostic direction. A prior history of heart failure or coronary artery disease can suggest a transudative hydrostatic pleural effusion secondary to volume overload, as can chronic kidney disease in a patient on hemodialysis. A history of cirrhosis with ascites suggests hepatic hydrothorax. Risk factors for deep venous thrombosis could lead to suspicion of pulmonary embolism.

Physical Examination

The physical exam can give important clues as to the presence, size, and etiology of a pleural effusion. A large pleural effusion results in decreased or absent breath sounds upon auscultation, as the fluid between the lung and the chest wall dampens normal respiratory sounds. Tactile fremitus will be decreased as well. Percussion of the chest yields a distinctive dullness corresponding to the level of the fluid. This allows you to estimate the size of the effusion, aids you in determining the proper location for thoracentesis, and allows you to differentiate pleural effusion from other causes of decreased breath sounds, such as pneumothorax or atelectasis.

It is important that you examine both sides of the chest to determine whether an effusion is unilateral or bilateral. Parapneumonic, traumatic, malignant, and pulmonary emboli effusions may occur on either side. Heart failure and volume overload states usually result in bilateral effusions, slightly greater on the right side than on the left. A right-sided effusion might suggest hepatic hydrothorax or Meigs syndrome (ovarian adenoma with associated pleural effusion). A left-sided effusion might be caused by pancreatitis, splenic infarction, aortic dissection, or esophageal rupture.

Labs and Tests to Consider

Key Diagnostic Labs and Tests

Bloody-appearing fluid is consistent with tuberculosis, pulmonary embolism, malignancy, and trauma. A pleural fluid hematocrit is useful to exclude a hemothorax from either trauma or iatrogenic complication; a pleural fluid hematocrit >50% of the peripheral hematocrit is diagnostic of a hemothorax. If malignancy is suspected, fluid should be sent for cytology and/or flow cytometry. Pleural fluid triglyceride levels >110 mg/dL or the presence of chylomicrons are diagnostic of chylothorax. A low pleural fluid glucose level (<60 mg/dL) or a low pH (<7.30) is highly suggestive of one of three entities: complicated parapneumonic effusion, empyema, or malignancy.

Imaging

While the physical exam can strongly suggest the presence of a pleural effusion, imaging studies are usually necessary to provide definitive evidence of that effusion. The most commonly used modalities are plain radiography, computed tomography (CT), and ultrasound.

Conventional chest radiography is inexpensive and readily accessible. An effusion is most usually manifest by an obscured costophrenic angle or a costophrenic angle medially displaced from the chest wall. However, plain radiography may miss a small effusion, or an effusion in a supine patient (i.e., in the intensive care unit). Upright and decubitus films are more sensitive and specific for the presence of an effusion. A chest radiograph can also provide other useful clinical information: a rough estimate of size of the effusion, whether the effusion is unilateral or bilateral, the presence or absence of an adjacent pulmonary infiltrate, signs of trauma (fractured ribs), and signs of heart failure (wided vascular pedicle, enlarged cardiac silhouette) (Fig. 22-1).

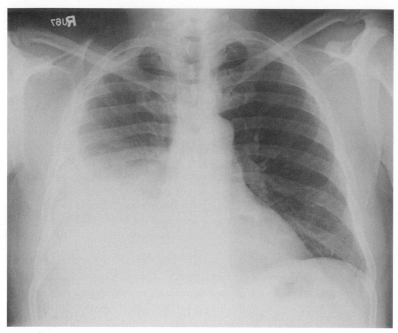

FIGURE 22-1: Large right-sided pleural effusion. (*Courtesy of Brian T. Garibaldi, MD, Division of Pulmonary and Critical Care Medicine, The Johns Hopkins Hospital.*)

Computed tomography (CT) is much more sensitive than conventional radiography for the detection of pleural effusions. CT also provides more information about the lung parenchyma itself, and thus can reveal pneumonias, masses, or other pulmonary pathology. Contrast-enhanced CT provides detailed images of the thoracic vasculature and can aid in the identification of lymphadenopathy, pulmonary emboli, and other potential causes of pleural effusions. In the case of a moderate to large pleural effusion that is easily visualized by chest radiography, it usually makes sense to get the CT after a large-volume thoracentesis so that the underlying lung parenchyma can best be visualized (Fig. 22-2). Downsides of CT scanning include expense, radiation exposure, contrast dye exposure, and identification of incidental findings.

Ultrasound is another imaging modality useful in the evaluation of pleural effusions. It is more sensitive than conventional radiography for the detection of pleural effusions, involves no radiation, and provides real-time imaging, which can be useful in the performance of thoracentesis. It may also help to distinguish exudative from transudative effusions based on certain fluid characteristics (Fig. 22-3). Table 22-2 lists some of the pleural fluid characteristics of exudative effusions.

A

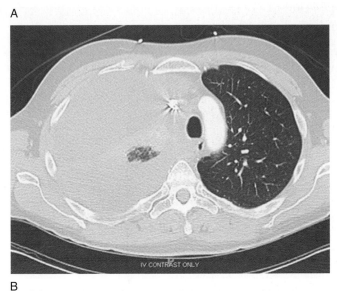

B

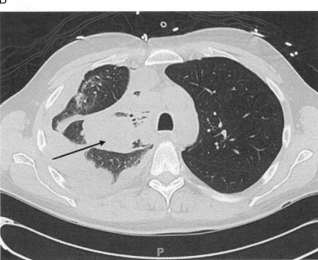

FIGURE 22-2: **A:** Large right-sided pleural effusion. **B:** Right upper lobe mass (*arrow*) discovered after large-volume thoracentesis. (*Courtesy of Brian T. Garibaldi, MD, Division of Pulmonary and Critical Care Medicine, The Johns Hopkins Hospital.*)

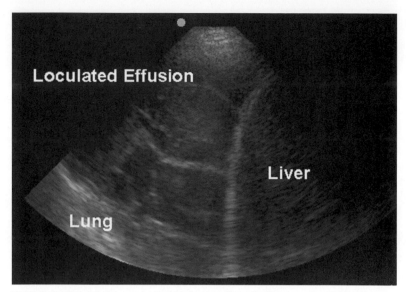

FIGURE 22-3: Ultrasound of a loculated pleural effusion. (*Courtesy of David Feller-Kopman, MD, Division of Pulmonary and Critical Care Medicine, The Johns Hopkins Hospital.*)

TABLE 22-2
Pleural Fluid Characteristics of Exudative Effusions

Light's Criteria (one or more of the following present)[a]

- Ratio of pleural fluid protein level to serum protein level >0.5
- Ratio of pleural fluid lactate dehydrogenase (LDH) to serum LDH >0.6
- Pleural fluid LDH more than two-thirds the upper limit of normal for serum LDH

Pleural Fluid Cholesterol (one or more of the following present)[b]

- Pleural fluid cholesterol >43 mg/dL
- Ratio of pleural fluid cholesterol to serum cholesterol >0.3

[a]Light RW, MacGregor MI, Luchsinger PC, et al. Pleural effusions: the diagnostic separation of transudates and exudates. *Ann Intern Med.* 1972;77:507–513.
[b]Light RW. Pleural effusion. *N Engl J Med.* 2002;346(25):1971–1977.

Treatment

Once a presumptive diagnosis has been made, treatment can begin. Unless the effusion is causing severe dyspnea, a transudative effusion can usually be managed conservatively. A transudative effusion due to congestive heart failure usually responds to diuresis. Likewise, a hepatic hydrothorax secondary to liver cirrhosis can be treated by measures aimed at reducing ascites (i.e., diuresis and salt restriction). Dyspneic patients can achieve symptomatic relief from large-volume thoracentesis, although unless the underlying cause of the effusion is treated, the effusion will quickly recur.

> ## CLINICAL PEARL
>
> *A chest tube should not be placed to treat a hepatic hydrothorax. It will prove nearly impossible to remove secondary to continued high-output drainage, placing the patient at risk for severe hypoalbuminemia and infection.*

Therapy for an exudate is more aggressive. If infection is suspected, as in the case of the patient at the beginning of the chapter, treatment depends on whether the effusion is thought to be an uncomplicated parapneumonic effusion, a complicated parapneumonic effusion, or an empyema. In the case of an uncomplicated parapneumonic effusion (pH >7.20, lactate dehydrogenase [LDH] <1,000 mg/dL), antibiotic therapy aimed toward causative organisms of pneumonia is sufficient, with repeat thoracentesis if the patient's clinical status worsens. A complicated parapneumonic effusion (pH <7.20, LDH >1,000 mg/dL, or glucose <50 mg/dL) should be drained in addition to therapy with antibiotics. This can be accomplished with serial thoracentesis or chest tube placement. An empyema (defined as frank pus in the pleural space or a positive pleural fluid culture) should be drained with a chest tube; the patient may also require surgical management. Appropriate antibiotics are mandatory for complicated parapneumonic effusions and empyema.

Other causes of exudative effusions are treated differently, with the caveat that most effusions with a pH <7.20 should be drained, usually with a chest tube. Malignant pleural effusion is a poor prognostic indicator; your treatment should be aimed at the underlying malignancy and may involve further pleural procedures for palliation. A chylothorax may require surgery for definitive repair, although conservative management by limiting oral fat intake to medium-chain fatty acids may be useful. A traumatic or iatrogenic hemothorax must be followed carefully. Chest tube placement allows for the monitoring of continued blood loss. Continuing hemorrhage or hemodynamic instability is an indication for surgical exploration.

EXTENDED IN-HOSPITAL MANAGEMENT

As described previously, management depends on the etiology of the effusion and the patient's response to therapy. You must rethink your diagnosis or the course of treatment if the patient's condition does not improve, suddenly changes, or worsens; pleural disease is a dynamic process. For example, a small effusion may progress to become symptomatic, an uncomplicated parapneumonic effusion may become an empyema, or a previously sterile effusion may become infected, either after a procedure or due to hematogenous spread from bacteremia. Keep an open mind, evaluate the patient each day, and always question whether the patient is responding to the prescribed therapy.

DISPOSITION

Discharge Goals

A patient is ready for discharge once the etiology of his or her pleural effusion has been explored and initial management has been initiated. For example, patients with complicated parapneumonic effusions or empyema should be afebrile and their chest tubes removed prior to considering discharge.

Outpatient Care

Depending on the etiology of the effusion, patients should be referred to the appropriate subspecialist including oncology, rheumatology, and pulmonology. Patients with exudative pleural effusions of unclear etiology should be referred to a pulmonologist or thoracic surgeon. Such patients may benefit from serial thoracenteses to increase diagnostic yield. Many patients will ultimately require pleural biopsy, usually by thoracoscopy or thoracotomy, to secure the diagnosis.

 WHAT YOU NEED TO REMEMBER

- A pleural effusion is an abnormal collection of fluid in the pleural space.
- Pleural effusions are either transudates or exudates. These are differentiated using Light's criteria.
- Common causes of transudates are heart failure and hepatic cirrhosis. Common causes of exudates are infection (parapneumonic effusion or empyema), malignancy, autoimmune disease, and trauma.
- A patient with a fever and pleural effusion should undergo thoracentesis as soon as safely possible.

- Causes of bloody effusions are trauma, tuberculosis, pulmonary embolism, and malignancy.
- Causes of massive pleural effusions are trauma, hepatic hydrothorax, malignancy, chylothorax, and occasionally empyema.
- Frank blood or pus in the pleural space and a pH <7.20 are indications for immediate drainage of the pleural effusion, usually with a chest tube.

REFERENCE

1. Light RW. Pleural effusion. *N Engl J Med.* 2002;346(25):1971–1977.

SUGGESTED READINGS

Collins TR, Sahn SA. Thoracentesis: complications, patient experience, and diagnostic value. *Chest.* 1987;91:817.

Feller-Kopman D. Ultrasound-guided thoracentesis. *Chest.* 2006;129(6):1709–1714.

Light RW, MacGregor MI, Luchsinger PC, et al. Pleural effusions: the diagnostic separation of transudates and exudates. *Ann Intern Med.* 1972;77:507–513.

Sahn SA. State of the art: the pleura. *Am Rev Respir Dis.* 1988;138:184–234.

Hemoptysis

THE PATIENT ENCOUNTER

A 57-year-old man arrives to the emergency department complaining of "spitting up blood." He has been coughing up streaks of bright red blood in his sputum for the last week, with an acute increase in the frequency and amount of blood leading to today's visit. His medical history is notable for chronic obstructive pulmonary disease, for which he is on "puffers." He continues to smoke one pack per day and while his vital signs are being obtained at triage, he develops a paroxysm of cough and produces about 15 mL of bright red blood mixed with thick sputum.

OVERVIEW

Definition

Hemoptysis is the expectoration of blood (or blood mixed with sputum) derived from the lower respiratory tract. Classification of "massive" hemoptysis varies among studies but has been defined as being between 100 mL and 600 mL of blood in 24 hours.

Pathophysiology

Hemoptysis can arise from vessels bleeding anywhere along the lower respiratory tract from the trachea to the alveolar space. The lung is supplied by two blood supplies: the low-pressure pulmonary circulation and the systemic bronchial circulation. Therefore, a wide variety of potential bleeding sources exist in hemoptysis. However, in most cases, bleeding arises from vessels of the bronchial circulation that supply the bronchi and bronchioles.

Epidemiology

The true incidence and prevalence of hemoptysis is unknown given that many cases go unreported. However, approximately 5% of patients who present to medical care for hemoptysis will experience massive hemoptysis.

Etiology

The most common etiologies for hemoptysis in the United States are bronchitis, bronchogenic carcinoma, and bronchiectasis. *Mycobacterium tuberculosis* is the most frequent cause worldwide. Even with a thorough evaluation,

TABLE 23-1
Etiologies of Hemoptysis

Infectious/Inflammatory

Bronchitis	*Mycobacterium tuberculosis*
Bronchiectasis	Mycetoma
Bacterial pneumonia	Lung abscess
Septic emboli	

Vascular

Pulmonary embolus	Mitral stenosis
Arteriovenous malformations	Congestive heart failure

Neoplastic

Bronchogenic carcinoma	Kaposi sarcoma
Metastatic disease	Bronchial adenoma

Autoimmune

Goodpasture syndrome	Systemic lupus erythematosus
Wegener granulomatosis	Idiopathic pulmonary hemosiderosis

Miscellaneous/Other

Cryptogenic	Foreign body
Coagulopathy	Trauma
Thrombocytopenia	Broncholithiasis
Iatrogenic (i.e., after biopsy)	Catamenial

up to 30% of cases of hemoptysis remain without a clear etiology and are labeled cryptogenic. The more common etiologies of hemoptysis can be grouped by category (Table 23-1).

ACUTE MANAGEMENT AND WORKUP

Coughing up blood can be quite frightening for both the patient and health care providers. It is important to proceed in a rapid yet meticulous way in order to triage the patient to the appropriate level of care.

The First 15 Minutes

Because hemoptysis can be a life-threatening emergency (with mortality rates as high as 80% with massive hemoptysis), your first impression of the patient's clinical status is critical. A patient who is in obvious respiratory distress or demonstrates inadequate gas exchange likely requires intubation and intensive care unit (ICU)–level care.

> ### CLINICAL PEARL
>
> *Death from hemoptysis usually results from asphyxiation, not exsanguination. Recall that our anatomic dead space is about 1 mL per body weight in pounds, so as little as 200 mL of hemoptysis can result in severe respiratory compromise.*

Initial Assessment

The initial assessment of a patient presenting with "coughing up blood" is to ensure that the symptom is really hemoptysis and not pseudohemoptysis (expectorated blood originating from the upper airway or gastrointestinal tract). The patient in our encounter likely has true hemoptysis because he had a witnessed episode of coughing up sputum mixed with blood. As noted previously, the very first evaluation should focus on the patient's clinical status and pulmonary reserve. The temporal nature of the hemoptysis should then be evaluated and it should be determined if there is ongoing hemoptysis. In general, patients and physicians alike tend to overestimate the amount of hemoptysis, so try to be specific. For example, ask the patient if he or she coughed up a soda cap or a shot glass full of blood. If at all possible, try to directly measure the amount of blood expectorated. A focused history and physical at this point will assist you in formulating a differential diagnosis and aid in triage decisions.

Admission Criteria and Level of Care Criteria

Patients with scant hemoptysis and very low risk (i.e., patient age younger than 40, no smoking history, no history suggestive of etiologies other than bronchitis) can be given empiric antimicrobials for presumptive bronchitis and arranged for outpatient follow-up. Patients with massive hemoptysis should be managed in an ICU with early pulmonary, thoracic surgery, and interventional radiology consultation. Patients with limited hemoptysis but without a history strongly suggestive of bronchitis should be monitored in an inpatient setting while his or her hemoptysis is being evaluated.

The First Few Hours

Once you complete the initial triage of a patient with hemoptysis, you can focus further efforts on obtaining the appropriate history, performing a physical examination, and determining the diagnostic studies to guide management.

History

A history of fevers and cough with thick sputum may indicate infection, such as bronchitis or pneumonia. The patient should be questioned about the presence of night sweats, weight loss, and the personal risks associated with *M. tuberculosis*. Past or current tobacco use or a personal history of cancer increases the pretest probability of a malignancy, either primary or metastatic, as the etiology of the hemoptysis. A medical history of a seizure disorder or other conditions that predispose a patient to an altered mental status may indicate a risk for aspiration events. The acute onset of pleuritic chest pain may suggest a pulmonary embolus. It is important to ask about known lung disease because patients with cystic fibrosis or bronchiectasis of any etiology are at higher risk for hemoptysis.

Physical Examination

A careful examination of the nasopharynx and oropharynx should be performed to evaluate for pseudohemoptysis from an upper airway source. Generalized lymphadenopathy may indicate tuberculosis or malignancy. Painful, unilateral lower extremity edema may suggest a deep venous thrombosis and the risk of a pulmonary embolism. The presence of a rash and polyarthritis may be signs of an autoimmune disorder. Examination of the cardiovascular system may reveal evidence of mitral stenosis or left ventricular dysfunction as a possible cause of the hemoptysis.

The pulmonary examination can be misleading in cases of hemoptysis. For example, while the source of hemoptysis may be an upper lobe airway lesion, the hemorrhage may pool in the dependent portions of the lung, producing signs of consolidation in the lower lobe.

Labs and Tests to Consider

Results of lab tests and radiographic studies can further assist with the initial differential diagnosis as well as help to guide management and therapeutic interventions.

Key Diagnostic Labs and Tests

Severely abnormal coagulation/clotting parameters may indicate a quickly correctable etiology of hemoptysis. In patients with massive hemoptysis, a type and cross should be sent to the blood bank in anticipation of the need for a blood transfusion. An elevated white blood cell count with a left-shifted differential suggests an infectious etiology. A purified protein derivative should be placed if tuberculosis is suspected along with the appropriate respiratory isolation measures. Sputum should be sent for culture and cytology.

If renal dysfunction is detected with basic chemistry/electrolyte labs, an evaluation for pulmonary-renal syndromes should proceed with urinalysis and autoimmune serologies such as antiglomerular basement membrane titers, antinuclear antibodies, and antineutrophil cytoplasmic antibodies. An arterial blood gas will help in the assessment of the adequacy of the patient's ventilation and oxygenation.

Imaging

A chest radiograph can help with the initial assessment of a patient with hemoptysis. A normal chest radiograph in a low-risk patient can be reassuring that the risk of malignancy is quite low. However, most patients will require further imaging in the form of a computed tomography (CT) scan to better characterize the nature of any abnormalities noted on the chest radiograph. Findings on CT scan of the chest may indicate an etiology of the hemoptysis (Fig. 23-1). The use of intravenous contrast for a CT angiogram may demonstrate a pulmonary embolus.

A

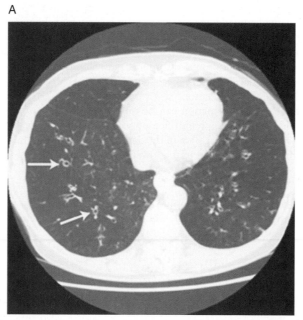

FIGURE 23-1: Abnormal chest imaging associated with hemoptysis. A: Computed tomography (CT) image of bronchiectasis with dilated, thickened bronchi demonstrating "signet ring sign" (*white arrow*).

B

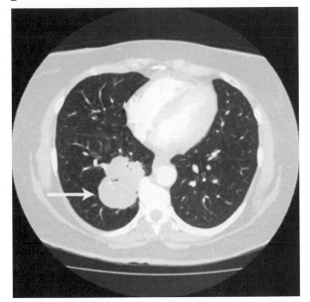

C

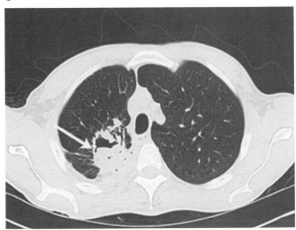

FIGURE 23-1: (Continued) **B:** CT image demonstrating dense right lower lobe mass; biopsy revealed non–small cell lung cancer. **C:** CT image of cavitary right upper lobe lesion with debris consistent with mycetoma. (*Images Courtesy of Matthew Pipeling, MD, Division of Pulmonary and Critical Care Medicine, The Johns Hopkins Hospital.*)

Treatment

Bronchoscopy is generally indicated as both a diagnostic and a therapeutic tool except in patients in whom a diagnosis is fairly certain or not amenable to bronchoscopic intervention (i.e., simple bronchitis or pulmonary embolism). The patient from the patient encounter likely has hemoptysis from bronchitis or pneumonia in the setting of his active tobacco use, although imaging studies would be necessary to rule out an underlying malignancy or cavitary lung lesion. If an actively bleeding site is seen during bronchoscopy, local control of the lesion may be possible with epinephrine, electrocautery, or cryotherapy. The highest diagnostic yield occurs with bronchoscopy in the first 24 hours. However, even with the increased diagnostic yield of early bronchoscopy, studies have not demonstrated a difference in outcomes between early and delayed bronchoscopy. If bronchoscopy cannot locate the bleeding source or efforts at hemostasis by bronchoscopic intervention are unsuccessful, arteriography of the bronchial circulation and catheter embolization may be attempted by an experienced interventional radiologist. In cases of massive hemoptysis, it may be better to proceed directly to angiography and possible embolization because bronchoscopy is unlikely to be able to localize a source if there is a tremendous amount of active bleeding.

CLINICAL PEARL

If the likely site of massive hemoptysis can be lateralized (i.e., known history of cavitary mass in left lower lobe), the nonbleeding lung may be selectively intubated by an experienced individual. This will help to prevent blood from entering the "good" lung and to preserve gas exchange. The patient can also be made to lie on the side of the bleeding lung to minimize blood pooling in the "good" lung by gravity.

If bleeding persists despite attempts at bronchoscopic or arteriographic control, or if diagnostic studies reveal a lesion at high risk of rebleeding such as a mycetoma, surgical resection should be considered in patients with sufficient pulmonary reserve and in whom the site responsible for hemoptysis has been localized to a specific, resectable region. However, the morbidity and mortality associated with surgical resection are not insignificant, particularly in an unstable patient with active bleeding or in a patient with severe underlying lung disease.

Serial hematocrits should be checked to help guide transfusion therapy, although, as in the case of gastrointestinal bleeding, there is no hematocrit goal in the setting of an active bleed. Any underlying coagulation abnormality should be aggressively corrected.

EXTENDED IN-HOSPITAL MANAGEMENT

As the diagnostic workup and management proceed, it is important to frequently reassess the patient's clinical status and level of care. A patient who appears to have a small amount of self-limited hemoptysis may present with a sentinel bleed and can suddenly develop massive hemoptysis that requires rapid intervention.

DISPOSITION

Discharge Goals

For patients requiring admission for hemoptysis, the disposition goals are cessation and, if possible, control of the bleeding source. As much as possible of the indicated diagnostic workup should be completed during the admission to help with further outpatient care.

Outpatient Care

Just as with any unplanned inpatient admission, the patient's primary care provider should be notified and close follow-up should be arranged for after discharge. Patients should be monitored for any recurrence of hemoptysis as this may warrant further diagnostic and therapeutic interventions. Certain diagnoses relating to the etiology of the hemoptysis warrant appropriate subspecialty outpatient follow-up, such as oncology, rheumatology, or pulmonology.

WHAT YOU NEED TO REMEMBER

- The bleeding of hemoptysis usually arises from the bronchial circulation.
- In developed countries the most common causes of hemoptysis are bronchitis, bronchiectasis, and bronchogenic carcinoma. Tuberculosis remains an important etiology in developing nations.
- Up to 30% of presentations of hemoptysis remain cryptogenic despite an appropriate assessment.
- Bronchoscopy is an important tool in the evaluation and management of hemoptysis.
- Massive hemoptysis accounts for only about 5% of cases of hemoptysis, but can be life-threatening with mortality rates as high as 80%.
- Patients with massive hemoptysis should be managed in an intensive care unit using a multidisciplinary approach with pulmonary, interventional radiology, and thoracic surgery.

SUGGESTED READINGS

Andersen PE. Imaging and interventional radiological treatment of hemoptysis. *Acta Radiol.* 2006;47:780–792.

Bidwell JL, Pachner RW. Hemoptysis: diagnosis and management. *Am Fam Physician.* 2005;72:1253–1260.

Cahill BC, Ingbar DH. Massive hemoptysis. Assessment and management. *Clin Chest Med.* 1994;15:147–167.

Dweik RA, Stoller JK. Role of bronchoscopy in massive hemoptysis. *Clin Chest Med.* 1999;20:89–105.

Tsoumakidou M, Chrysofakis G, Tsiligianni I, et al. A prospective analysis of 184 hemoptysis cases: diagnostic impact of chest X-ray, computed tomography, bronchoscopy. *Respiration.* 2006;73:808–814.

Approach to the Infectious Diseases Evaluation

Infectious diseases span not only all organ systems and specialties, but also all types of patients from the healthy to the chronically ill and immunosuppressed. In this section, we will discuss pathogen and host factors that determine the types and severity of infection; an understanding of these is paramount to an understanding of the presentations and diagnoses of infectious diseases. We will also address key elements of the history and physical examination as they pertain to the evaluation of infectious diseases. We will end with a basic discussion of use of the laboratory in investigation and diagnosis of infectious diseases.

MICROBIAL PATHOPHYSIOLOGY

Virulence is the ability of an organism to cause disease. An organism's virulence depends on multiple factors, including the ability to adhere to and enter a host, followed by growth and multiplication within that host, the evasion of the immune system, the ability to invade tissue and cause tissue damage, and, ultimately, the replication and dissemination to new hosts. An understanding of these basic principles facilitates understanding of the predominant signs and symptoms of most infectious diseases.

The manifestations of disease caused by an organism depend on the site of entry of that organism into the host. For example, varicella zoster virus usually becomes dormant in the dorsal root ganglia after primary varicella infection (chickenpox). It then reactivates with suppression of the immune system in a predictable dermatomal pattern as it travels from the nerve ganglion along the nerve and ultimately to the skin. The most common sites of entry for organisms are the skin and mucosal surfaces such as the respiratory, gastrointestinal, and urogenital tract.

After entry into a host, a microbe must be able to adhere to host tissue. Once anchored on host tissue, organisms must then replicate. Many viruses replicate within host cells and use the host cell's genetic machinery for transcription and translation of viral proteins and then processing of new viruses. The classic example of this is the human immunodeficiency virus (HIV). Many bacteria and fungi grow in biofilms, which are essentially large masses of slowly growing organisms. Growth in biofilms leads to the ability of organisms to evade host defenses as well as antimicrobial agents. Bacteria and viruses also possess extracellular proteins, which facilitate tissue invasion. Tissue invasion as well as further tissue damage through organism replication and microbial toxin production contribute to disease. Most pathogenic organisms are transmitted in the same mode that they enter a host.

For example, respiratory pathogens are usually spread in respiratory secretions. Once out of the host, the ability to resist a hostile environment is another factor that promotes the spread of pathogenic organisms.

Host Factors

A multitude of host factors determine the scope of infectious diseases to which a particular host is susceptible. Basic information, such as the age of the host, the immunization history, nutritional status, and prior and coexisting illnesses, can alter the likelihood of infection. Those at the extremes of age are more susceptible to infections overall, and those with more complicated preexisting conditions, such as diabetes mellitus and renal insufficiency, are also at increased risk.

Other important yet often forgotten host factors include geography, the environment in which the host resides or travels, and the behaviors of the host. For example, those residing or traveling in the North American Southwest are at risk of coccidiomycosis. Another example of a high-risk but sometimes forgotten environment is the health care environment. Medical care places patients at risk for infections through contact with hospital pathogens that are often different from pathogens in the community. Breaches in skin integrity due to intravenous catheters and other foreign objects, antibiotic-associated alterations in normal host flora, and drug-induced immunosuppression are other health care–associated risks for infection.

Host behaviors are important as well. For example, we know that intravenous drug users are at increased risk for bacterial endocarditis due to introduction of bacteria through the skin into the bloodstream.

The role the host immune system plays in defending against infections becomes most apparent when it is compromised in states such as medication-induced immunosuppression or in those with HIV. The host's ability (or inability) to mount an inflammatory response to an invasive pathogen also contributes to the clinical signs and symptoms of disease as well as the ability to clear an infection.

PATIENT EVALUATION

Infected patients commonly present with nonspecific signs and symptoms, so developing a consistent approach is important.

History

Many infectious diseases have characteristic durations as well as a characteristic progression of symptoms that are important to elicit. The history should include a detailed search for a possible preceding nidus of infection, such as prior trauma, lacerations, or burns, and symptoms of a viral infection, such as influenza, which can predispose to a bacterial superinfection. A history of recent or current foreign objects, such as intravenous catheters and prosthetic joints, should always be obtained. A detailed travel history, if present, should always be taken and should include details about the location, the duration of travel, animal exposure, the types of food and water ingested, activities, and a history of any prophylaxis or vaccines taken prior to travel.

CLINICAL PEARL

Regardless of travel, an exposure history is of key importance and questions should focus on exposure to animals, insects, potentially contaminated food and water supplies, and other people with a potentially transmissible infection.

A review of systems should focus on the presence of fever, rigors, weight loss, and a detailed neurologic review, including any evidence of meningismus or altered sensorium. Thorough questions detailing possible rheumatologic symptoms, such as rashes, joint complaints, and weakness, are important because infectious diseases and rheumatologic diseases can often present similarly. A thorough sexual and menstrual history is important not only when genitourinary complaints are present, but also to assess for risk of HIV infection and other sexually transmitted diseases.

The past medical history should focus on a history of any previous infections as well as a history of any immunocompromising conditions such as HIV, organ transplantation, diabetes mellitus, significant liver or renal disease, malignancy, or asplenia.

A detailed medication and allergy history is important to rule out any new medications that may be causing a hypersensitivity reaction, but also to assess for medications that may predispose to infection. You should elicit details of how long the patient has been on any potentially immune-suppressing medications, and any recent changes to his or her medication list.

The social history should focus on smoking and alcohol consumption patterns because the heavy use of both can predispose to respiratory infections and represent risk factors for malignancy. A thorough history detailing any illicit drug use, including the route, quantity, and date and type of most recent use, are important because, depending on these factors, patients will be susceptible to different types of infection. Other important aspects of the social history include an occupational history, travel history, sexual history, history of incarceration, and any current or past history of homelessness. Homelessness and incarceration are risk factors for *Mycobacterium tuberculosis* infection.

The family history should focus on sick contacts and a family history of immunodeficiency, malignancy, tuberculosis, or rheumatologic diseases.

Physical Examination

The first and most important task is assessing the general appearance of the patient. This includes looking for signs of toxicity that can range from anxiety and agitation to apathy and stupor. Tachypnea, hyper- or hypothermia, and tachycardia are all signs of systemic inflammation and are often the first signs of impending septic shock prior to changes in blood pressure (see Chapter 29).

In addition to a thorough, symptom-based examination, special attention should be paid to several areas. A head and neck examination should search for signs of dental, sinus, or ear infections, as well as examination of the mucous membranes for evidence of lesions or petechiae, sometimes seen with systemic infection such as endocarditis or meningococcemia. The conjunctiva and fundi should be examined for evidence of petechiae or Roth spots, sometimes seen in endocarditis, and to look for papilledema.

Lymph Node Examination

A full lymph node examination should be performed, including assessment of cervical, axillary, supraclavicular, epitrochlear, and groin lymph nodes. Enlargement of any or all of these can be seen in HIV, lymphoma, syphilis, mononucleosis, or sarcoidosis, or in more common bacterial or viral infections.

Cardiac and Pulmonary Examinations

The cardiopulmonary examination should focus on evaluating for new murmurs that may be indicative of endocarditis, as well as pericardial rubs, which may be heard with pericarditis. The pulmonary examination should look for signs of a focal consolidation or pleural effusion.

Abdominal and Genital Examination

The abdominal and genital examination should focus on any symptoms that were elicited in the history. A pelvic examination should be performed in all women (especially those that are sexually active) with lower abdominal complaints.

Skin Examination

The skin examination should always be thorough and focus on any evidence of abnormal rashes or localized abnormalities that may be consistent with infection. Look for signs of trauma or insect or animal bites that may be the nidus of infection. Petechial rashes may be seen with Rocky Mountain spotted fever or meningococcemia. Diffuse erythroderma is commonly seen with drug reactions and toxic shock syndromes. Intravenous drug users should be asked where they most recently injected, as these areas are prone to cellulitis and abscess formation. Be sure to look for stigmata of endocarditis on the examination of the skin and nails (see Chapter 28). Soft tissue and muscle examination is important as localized areas of tenderness, erythema, duskiness, and edema may represent necrotizing fasciitis or myositis. All joints should be examined for evidence of effusions or a decreased range of motion, which may be consistent with septic arthritis.

Neurologic Examination

Finally, the neurologic examination should focus on a thorough mental status evaluation to assess for subtle signs of encephalopathy. If meningitis is a concern, assess for photophobia and meningismus. The neurologic examination should also look for evidence of focal neurologic signs as well as evidence of localized spinal tenderness, which may represent vertebral osteomyelitis or an epidural abscess.

Key Diagnostic Evaluations

The basic diagnostic workup for patients who are likely infected includes a complete blood count with differential and a complete metabolic panel to assess renal and liver function.

Laboratory Tests

A complete blood count will likely show leukocytosis (although leukopenia may occur). The differential may be useful as bacterial infections usually show a predominance of neutrophils or band forms, viral infections show a predominance of mononuclear cells, and parasitic infections or allergic reactions show a predominance of eosinophils.

Having a microbiology laboratory is imperative in the diagnosis of infectious diseases. For anyone suspected of having a bloodstream infection, and specifically endocarditis, collection of blood cultures are the first step in the diagnosis and should precede the administration of antibiotics (see Chapter 28). Anyone with symptoms likely secondary to a urinary tract infection should have a complete urinalysis with microscopic evaluation and urine culture. The rapid collection of cerebrospinal fluid is critical in any patient with suspected meningitis or encephalitis (see Chapter 26).

Imaging

Other important diagnostic tests include radiologic imaging, specifically chest roentgenogram to look for evidence of pneumonia, and computed tomography or ultrasound of potentially deep-seated soft tissue infections.

WHAT YOU NEED TO REMEMBER

- Understanding the basics of virulence and host–organism interactions will help to frame your understanding of most infectious diseases.
- The immune status of a patient helps to determine the types of infections to which they are susceptible as well as the manner in which those infections present.

- An exposure history is critical when formulating a differential diagnosis for a patient with a possible infectious disease.
- A thorough skin and lymph node examination is critical to identifying a variety of infectious diseases.
- Cultures are crucial to identifying specific pathogens and, when possible, should be drawn prior to the administration of antibiotics.

SUGGESTED READINGS

Betts RF, Chapman SW, Penn RL, eds. *A Practical Approach to Infectious Diseases.* 5th ed. Philadelphia: Lippincott Williams & Wilkins; 2003.

Gladwin M, Trattler B. *Clinical Microbiology Made Ridiculously Simple.* 3rd ed. Miami, FL: MedMaster, 2007.

Mandell GL, Bennett JE, Dolin R. *Principles and Practice of Infectious Diseases. Part I – Basic Principles in the Diagnosis and Management of Infectious Diseases.* 6th ed. Philadelphia: Churchill Livingstone, Elsevier; 2005.

Pneumonia

A 63-year-old woman is brought to the emergency department by her family with acute-onset chest pain, fever, productive cough, and shortness of breath. She is confused, febrile, tachycardic, and markedly short of breath. Chest radiography reveals a right lower lobe consolidation.

OVERVIEW

Definition

Pneumonia is defined as inflammation of one or both lungs with consolidation of the lung parenchyma. There are a number of processes that can cause pulmonary inflammation and consolidation. This chapter will focus on the approach to and management of inpatients with infectious pneumonia.

Pathophysiology

Microaspiration from the upper respiratory tract is the most common way that pathogens reach the lung. Macroaspiration, such as aspiration of gastric contents, is also a portal of entry for organisms. Hematogenous spread from a distant site or direct spread from an adjacent focus of infection can also allow pathogenic organisms to reach the lungs. Infection results when host defense mechanisms falter, the pathogen has a specific virulence factor that is able to evade the immune system, or the size of the inoculum is high enough to overwhelm host defenses.

Epidemiology

Pneumonia is the seventh leading cause of death in the United States, with mortality being highest among the elderly and patients with other comorbid conditions (1). Rates of infection are higher in the winter months, with a higher predilection for men and the elderly.

Etiology

The most common causes of community-acquired pneumonia vary by age group but include *Streptococcus pneumonia*, *Haemophilus influenza*, and *Chlamydia pneumonia*. Viral pathogens such as influenza, parainfluenza, and respiratory syncytial virus may account for as many as 20% of cases. In clinical practice, the etiologic agent is identified in <50% of cases.

ACUTE MANAGEMENT AND WORKUP

The first few hours are critical in the evaluation and management of a patient with pneumonia.

The First 15 Minutes

The timely administration of antibiotics and the rapid assessment of illness severity can make the difference between a short inpatient stay or a prolonged hospitalization.

Initial Assessment

Pneumonia is the most common cause of sepsis in the United States. As a result, it is important to look for evidence of sepsis because recognizing this syndrome early is the key to improving the patient's outcome (see Chapter 29). The patient in the clinical encounter is likely septic because she is tachypneic, tachycardic, and febrile and has signs of likely cerebral hypoperfusion.

> ### CLINICAL PEARL
>
> *Remember that a patient can be septic without being hypotensive. Do not be falsely reassured by a "normal" blood pressure in a patient with pneumonia.*

Pneumonia is also one of the most common causes of acute respiratory distress syndrome (ARDS), so it is important to carefully examine your patient for evidence of impending respiratory failure (see Chapter 17). Even in the absence of ARDS, pneumonia can cause both profound hypoxia and hypercarbia, so a thorough pulmonary exam early on provides valuable information about a patient's likely clinical trajectory.

Admission Criteria and Level of Care Criteria

Older patients, patients with multiple comorbidities such as diabetes and heart disease, and patients with new oxygen requirements deserve admission to the hospital. Scoring systems like the Pneumonia Severity Index (PSI) or CURB-65 score can be helpful but should not be used as a triage tool by themselves. The CURB-65 score is relatively easy to remember. Assign one point for each of the following: *C* for confusion, *U* for uremia (blood urea nitrogen >19 mg/dL), *R* for respiratory rate >30, *B* for systolic blood pressure <90, and *65* for patient age >65. Higher scores predict higher mortality (1).

The American Thoracic Society (ATS) and Infectious Diseases Society of America (IDSA) have published major and minor criteria for classifying "severe pneumonia" (2). Although these criteria have yet to be prospectively validated, they can be used as a rough guide to help determine which patients may benefit from closer monitoring. Major criteria include the need for vasopressor therapy or mechanical ventilation. Minor criteria include the use of noninvasive ventilation, a respiratory rate >30, multilobar infiltrates, hypotension that requires aggressive fluid resuscitation, hypothermia, thrombocytopenia, leukopenia, delirium, uremia, a PaO_2/FiO_2 <250, and hypoglycemia in a nondiabetic patient. In general, the presence of one major and/or three minor criteria likely warrants admission to an intensive care unit.

The First Few Hours

Once a patient is clinically stable, you can turn your attention to gathering more detailed information that will help guide further management.

History

Determining the onset and character of symptoms provides clues about the possible pathogen. Patients with pneumococcal pneumonia often describe the acute onset of fevers and chills, followed closely thereafter by productive cough with rusty sputum and pleuritic chest pain. Patients with atypical pathogens often describe a more insidious onset (e.g., dry cough and dyspnea with exertion that lasts several days to weeks). Abdominal pain, nausea, vomiting, and diarrhea may point to *Legionella* pneumonia, but these are by no means specific findings. Hemoptysis can be seen with any pneumonia, but massive hemoptysis (defined usually as >300 mL of blood) may suggest infections such as *Mycobacterium tuberculosis* or other etiologies such as pulmonary embolism or malignancy. Likewise, pleuritic chest pain may be caused by pneumonia, a pulmonary embolism, or pleural effusion of any etiology.

Immunocompromised patients are at risk for a host of pathogens that are not normally empirically treated and may therefore require aggressive diagnostic testing to rule out more serious infections. Patients who have recently been hospitalized are at risk for nosocomial pathogens in addition to the more common organisms. A preceding upper respiratory infection, such as influenza, can result in a more severe bacterial postinfection, such as *Staphylococcus aureus*. Smokers are more likely to acquire *Legionella pneumophila* or *H. influenza* but may also present with respiratory symptoms and fever in the setting of malignancy. A travel history or history of incarceration is important because it may provide clues to such infections as tuberculosis, atypical mycobacterial infection, or other endemic infections. Occupational history is likewise important because certain professions predispose to infections like brucellosis but also make interstitial lung disease a possible cause of cough, dyspnea, and pulmonary infiltrates. A history of stroke, alcohol use, or previous aspiration raises the possibility of anaerobic infection from aspiration, although most aspiration pneumonias are gram negative or polymicrobial. Recent dental work may predispose to infection with *Streptococcus viridans*. Intravenous drug users are more likely to develop *S. aureus* pneumonia but may also be at risk for septic pulmonary emboli from right-sided endocarditis.

Recurrent pneumonias may indicate an underlying immunocompromised state, such as human immunodeficiency virus. Pneumonia occurring in the middle lobe or recurrent pneumonia in the same area of the lung might be a sign of a postobstructive process secondary to an airway lesion or malignancy.

It is also important to search for other causes of shortness of breath, cough, and pulmonary infiltrates. For example, a patient with orthopnea, dyspnea on exertion, and pulmonary infiltrates may very well have a heart failure exacerbation and not an acute pneumonia.

Physical Examination

In addition to indicating signs of respiratory failure and sepsis, the physical examination can provide other useful information. The presence of clubbing suggests a chronic condition, such as a malignancy or prolonged hypoxemia from an underlying chronic lung disease. Cyanosis likewise suggests severe hypoxemia from either an acute process or a chronic condition such as congenital right-to-left shunt. An elevated jugular venous pressure may suggest an alternative cause of the patient's shortness of breath, such as cardiac tamponade, heart failure, pulmonary embolism, or pulmonary hypertension, although remember that pneumonia itself can precipitate a worsening of these underlying conditions. An undetectable or low jugular venous pressure may suggest that a patient is intravascularly volume depleted and may require aggressive fluid resuscitation.

The cardiac examination should focus on detecting signs of heart failure. Extremity warmth and distal pulses should also be assessed to look for signs of hypoperfusion or excessive vasodilation. Poor dentition can be a marker for anaerobic infections related to aspiration.

Finally, you should perform a lung exam to search for focal consolidations, effusions, and pleural inflammation. Remember that listening to the lung fields should be the last part of the pulmonary examination because observation, percussion, and palpation oftentimes provide enough information to localize a consolidation.

CLINICAL PEARL

Both consolidation and effusion will result in dullness to percussion, but only effusion will decrease tactile fremitus.

Labs and Test to Consider

It is only possible to identify the pathogen about 50% of the time in cases of community-acquired pneumonia. Certain tests can improve the likelihood of obtaining a diagnosis but can also help to risk-stratify patients as far as illness severity.

Key Diagnostic Labs and Tests

Blood cultures should be sent in all patients who are ill enough to be admitted to the hospital, preferably before the administration of antibiotics. Sputum Gram stain and culture can be helpful but may also be misleading if the patient is colonized with an organism, if the specimen is of poor quality, or if the patient has already received antibiotics. A quality sputum culture that does not yield gram-negative organisms or *Staphylococcus* is usually adequate evidence that these infections are not present. Nasopharyngeal aspirates to look for viral pneumonias are indicated during influenza season and have high specificities. Sputum induction does not increase the diagnostic yield for normal pathogens but may be useful in diagnosing tuberculosis and pathogens more common in immunocompromised patients, such as *Pneumocystis jiroveci* (see Chapter 30). Bronchoscopy is rarely indicated in patients with community-acquired pneumonia but may be necessary in immunocompromised patients or in patients who do not respond to empiric therapy. Urine testing for pneumococcal and legionella antigens are relatively inexpensive tests and are fairly specific in adult populations. They also maintain their sensitivity in patients who have already received antibiotics.

Laboratory evaluation should be conducted to search for signs of systemic hypoperfusion and end-organ dysfunction. A complete blood count should be sent to look for an elevated or low white blood cell count, either of which can be a sign of a serious infection. A differential should also be obtained to look for signs of a left shift. Thrombocytopenia may also be a sign of severe infection. Arterial blood gas analysis should be performed in any patient with signs of respiratory distress or a significant oxygen requirement. It should also be sent in any patient with hypotension or a low bicarbonate level in order to assess acid–base status. A serum lactate level may be useful to assess for hypoperfusion.

About half of all patients hospitalized with pneumonia will have a pleural effusion, but only a small percentage of patients will go on to develop a complicated parapneumonic effusion or empyema. Thoracentesis should be considered if the collection is moderate to large, the patient is severely ill, or the patient has persistent signs of infection despite appropriate antibiotics (see Chapter 22).

Imaging

Because, by definition, pneumonia implies consolidation, all patients suspected of having pneumonia should have chest radiography. If an infiltrate is not present on plain radiograph, computed tomography scanning of the chest may be useful to search for an infiltrate and, more importantly, to explore other etiologies of shortness of breath, fever, and chest pain. Some clinicians believe that an infiltrate may blossom after a patient is volume resuscitated. There is some controversy surrounding this issue but repeat chest radiography may be in order after fluid resuscitation if the initial chest radiograph was negative and the clinical picture otherwise suggests pneumonia. This may also

TABLE 25-1
Radiologic Findings of Pneumonia and Their Possible Significance

Radiologic Finding	Significance
Lobar infiltrate with air bronchograms (see Fig. 25-1A)	Possible *Pneumococcus*
Diffuse interstitial pattern or a combined alveolar/interstitial pattern (see Fig. 25-1B)	Atypical pathogens
Diffuse alveolar infiltrates (see Fig. 25-1C)	Possible acute respiratory distress syndrome
Upper lobe infiltrates	Possible tuberculosis
Cavitary lesions	Tuberculosis or other mycobacterial infections, anaerobic or necrotizing infections, malignancy, autoimmune disease, or septic pulmonary emboli
Bronchiectasis	Chronic infections such as atypical mycobacteria; chronic lung disease such as cystic fibrosis or ciliary dyskinesia
Superior segment of the lower lobes or posterior segment of the right upper lobe	Aspiration pneumonia

be the case in patients who are granulocytopenic because they may not be able to mount enough of an inflammatory response to create an infiltrate.

The pattern of infiltrate may provide valuable diagnostic information (Table 25-1).

Chest radiography may also provide information about the presence and character of pleural effusions and help to inform the decision about whether or not a thoracentesis is indicated. An enlarged cardiac silhouette may signify a pericardial effusion or an enlarged heart secondary to a dilated cardiomyopathy. An enlarged vascular pedicle width may signify volume overload. Enlarged pulmonary arteries may indicate pulmonary hypertension.

A

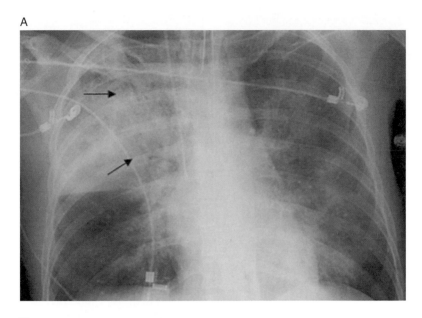

B

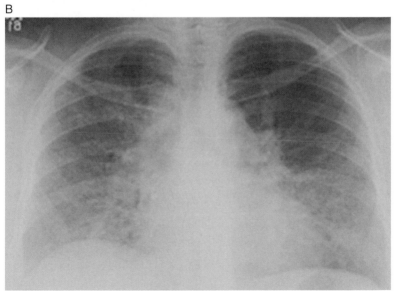

FIGURE 25-1: Common radiographic patterns of pneumonia. **A:** Right upper lobe infiltrate with air bronchograms (*arrows*). **B:** Diffuse interstitial infiltrates.

(continued)

C

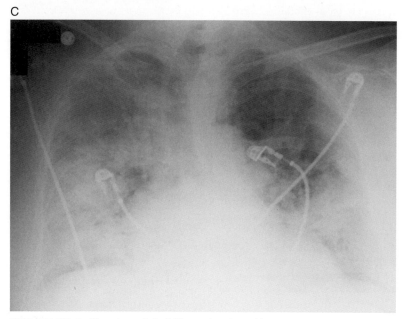

FIGURE 25-1: (Continued) **C:** Diffuse alveolar infiltrates. (*Images courtesy of Brian T. Garibaldi, MD, Division of Pulmonary and Critical Care Medicine, The Johns Hopkins Hospital.*)

If at all possible, you should review the films with the radiologist because you can provide contextual information and learn how to read radiographs from an expert at the same time.

Treatment

Early administration of antibiotics is probably the single most important intervention in a patient with pneumonia as it is one of the few interventions that has been shown to reduce mortality. A fluoroquinolone by itself or a macrolide plus a third-generation cephalosporin is usually the regimen of choice for inpatients. The IDSA recommends a minimum 5-day course. Treatment should continue until the patient is afebrile for 48 to 72 hours and is clinically stable.

If a patient is severely ill or at risk for a nosocomial pathogen, either piperacillin/tazobactam or cefepime at pseudomonal dosing plus a macrolide (to cover *Legionella* and atypical pathogens) should be used. With the recent rise of community-acquired methicillin-resistance *S. aureus* (MRSA) infections, vancomycin should be added empirically in patients who are severely ill or who have evidence of a necrotizing infection. Severe infections such as MRSA and *Pseudomonas* may require as many as 14 to 21 days of intravenous antibiotics.

If a patient is exhibiting signs of sepsis, then aggressive fluid resuscitation should be started while contacting the intensive care unit for closer observation and possible invasive hemodynamic monitoring. If a patient is demonstrating signs of respiratory distress or has a low oxygen saturation despite high levels of oxygen, noninvasive positive-pressure ventilation or intubation and mechanical ventilation may be indicated.

EXTENDED IN-HOSPITAL MANAGEMENT

A number of patients will deteriorate and require either intermediate-level or intensive care unit (ICU)–level care after admission. Persistent fever, worsening oxygen requirement, respiratory distress, deterioration in mental status, increasing white blood cell count, and even persistent/worsening sinus tachycardia may all be signs that a patient's infection is progressing to sepsis, ARDS, or both, despite appropriate therapy. Parapneumonic effusions are a common occurrence and can oftentimes lead to persistent infection. Repeat imaging should be performed in patients who fail to improve in order to evaluate for the presence of a fluid collection that will need to be sampled and possibly drained.

It is also important to look for other potential causes of deterioration. Common problems in a sick, immobile patient are pulmonary embolism, nosocomial infections, and symptomatic heart failure after fluid resuscitation. Again, the key is recognizing these patients early and getting them to an intermediate-care unit or ICU-level setting for aggressive monitoring and treatment.

Elderly patients and severely ill patients should have physical and occupational therapy to shorten their inpatient rehabilitation stay after their hospitalization. Even in patients who do not require rehabilitation, getting them up and out of bed early will help them mobilize their secretions and reduce the risk of feared complications, such as pressure sores, decubitus ulcers, and venous thromboembolism.

DISPOSITION

Discharge Goals

In general, patients are ready to go home when their fever has resolved and they are once again maintaining an acceptable oxygen saturation while breathing ambient air. They also need to be able to tolerate a diet by mouth so that they can remain hydrated and take oral antibiotics if they have not already completed their treatment course. Sometimes it is possible to arrange for home oxygen with close outpatient follow-up, but this depends in part on the particular patient and whether or not insurance will cover that level of home care.

At discharge, all patients should receive vaccination against influenza if it is during the influenza season. Patients over the age of 65 or with comorbidities such as lung disease, diabetes, or immunosuppression should also receive the adult pneumococcal vaccine.

Outpatient Care

Most patients can follow up with their primary care physician in 1 to 2 weeks after discharge from the hospital. Be sure to contact the patient's primary care physician during his or her hospitalization. The primary care physician can often be a helpful resource about the patient's past medical history and may be able to assist in scheduling outpatient follow-up.

 WHAT YOU NEED TO REMEMBER

- Community-acquired pneumonia is a common diagnosis that often requires admission to the hospital.
- In general, elderly patients and patients with comorbid conditions are likely to be sicker and require a higher level of care.
- Recognize patients with respiratory failure and/or sepsis early and refer to the intensive care unit as soon as possible.
- Chest radiography is essential and may provide important clues to the diagnosis and severity of the pneumonia.
- Early administration of antibiotics is a critical intervention that may reduce mortality.
- Monitor your patients closely for signs of clinical deterioration, such as an increased work of breathing, persistent fever, confusion, and tachycardia.

REFERENCE

1. Lim WS, van der Eerden MM, Laing R, et al. Defining community acquired pneumonia severity on presentation to hospital: an international derivation and validation study. *Thorax.* 2003;58:377–382.
2. Mandell LA, Wunderink RG, Anzueto A, et al.; Infectious Diseases Society of America. Infectious Diseases Society of America/American Thoracic Society consensus guidelines on the management of community-acquired pneumonia in adults. *Clin Infect Dis.* 2007;44(Suppl 2):S27–72.

SUGGESTED READINGS

Bartlett JG. Diagnostic test for etiologic agents of community-acquired pneumonia. *Infect Dis Clin North Am.* 2004;18(4):809–827.
Fine MJ, Auble TE, Yealy DM, et al. A prediction rule to identify low-risk patients with community-acquired pneumonia. *N Engl J Med.* 1997;336:243–250.
Washington L, Palacio D. Imaging of bacterial pulmonary infection in the immunocompetent patient. *Semin Roentgenol.* 2007;42(2):122–145.

Meningitis

THE PATIENT ENCOUNTER

A 68-year-old man develops cough, fever, headache, and confusion. While his wife is driving him to the emergency room, he has a generalized seizure. A chest radiograph shows a right lower lobe consolidation. Cerebrospinal fluid from lumbar puncture is remarkable for 1,120 white blood cells (72% neutrophils), 0 red blood cells, glucose of 15 mg/dL, protein of 120 mg/dL, and gram-positive diplococci on Gram stain.

OVERVIEW

Definition

Meningitis describes meningeal inflammation secondary to infection, chemical irritation, or neoplasm. This chapter will focus predominantly on infectious meningitis.

Pathophysiology

Meningitis occurs when an irritant, typically infection, gains access to the central nervous system (CNS) through one of four mechanisms:

1. *Hematogenous spread* requires host aberrations, pathogenic virulence factors, or a combination of the two.
2. *Direct extension* most commonly occurs with spread from sinusitis, otitis, or mastoiditis into the CNS, but can arise from epidural abscess, tumor, or other adjacent sources of irritants.
3. *Invasive procedures* may seed the CNS space directly.
4. *Retrograde infection* along a nerve into the CNS is a specific feature of a limited number of viruses, including herpes simplex virus (HSV).

Regardless of the mechanism of entry, meningeal inflammation can contribute to vasculitis, ischemia, and direct cytotoxicity. This can lead to infarction or, more commonly, swelling and elevated intracranial pressure (ICP). With increasing age, patients are also at increased risk for mortality from systemic manifestations of their infection including sepsis, adult respiratory distress syndrome (ARDS), and disseminated intravascular coagulation.

Epidemiology

In the United States, bacterial meningitis occurs in approximately 3 cases per 100,000 people. Viral meningitis likely affects 1 of 10,000 people annually (1).

TABLE 26-1
Common Etiologies of Bacterial Meningitis Arranged by Host Factors

Host Factor	Common Organisms
Age <50	*Streptococcus pneumoniae, Neisseria meningitidis*
Age >50	*S. pneumoniae, N. meningitidis, Listeria monocytogenes,* GBS
Presence of diabetes, cirrhosis, alcoholism at any age	*S. pneumoniae, N. meningitidis, L. monocytogenes,* GBS, GNR, *Enterococcus, Staphylococcus aureus*
Pregnancy	*S. pneumoniae, N. meningitidis, L. monocytogenes,* GBS
AIDS or immunosuppression	*S. pneumoniae, N. meningitidis, L. monocytogenes,* GBS, GNR, *S. aureus,* CoNS
Recent neurosurgical procedure	*S. pneumoniae,* GBS, GNR, *S. aureus,* CoNS

AIDS, acquired immunodeficiency syndrome; CoNS, coagulase-negative *Staphylococcus*; GBS, group B *Streptococcus*; GNR, gram-negative rod.

Etiology

The etiology of infectious meningitis is heavily dependent on host factors as shown in Table 26-1. In adults, about 50% are due to *Streptococcus pneumoniae*, 25% from *Neisseria meningitidis*, 15% from group B *Streptococcus*, and 10% from *Listeria monocytogenes*. Although markedly fewer cases of *Haemophilus influenzae* are seen since comprehensive childhood vaccination was started, there are still occasional cases in unvaccinated adults.

Viral meningitis is typically secondary to enteroviruses (up to 75% of cases), although HSV, arboviruses, Ebstein-Bar virus (EBV), human immunodeficiency virus (HIV), and varicella zoster virus (VZV) are common.

ACUTE MANAGEMENT AND WORKUP

Bacterial meningitis should be suspected whenever the triad of headache, fever, and nuchal rigidity is present. The full triad is found 40% to 70% of the time and nearly all patients with bacterial meningitis have at least one component. In an immunocompetent patient, the absence of all three components of the meningitic triad during an acute illness nearly negates the possibility of bacterial meningitis.

The First 15 Minutes

Morbidity in adults with meningitis is shared by neurologic and systemic complications. Seizures, a diminished Glasgow Coma Scale (GCS) Score, and focal neurologic signs should be noted. Systemically, signs of sepsis as well as respiratory distress must be recognized early.

Initial Assessment

Preparation for lumbar puncture (LP) should begin during the initial encounter. Acute, pre-LP head imaging should be considered for any patient with a decreased level of consciousness, recent seizure, cranial nerve palsy, papilledema, or evidence of Cushing's triad (increased blood pressure, decreased heart rate, and somnolence). A head computed tomography (CT) scan should also be obtained in immunocompromised patients, in those with head trauma or cancer, and in any patient older than age 65.

Timely administration of antibiotics is critical. If bacterial meningitis is suspected and any factors, including head imaging, result in a delay of the LP, then blood cultures should be drawn and empiric antibiotics should be started before the LP.

Admission Criteria and Level of Care Criteria

Patients with meningitis almost always require admission. Intensive care unit consultation should be obtained for patients with the following risk factors: decreased GCS score, the presence of cranial nerve palsies, the presence of organisms on Gram stain, seizures, focal neurologic findings, sepsis, or ARDS. Stigmata of increased ICP on the physical, history, or head imaging should lead to neurosurgical consultation for management and/or invasive pressure monitoring.

The First Few Hours

Once the diagnosis of meningitis is considered and the LP is obtained, you can begin to gather additional information to help further guide diagnosis and management.

History

One initial branch point in the differential diagnosis of meningitis is illness tempo. Chronic meningitis is frequently related to tuberculosis (TB), neoplasm, fungus, or medications. Subacute meningitis evolves over several days to weeks and shares etiologies with chronic meningitis, but also includes partially treated bacterial meningitis and persistent viral illness. Acute meningitis develops over 1 to 3 days and is most typically from a virus or bacteria. Fulminant meningitis progresses over 24 hours and strongly suggests a bacterial etiology. Instantaneous or stuttering progression is worrisome for subarachnoid hemorrhage, which can symptomatically masquerade as meningitis.

In addition to the tempo and cerebrospinal fluid (CSF) profile, the severity of the illness can suggest the etiology. A history of profound neurologic change including seizure, focal weakness, cranial nerve palsy, confusion, or significant somnolence should never be attributed to viral meningitis and suggests bacterial, amebic, or rickettsial meningitis or viral encephalitis.

Conditions such as asplenia, complement deficiency, or hypogammaglobulinemia suggest increased risk of infection with encapsulated organisms. A number of other host risk factors should be investigated (see Table 26-1).

Further questioning should be directed toward clinical manifestations of specific organisms. For example, a maculopapular rash or petechiae is commonly the herald of *N. meningitidis*, but can also be seen in rickettsial disease. Recent basilar skull fracture, sinusitis, ear infection, or pneumonia is characteristic of *S. pneumoniae* infection, a likely diagnosis in our patient from the encounter.

A more indolent and benign course is suggestive of a viral process and may include constitutional symptoms such as myalgia, arthralgia, abdominal pain, diarrhea, and pharyngitis. Furthermore, viral etiologies are more likely during the summer and fall. The history should search for regional clusters, suggesting an arbovirus outbreak. Patients should also be asked about history of HSV or VZV, although up to 50% of cases with meningitis have no rash. In addition, HIV risk factors should be assessed given the high prevalence of viral meningitis in primary HIV infection.

Given the potential for rickettsial infections, all patients should be asked about camping, hiking, or other activities that may have led to tick or mosquito exposure. Lastly, a careful medication history should be taken, including recent changes and known chemical irritants (isoniazid, sulfa moieties, nonsteroidal anti-inflammatory medications, and epidural injections).

Patients with subacute or chronic meningitis may present with more nonspecific findings. For these patients, a more thorough history involving changes in personality, indolent cranial nerve palsies, numbness or weakness in the arms or legs, or clumsiness might suggest CNS inflammation. Because of the increased risk of TB, syphilis, and partially treated or parameningeal infection in this group, further questions should search for risk factors or a history of these infections.

Causes of chronic meningitis particular to acquired immunodeficiency syndrome and immunocompromised patients are broad. However, a travel history is particularly worthwhile (American Southwest, *Coccidioides*; Mississippi River Valley, *Histoplasmosis*; American Midwest, *Blastomycoses*). Skin manifestations may point toward *Cryptococcus*, while oral ulcers point toward histoplasmosis.

In difficult cases, unusual exposures may be elicited, including bat exposure or animal bites (rabies), bird exposure (psittacosis), cat exposure (*Bartonella*), and the ingestion of unpasteurized dairy products (*Brucella*). Patients should be asked about B symptoms, weight loss, carcinogenic exposures/known cancers, and completion of age-appropriate cancer screening. Other unusual inflammatory causes may include Behçet or CNS lupus. CNS sarcoidosis should be considered in patients with a history of abnormal chest radiography or erythema nodosum.

Physical Examination

You should begin the exam by looking for the stigmata of increased ICP. The level of consciousness, including a GCS score, should be documented. A funduscopic exam, cranial nerve exam, and global assessment of strength and sensation should be performed. When time permits, a thorough neurologic examination should be conducted given the potential for complications of meningitis, including stroke, myelopathy, and radiculopathy. The assessment of meningeal irritation can often be elicited simply with resistance or pain on neck flexion; however, Kernig's sign (extension of the leg at the knee with the hip flexed, leading to pain) and Brudzinski's sign (involuntary leg flexion during neck flexion) should also be checked. It is important to realize that these maneuvers are <50% accurate in adults and even less accurate in immunosuppressed, somnolent, and elderly patients.

The head, neck, and chest examination should look for the stigmata of otitis, sinusitis, pharyngitis, and pneumonia, which might suggest pneumococcal infection. A thorough skin exam should look for zoster rash, herpetic vesicles, or evidence of cutaneous *Cryptococcus*. Maculopapular or petechial rash, while present in Rocky Mountain spotted fever (RMSF), ehrlichiosis, and several viral illnesses, should always raise concern for fulminant meningococcemia. The musculoskeletal exam should include palpation of the entirety of the spine and paraspinal regions to look for evidence of vertebral osteomyelitis or a paraspinal abscess. Arthritis may suggest *Neisseria*.

Labs and Tests to Consider

The importance of CSF analysis cannot be overstated. However, it should be recognized that CSF profiles change over time and that diagnosing the etiology of the meningitis often relies on additional lab tests.

Key Diagnostic Labs and Tests

LP should be performed as early as possible (Table 26-2). An initial hematologic profile, coagulation panel, blood cultures, urinalysis/culture, and sputum culture should also be performed.

Bacterial etiologies can be evaluated with *S. pneumoniae* urinary antigen, latex agglutination testing for common bacterial etiologies in the CSF, or broad-array polymerase chain reaction (PCR) in both CSF and blood. Serologies can be sent for *Chlamydia psittaci*, *Brucella*, and Q fever. RMSF or ehrlichiosis can be detected by immunofluorescence, PCR, or serology. Rapid plasma reagin should be sent from the blood and Venereal Disease Research Laboratories from the CSF if syphilis is suspected. Skin lesions should be biopsied to look for meningococcus at the dermal interface. If

TABLE 26-2
Classic CSF Abnormalities in Meningitis

Process	Opening Pressure	Protein (mg/dL)	Glucose (mg/dL)	Cell Count/ Differential	Stain
Normal	6–20 cm H$_2$O	18–58	>6/10 of serum or >40 mg/dL	RBC: <2 WBC: <5 PMN: ~70%	No organism on stain and sterile culture
Bloody tap	Normal	Up by 1 mg/dL: 1K RBCs	Normal to decreased	1 WBC:700 RBCs RBCs clearing between tubes	Normal
Bacterial	>18 cm H$_2$O	Elevated	Normal to very decreased	WBC: >1,000 or 100–1000 PMN: >50%	Gram stain positive in 60%–80% of untreated cases
Viral	Normal to elevated	Normal to elevated	Typically normal	WBC: 5–2,000 PMN: <50%	No organism on stain, viral PCRs may be positive
Fungal	Increased	May be markedly increased	Normal to decreased	WBC: 10–500 Monocyte: >50%	India ink stain: 80% sensitive on large volumes of CSF
TB	Usually increased	Mildly to markedly elevated	Mildly to markedly decreased	WBC: 10–500 Early: PMN >50% Late: PMN <50%	Acid fast stain positive in 10%–40%
Neoplasm	Variable	Increased	Normal to decreased	Variable	Flow cytometry often positive

CSF, cerebrospinal fluid; PCR, polymerase chain reaction; PMN, polymorphonuclear leukocyte; RBC, red blood cell; TB, tuberculosis; WBC, white blood cell.

viral meningitis is suspected, tests should include CSF/serum PCR and serologies for HSV, VZV, West Nile virus, HIV, EBV, enterovirus, adenovirus, or influenza, if suspected.

A workup for fungal infection should begin with a CSF fungal culture and smear but should also include a search for possible immunodeficiency. Specific tests are available for CSF/serum cryptococcal antigen, urinary/CSF/serum histoplasma antigen or antibody, and CSF/serum coccidioidal antibody. If TB is strongly suspected, a purified protein derivative should be placed and multiple cultures, including CSF, serum, urine, and sputum mycobacterial cultures, should be obtained to increase the yield. If there is a concern for malignancy, CSF and peripheral blood flow cytometry and cytopathology should be ordered.

Imaging

In addition to performing an initial noncontrast CT before LP in selected patients, nearly all patients with meningitis warrant neuroimaging. This is particularly true with any change in neurologic status or focal neurologic signs. Magnetic resonance imaging (MRI) will detect small lesions or complications, but a head CT scan is often an appropriate first choice to assess for catastrophic conditions such as a large bleed, a mass lesion, or diffuse cerebral edema, as well as to evaluate for sinusitis or mastoiditis. Patients should also have chest radiography given the association of meningitis in adults with ARDS and pneumonia.

> **CLINICAL PEARL**
>
> *HSV encephalitis commonly demonstrates temporal enhancement on MRI with gadolinium.*

A spinal MRI should be obtained if there is suspicion for an epidural abscess. Lastly, electroencephalography is occasionally used to look for a temporal focus that is suggestive of HSV encephalitis.

Treatment

Empiric treatment is chosen based on host factors, clinical suspicion, and initial testing, including Gram stain. Therapy can then be refined based on test results and clinical response.

In bacterial meningitis, the backbone of therapy is a third-generation cephalosporin. Vancomycin is added to address increasing resistance of *S. pneumoniae* to penicillin. If the patient is at risk for *L. monocytogenes*, then ampicillin should be added. In neurosurgical patients, it is important to select a cephalosporin with good coverage of *Pseudomonas*.

If viral encephalitis, especially HSV, is a concern, empiric acyclovir should be started pending results of PCR and culture. If a CNS abscess is found, metronidazole should be added and infectious disease/surgical consultation obtained. Fungal meningitis is typically treated with liposomal amphotericin B. Lifelong suppressive therapy with fluconazole may be necessary. If TB is suspected, four-drug therapy with isoniazid, rifampin, pyrazinamide, and ethambutol should be started and an infectious disease specialist should be consulted.

Steroid use is the subject of long-standing debate, but the current weight of the literature appears to support steroid use in proven or nearly certain cases of bacterial meningitis. Steroids should be given with the first dose of antibiotics and for 4 days in immunocompetent hosts, with the most benefit in *S. pneumoniae* infections. Steroid critics note decreased CSF antibiotic penetration and lack of validation in special populations. Steroids are also likely useful with antimicrobial therapy in patients with TB, especially in the setting of a decreased GCS. Increased morbidity and mortality have been suggested when patients receive steroids in the absence of appropriate antimicrobial therapy. The patient in our encounter should probably receive corticosteroids with his first dose of antibiotics.

A neurologist or neurointensivist should be involved in the treatment of neurologic complications of meningitis. No role has been shown for primary prophylaxis with antiseizure medications, but they should be considered for secondary prophylaxis. With increased ICP, hyperventilation may be used for very brief intervals as a bridge to other therapies, but ultimate control may require mannitol, hypertonic saline, or surgical decompression. In general, antihypertensive medications should be avoided given the potential for later sepsis and possible insult to the cerebral perfusion pressure if the ICP is elevated.

EXTENDED IN-HOSPITAL MANAGEMENT

Long hospital stays should include vigilance for nosocomial complications and early aggressive rehabilitation. For persistent meningitis that defies diagnosis, serial LPs have value given the evolution of CSF profiles over time. Repeat CSF examination for mycobacteria, flow cytometry, and cytology can improve sensitivity of these low-yield tests. Broader imaging for occult neoplasm can be considered.

DISPOSITION

Discharge Goals

Patients can be discharged once an etiology for their meningitis is identified and they show neurologic improvement or stability. Oral antibiotics are not used for acute meningitis, so patients must either stay in the hospital to complete their antibiotic course or have a special catheter placed that is appropriate for home or skilled nursing facility use.

Outpatient Care

Viral meningitis is an acute and self-limited illness and requires standard follow-up with an outpatient physician to ensure continued improvement. Bacterial meningitis often leaves patients with significant long-term morbidity, and rehabilitation is often an important component of outpatient care. Importantly, contacts of patients with *N. meningitidis* (including hospital staff and health care providers) should complete a course of rifampin or ciprofloxacin prophylaxis. Patients with fungal, tuberculous, or other infections requiring a prolonged treatment course should follow up with an infectious disease specialist regularly after discharge.

WHAT YOU NEED TO REMEMBER

- Bacterial meningitis is a life-threatening neurologic emergency and warrants rapid evaluation, urgent antibiotics, and close monitoring.
- Even with optimal treatment, mortality for bacterial meningitis is about 25%.
- The stigmata of increased ICP, especially with an abnormal head CT, should prompt intensive care unit admission and neurosurgical consultation.
- CSF profiles change over time in many infections.
- CSF profile results are fallible. Sick patients should receive broad therapy until Gram stain, culture, and PCR results are available.

REFERENCE

1. Roos KL, Tyler KL. Meningitis, encephalitis, brain abscess and empyema. In: Fauci AS, Braunwald E, Kasper DL, et al., eds. *Harrison's Principles of Internal Medicine*. 17th ed. New York: McGraw-Hill; 2008.

SUGGESTED READINGS

Fitch M, van de Beek D. Drug insight: steroids in CNS infectious disease-new indications for an old therapy. *Nat Clin Pract Neurol*. 2008;4:97–104.

Kastenbauer S, Pfister H. Pneumococcal meningitis in adults. *Brain*. 2003;126: 1015–1025.

van de Beek D, de Gans J, Tunkel AR, et al. Community-acquired bacterial meningitis in adults. *N Engl J Med*. 2006;354(1):44–53.

Urinary Tract Infections and Pyelonephritis

THE PATIENT ENCOUNTER

A 75-year-old woman is brought to the emergency room by ambulance from a local nursing home because she was found by the staff to be febrile, mildly confused, and incontinent. She is indicating that she has suprapubic and left flank pain and she has vomited once. A urinalysis demonstrates white blood cells too numerous to count, a moderate amount of red blood cells, positive nitrite, and positive leukocyte esterase.

OVERVIEW

Definition

A urinary tract infection (UTI) may involve only the lower urinary tract or both the upper and lower tracts. Two common presentations are acute cystitis, defined as an infection of the bladder epithelium, and acute pyelonephritis, defined as an infection of the renal parenchyma and collecting system.

Pathophysiology

Infections of the urinary tract commonly occur when bacteria migrate from the rectum and enter through the distal urethra, thereafter ascending to the bladder or kidneys. Infection results when the bacteria overcome the normal anticolonization and antiadherence host defenses, such as urine flow, urea concentration, specialized bladder epithelium, the presence of the ureterovesical valves, and urine osmolarity and pH. Rarely, pyelonephritis can occur through hematogenous spread, especially with *Staphylococcus aureus*.

Epidemiology

The majority of UTIs occur in women (30:1 female-to-male ratio), mainly due to the proximity of the female urethra to the perianal areas and the shorter length of the female urethra. Almost 50% of women report having had at least one UTI in their lifetime. Men experience an increase in the rates of UTIs starting in their 40s and approach an incidence rate similar to women in their 60s, likely due to the increase in prostate gland hypertrophy. Each year in the United States, UTIs account for approximately 7 million doctor visits with an average cost per year of $1.6 billion (1).

Etiology

Most UTIs are caused by *Escherichia coli*, followed by *Proteus*, *Klebsiella*, and *Staphylococcus saprophyticus* for uncomplicated UTIs and enterococci, and *Pseudomonas*, *Staphylococcus epidermidis*, and other gram-negative rods for complicated UTIs. Catheter-associated UTIs are commonly caused by yeast (30%).

ACUTE MANAGEMENT AND WORKUP

The most important distinction in approaching a UTI is determining whether it is limited to acute lower tract disease, such as acute cystitis, urethritis, and prostatitis, or whether it involves the upper tract, such as pyelonephritis and renal abscess. The prompt treatment of pyelonephritis with intravenous (IV) antibiotics can help prevent progression to abscess formation, parenchymal scarring, and renal failure.

The First 15 Minutes

The initial management of a patient with a UTI centers on how far the infection has progressed.

Initial Assessment

A communicative, afebrile, well-appearing patient often has limited disease, whereas a febrile, confused, toxic-appearing patient, such as the one in our patient encounter, likely has a disseminated infection. This distinction is important because a patient with simple acute cystitis can be managed at a more leisurely pace than can a patient with a more serious pyelonephritis. At times, a UTI can lead to bacteremia and urosepsis, which need prompt treatment to prevent morbidity and mortality.

It is important to keep UTI in the back of your mind when evaluating patients with altered mental status because it is a very common cause of delirium, especially in patients with poor reserve.

Admission Criteria and Level of Care Criteria

A patient with an acute cystitis can almost always be managed as an outpatient, whereas patients with severe pyelonephritis or bacteremia likely require an inpatient admission for treatment with IV antibiotics and close observation. A compliant patient with acute uncomplicated pyelonephritis can often be stabilized with rehydration and antibiotics in an outpatient facility or emergency room and then sent home with oral antibiotics. Patients with high fevers, pain, and debilitation will likely need an inpatient admission for IV antibiotics. You should also consider extenuating circumstances, such as a previous renal transplant, an immunosuppressed state, diabetes mellitus, or pregnancy, because these will lower your threshold for admission.

> ### CLINICAL PEARL
>
> *The absence of upper tract symptoms in no way excludes upper tract infection.*

Urosepsis is commonly described as clinical evidence of a urinary tract infection plus two or more of the systemic inflammatory response syndrome criteria (see Chapter 29 for a more detailed discussion). Patients with evidence of urosepsis need prompt intensive care unit (ICU) consultation and management.

The First Few Hours

Once the patient has been stabilized, you can then proceed to take a proper history and perform a physical exam to help confirm your diagnosis and guide your management.

History

The diagnosis of an acute uncomplicated cystitis can essentially be made on the history alone. Acute cystitis commonly presents with a few days of dysuria, increased frequency, urgency, the production of small amounts of cloudy urine with or without blood, and occasionally suprapubic tenderness. In women who present with at least one symptom of a UTI, the probability of having an infection is approximately 50%. Certain combinations of symptoms (such as dysuria and frequency without vaginal discharge or irritation) increase the likelihood of infection.

Complicated cystitis is sometimes defined as a clinical syndrome that includes the previously mentioned symptoms of acute cystitis with the addition of fever, chills, flank pain, back pain, costovertebral angle (CVA) tenderness, or malaise. Patients with indwelling catheters, multidrug-resistant organisms, immunosuppression, and other risk factors for poor outcomes are also said to have complicated cystitis.

The signs and symptoms of complicated cystitis are very similar to those seen in acute uncomplicated pyelonephritis, which commonly presents with fever, chills, flank pain, and CVA tenderness. It is occasionally accompanied by nausea, vomiting, and diarrhea. The symptoms of lower tract disease may or may not be present. Pyelonephritis is frequently associated with bacteremia caused by the same organism as in the urine. Complicated pyelonephritis can be associated with underlying anatomic or functional abnormalities and may be associated with months of insidious signs, such as malaise, fatigue, nausea, and abdominal pain.

Once you have determined that the patient has a UTI, ask about any functional or anatomic abnormalities that would classify a UTI as complicated, such as urinary catheterization, a neurogenic bladder, obstructive uropathy with nephrolithiasis or fibrosis, azotemia due to intrinsic renal disease, and the presence of prostatic hypertrophy or other causes of urinary retention in men. Make sure to identify risk factors for UTIs, as modification of these factors may help to prevent recurrent infections. Common risk factors in all patients include diabetes, human immunodeficiency virus, lower socioeconomic group, and functional or cognitive impairment. Female-specific risk factors include pregnancy, sexual intercourse, lack of urination after intercourse, spermicidal jelly, diaphragm use, estrogen deficiency, and bladder prolapse. Male-specific risk factors include lack of circumcision, insertive rectal intercourse, condom catheters, and prostatic enlargement. Specific attention should also be given to any history of previous UTIs and any underlying diseases that would affect the management and decision to admit, such as an immunosuppressed state or renal transplantation.

Lastly, make sure to question the patient about other potential causes of his or her symptoms. Sexually transmitted diseases can cause urethritis, but are often accompanied by a history of a foul-smelling discharge, unprotected intercourse with an infected partner, and, occasionally, pelvic pain. Kidney stones often present with the predominant complaints of severe colicky flank pain and hematuria. Atrophic vaginitis classically presents in postmenopausal women with complaints of itching, soreness, and dyspareunia, in addition to dysuria. Benign prostatic hypertrophy is usually described as causing hesitancy, straining, weak flow, dribbling, dysuria, and nocturia. In patients who are unable to provide a good history, it may be necessary to contact family members or other care providers.

Physical Examination

Once it is determined that the patient is clinically stable, specific attention should be given to the abdominal exam, mainly evaluating the patient for suprapubic tenderness and CVA tenderness. CVA tenderness is described as pain elicited with fist percussion over the kidneys. Generally, the tenderness is not subtle and the patient will often jump when percussed.

CLINICAL PEARL

Start percussing for CVA tenderness well above the costovertebral angles and slowly work your way down. Sometimes the patient can be startled by the initial percussion and will jump, thereby clouding the accuracy of your exam.

A pelvic exam may be required if there are concurrent symptoms of a sexually transmitted disease. The cardiopulmonary exam can help identify any important comorbidities or signs of sepsis that would affect treatment. It is also useful to assess the patient's volume status as many older patients with UTIs, particularly those in long-term care facilities, may be dehydrated and will need IV fluids.

Labs and Test to Consider

In healthy women with symptoms of an uncomplicated cystitis, usually only a urinalysis is necessary. Any failure of treatment will necessitate a urine culture to evaluate for the causative organism and resistance patterns. If the patient has a complicated UTI or any other confounding variables, a urine culture and additional studies may be necessary.

Key Diagnostic Labs and Tests

Microscopic examination of a midstream voided urine specimen or a catheterized specimen is the first test to order when evaluating a patient for a UTI. Often it will show pyuria (defined as 8 to 10 leukocytes/mm^3) and bacteriuria with or without hematuria and proteinuria. A high number of epithelial cells indicates that the sample is contaminated and may yield false-positive results. The dipstick leukocyte esterase test, a rapid screening test for pyuria, is often positive. A positive nitrite test usually indicates the presence of Enterobacteriaceae, which convert nitrate to nitrite. A Gram stain of the urine specimen can also help with the diagnosis and can be correlated with the urine culture. A urine culture is considered positive if it yields $>10^5$ colony forming units (CFU)/mL in asymptomatic women, 10^3 CFU/mL in men, or 10^2 CFU/mL in symptomatic women with pyuria. Any patient with *S. aureus* recovered from the urine should be carefully screened for bacteremia and possible endocarditis, because *S. aureus* oftentimes seeds the kidney during active bacteremia.

In patients with suspected pyelonephritis, further evaluation requires a complete blood count with differential, renal function panel, and blood cultures. Patients who appear septic will need additional tests to evaluate for end-organ damage and acid–base status, such as liver function tests, lactate, bicarbonate, coagulation tests, and possibly an arterial blood gas.

Imaging

Most patients with cystitis or pyelonephritis do not need imaging. The failure of a patient to defervesce after appropriate antibiotics or recurrent infections should prompt some form of diagnostic imaging, usually a computed tomography scan with contrast to look for urinary tract pathology, such as an abscess, an obstruction, or a kidney stone. If the patient has evidence of renal failure, an ultrasound can also be used, although it is less sensitive. Because urinary tract infections are less common in men with normal anatomy, some clinicians argue that all men with urinary tract infections should undergo some form of imaging.

Treatment

The treatment of cystitis is based on whether it is uncomplicated or complicated. Forty to seventy percent of uncomplicated cystitis infections clear spontaneously. However, patients should still be treated with antibiotics to prevent possible progression to pyelonephritis. Women with acute uncomplicated cystitis can be treated as outpatients with 3 days of antibiotics, usually trimethoprim-sulfamethoxazole (TMP-SMX), cefpodoxime, or a fluoroquinolone, usually ciprofloxacin. Nitrofurantoin has been associated with lower cure rates and is often prescribed for 5 days. Patients with complicated cystitis should be treated for 7 to 14 days with a fluoroquinolone. TMP-SMX or nitrofurantoin should be avoided because of the high prevalence of resistance in patients with complicated cystitis. Parenteral antibiotics should be considered in patients with a history of previous UTIs with multiply-resistant organisms or those who are allergic to fluoroquinolones. These patients can be switched to oral therapy after clinical improvement. Symptoms of acute cystitis should resolve in 1 to 3 days; any patient who fails to respond to treatment or develops a recurrent UTI needs further investigation. For patients with severe dysuria, urinary analgesia can be provided with phenazopyridine for 1 to 2 days.

Patients with uncomplicated pyelonephritis should be treated with 7 days of antibiotics. First-line therapy should be with a fluoroquinolone or ceftriaxone. If gram-positive cocci are observed on the Gram stain, then amoxicillin should be added to cover *Enterococcus* until the causative agent is identified. Complicated pyelonephritis should be managed as an inpatient with broad-spectrum antibiotics, such as piperacillin-tazobactam, cefepime, meropenem, or ticarcillin-clavulanate. Underlying anatomic or functional abnormalities of the urinary tract should be managed in conjunction with a urologist.

The patient in our encounter has features suggestive of urosepsis, with possible complicated pyelonephritis. She will need IV antibiotics and aggressive fluid resuscitation. Further management will be dictated by how she responds over the first 1 to 2 days of treatment.

CLINICAL PEARL

In a patient with a previous history of UTIs, reviewing any known culture data for causative organisms and resistance patterns can help tailor therapy.

EXTENDED IN-HOSPITAL MANAGEMENT

Most patients admitted with acute pyelonephritis will improve within 24 to 48 hours if administered appropriate antibiotics. If a patient is not improving, consider possible antibiotic resistance or an alternative diagnosis. One possibility to consider is a renal abscess, which presents similarly to acute pyelonephritis except that the fever persists despite appropriate antibiotics. In patients with bacteremia, it is appropriate to send surveillance blood cultures to demonstrate clearance of the pathogen. Patients with urosepsis will need the appropriate supportive measures, often in an ICU, until the infection has resolved and the hemodynamic parameters have stabilized.

DISPOSITION

Discharge Goals

Patients can be discharged once their infection has resolved, indicated by resolution of their fever, pain, and any hemodynamic instability. They also need to be able to tolerate adequate fluids and oral antibiotics to finish the recommended length of treatment. Any underlying anatomic or functional abnormalities should be addressed in conjunction with a urologist, and any identified risk factors modified.

Outpatient Care

For patients being treated as outpatients for acute cystitis, a follow-up call in 2 to 3 days to ensure resolution of symptoms is recommended. A follow-up urinalysis or culture is not indicated unless symptoms persist. Patients discharged after an admission for pyelonephritis or urosepsis should follow up with their primary care physician in 1 to 2 weeks. Any necessary follow-up appointments with urology or follow-up imaging should be arranged prior to discharge.

WHAT YOU NEED TO REMEMBER

- Urinary tract infections constitute a spectrum of diseases ranging from acute uncomplicated cystitis to severe pyelonephritis with abscess formation.
- The severity of the disease, comorbidities, and risk factors help guide whether the patient requires parental or oral antibiotics and whether the condition can be managed as an inpatient or outpatient.
- Any patient with evidence of urosepsis needs to be managed aggressively, and those who are unstable require an early referral to the ICU.
- With appropriate antibiotics, the patient should improve within 24 to 48 hours.

REFERENCE

1. Bent S, Nallamothu BK, Simel DL, et al. Does this woman have an acute uncomplicated urinary tract infection? *JAMA*. 2002;287(20):2701–2710.

SUGGESTED READINGS

Fihn SD. Acute uncomplicated urinary tract infection in women. *N Engl J Med*. 2003;349:259.

Sobel JD, Kaye D. Urinary tract infections. In: Mandell GL, Bennett JE, Dolin R, eds. *Principles and Practice of Infectious Diseases*. 6th ed. Philadelphia: Churchill Livingstone Elsevier; 2004.

28

Endocarditis

THE PATIENT ENCOUNTER

A 34-year-old African American man presents to the emergency department with fevers, chills, loss of appetite, and malaise over the past several weeks. He has no history of heart disease but uses intravenous heroin daily. Pertinent physical findings include a temperature of 38.4°C (101.1°F), a heart rate of 112 bpm, respiratory rate of 30 breaths per minute, and a 3/6 systolic ejection murmur radiating to the axilla.

OVERVIEW

Definition

Infective endocarditis is a microbial infection of the endocardial surface of the heart, classically manifesting as a discrete lesion or "vegetation," which is composed of platelets, fibrin, and bacteria that adhere to the heart valves. Although there are some noninfectious causes of valvular vegetations, such as nonbacterial thrombotic endocarditis or marantic endocarditis, this chapter will focus on the approach to and management of inpatients with infective endocarditis.

Pathophysiology

Infective endocarditis requires both a source of bacteremia and an abnormal endothelial surface, which allows for adhesion of the bacteria. Bacteremia occurs daily with microbial translocation across mucosal surfaces as a part of normal activities, such as routine dental hygiene or bowel movements. More directly, the injection of drugs or dialysis catheter access can introduce bacteria into the bloodstream. In a normal individual with a healthy cardiovascular system, transient bacteremia will not lead to endocarditis. However, in patients with valvular prostheses or who have sustained prior endothelial damage due to vascular disease or extrinsic factors (e.g., repetitive exposure to impurities found in street drugs), even transient bacteremia may lead to endocarditis.

Epidemiology

The incidence of endocarditis is between 2 and 6 per 100,000 patients and is higher in intravenous drug abusers (1).

Etiology

In cases where a blood culture is positive, 80% of bacterial endocarditis is caused by *Streptococcus*, *Enterococcus*, or *Staphylococcus* species. Culture-negative endocarditis can be caused by bacterial species from the HACEK group (*Haemophilus*, *Actinobacillus*, *Cardiobacterium*, *Eikenella*, and *Kingella*); intracellular organisms, such as *Coxiella brunetii* (referred to as Q fever), *Bartonella*, *Chlamydia*, *Tropheryma whipplei*, *Legionella*, and *Brucella* species; and in rare cases, fungi.

ACUTE MANAGEMENT AND WORKUP

A focused history and physical exam in the emergency department should alert you to the possible diagnosis of endocarditis.

The First 15 Minutes

Quickly assess for the most catastrophic complications and determine the level of care the patient will require in the short term.

Initial Assessment

First, assess the overall appearance of the patient to get a general sense of how ill or "toxic" he or she appears. It is important to recognize septic patients, such as the one in our patient encounter, early in the course of their illness in order to improve outcomes (see Chapter 29).

Pay special attention to the cardiac exam. A new cardiac murmur is an important part of the diagnostic criteria for endocarditis and may provide clues to the site of the infection as well as guide further diagnostic studies. Even more important to determine in your initial assessment is whether there is evidence of cardiac complications of endocarditis such as heart failure or, in some cases, heart block, because these patients will require a higher level of care. The pulmonary exam is also critical because patients may develop respiratory failure from acute respiratory distress syndrome or have evidence of septic pulmonary emboli detectable as either focal consolidations or pleural inflammation. Finally, look for any neurologic abnormalities suggestive of meningeal irritation, thrombotic or hemorrhagic stroke, or hypoperfusion from sepsis.

Admission Criteria and Level of Care Criteria

Any patient with suspected endocarditis will require a hospital admission for blood cultures and an echocardiogram. Oral antibiotics are not the standard of care. Therefore, the diagnosis must be certain and a plan for long-term intravenous antibiotic treatment must be established before the patient can be safely monitored as an outpatient.

Patients who meet criteria for sepsis or show signs of cardiac, respiratory, or neurologic complications will need close observation in an intermediate care–or intensive care unit–level setting.

The First Few Hours

Once the patient is clinically stable, you can begin to gather more detailed information to help guide diagnostic testing and management.

History

It is critical to ask about predisposing factors to endocarditis, including intravenous drug use, indwelling hardware such as a pacemaker or hemodialysis catheter, and certain high-risk heart conditions, including previous endocarditis, prosthetic valves, degenerative aortic or mitral valve disease, a history of rheumatic fever, congenital heart disease, and aortic coarctation.

The time course of symptoms provides important information. Traditionally, streptococcal endocarditis has a more gradual course compared to *Staphylococcus aureus*, which is generally abrupt in onset. In addition to general symptoms like fever, anorexia, weight loss, malaise, and night sweats, specifically ask about symptoms indicative of associated complications: chest pain (pericardial involvement), cough or shortness of breath (congestive heart failure/pulmonary edema or septic pulmonary emboli), visual changes, focal weakness, headache (central nervous system emboli), abdominal pain, nausea, vomiting and diarrhea (systemic embolic involving liver, spleen, or mesenteric arteries), and decreased urine output or hematuria (renal emboli or immune complex glomerulonephritis). Whole body aches and pains, especially back pain, can also be a predominant feature of endocarditis and may reflect either systemic inflammation or septic thromboembolism.

Be aware of risk factors for certain pathogens. Injection drug users are at highest risk for methicillin-resistant *S. aureus* (MRSA) and fungal endocarditis. Recent dental work may predispose to infection with *Streptococcus viridans*. Cystoscopy or urinary tract manipulation is associated with enterococcal endocarditis.

In forming a broader differential, consider other causes of fever, anorexia, and malaise that may mimic endocarditis.

CLINICAL PEARL

Particularly in intravenous drug users, acute human immunodeficiency virus infection can often manifest with generalized signs and symptoms similar to infective endocarditis.

Malignancy can cause nonbacterial thrombotic endocarditis. Other valvular vegetations can also mimic the syndrome of infective endocarditis such as atrial myxoma, systemic lupus erythematosus, and rheumatic fever.

Physical Examination

In addition to a primary focus on signs of sepsis, shock, heart failure, and neurologic or respiratory involvement, a detailed physical examination can provide other classic clues.

Cardiac examination should focus on the type and the location of any murmurs. Is the murmur right-sided or left-sided? Right-sided endocarditis almost always affects the tricuspid valve and is common in intravenous drug users. Left-sided lesions in endocarditis commonly include mitral regurgitation and aortic insufficiency.

The skin exam should focus on identifying vascular and immunologic phenomena, such as petechiae, purpura, splinter hemorrhages (often seen under the fingernails and toenails), Osler nodes (painful nodules on the fingerpads and toepads), and Janeway lesions (painless pustular or hemorrhagic lesions on the palms and soles). Other pertinent physical exam findings include poor dentition, which can be a marker for streptococcal infections.

A thorough neurologic and ophthalmologic exam should be performed because up to 65% of embolic events in endocarditis involve the central nervous system (CNS). Patients may develop meningitis and display signs of meningeal irritation. Focal weakness or sensory loss is concerning for embolic stroke. Retinal lesions or hemorrhages such as Roth spots are suggestive of microemboli. Any of these signs would indicate a left-sided lesion or right-sided lesion with a shunt and subsequent "paradoxical emboli" (i.e., through a patent foramen ovale).

Labs and Test to Consider

The diagnostic criteria for bacterial endocarditis rely heavily on laboratory and imaging data (Table 28-1); as a result, ordering the proper tests is critical.

Key Diagnostic Labs and Tests

Before administering antibiotics, blood cultures should be sent from at least two separate sites in all patients in whom you suspect endocarditis. These cultures should be repeated at least 12 hours later and then daily until bacteremia clears. Some organisms are particularly fastidious and may not grow in culture (e.g., HACEK organisms).

Electrocardiography (ECG) should be performed on admission and periodically thereafter as valvular lesions can cause new atrioventricular, fascicular, or bundle branch blocks, classically with aortic valve lesions. Such ECG abnormalities are highly suggestive of an aortic valve-ring abscess, which will usually require surgical therapy.

A complete blood count with differential should be sent to look for an elevated or low white blood cell count with a left shift, which could suggest sepsis. Anemia is also found in more than 70% of patients. Other common findings include an elevated erythrocyte sedimentation rate, positive rheumatoid factor, proteinuria, and hematuria.

TABLE 28-1
Modified Duke Criteria for the Diagnosis of Infective Endocarditis

Diagnosis = **2 major** OR **1 major + 2 minor** OR **5 minor criteria**

Major Criteria

- Two positive blood cultures with endocarditis-specific organisms (*Streptococcus viridans, Staphylococcus aureus, Enterococcus,* HACEK) in absence of primary focus (i.e. line, abscess)
- Persistently positive blood cultures (>12 h apart)
- Positive serology or PCR for specific endocarditis organism (e.g., *Coxiella brunetii*)
- New regurgitant murmur on cardiac exam OR echocardiogram with oscillating valvular lesions, abscess, new valvular regurgitation, or prosthetic valve dehiscence

Minor Criteria

- Predisposing heart disease or risk factor
- Fever >38°C (100.4°F)
- Immunologic phenomena (Osler nodes, Roth spots, glomerulonephritis)
- Vascular phenomena (major arterial emboli, septic pulmonary emboli, Janeway lesions)
- Microbiologic evidence not fitting major criteria

HACEK, *Haemophilus, Actinobacillus, Cardiobacterium, Eikenella,* and *Kingella*; PCR, polymerase chain reaction. Adapted with permission from Li J, Sexton D, Mick N, et al. Proposed modifications to the Duke criteria for the diagnosis of infective endocarditis. *Clin Infect Dis.* 2000;30:633–638.

Imaging

Transthoracic echocardiography (TTE) is the first test of choice to identify vegetations and is highly specific (98%). However, technical limitations in obese patients or patients with chronic obstructive pulmonary disease result in a sensitivity for endocarditis of only 60% to 70%. TTE is also not as accurate at characterizing perivalvular extension and the presence of a perivalvular abscess. In patients in whom TTE is negative or who have signs of cardiac complications, a transesophageal echocardiogram (TEE) should be performed.

For patients with meningeal signs or focal neurologic deficits, contrast-enhanced computed tomography (CT) or magnetic resonance imaging can identify an intracranial mycotic aneurysm, hemorrhage, or infarct. If pulmonary emboli or edema is suspected, order a chest radiograph or noncontrast chest CT. Contrast-enhanced abdominal CT may diagnose other systemic emboli to the liver, spleen, kidneys, or mesentery if the patient presents with any concerning signs or symptoms.

Treatment

A prolonged course of intravenous antibiotics is the mainstay of treatment and is guided by the type of endocarditis and the specific pathogen isolated. The most important determination to make will be whether or not the patient is at risk for MRSA and requires vancomycin. In addition, for prosthetic valves, rifampin and gentamicin are usually added to the primary regimen and the duration of therapy is longer. Surgical consultation will be required for patients who have cardiac complications such as perivalvular extension and abscesses. A summary of the most common clinical scenarios and recommended antibiotic regimens is included in Table 28-2. (More specific regimens and alternative regimens can be found in the American College of Cardiology/American Heart Association guidelines listed in the Suggested Readings section.)

In certain cases, antibiotic therapy alone is not sufficient to clear the infection. Patients with heart failure, perivalvular abscess, large vegetations, failure to clear bacteremia after 1 week of treatment, multiple thromboembolic complications, mechanical valves, and certain pathogens, such as fungal or resistant gram-negative organisms, will likely require surgical intervention. It is important to always search for other sources of infection, such as abscesses, in patients who do not clear their bacteremia after appropriate antibiotic therapy.

EXTENDED IN-HOSPITAL MANAGEMENT

The patient does not need to be hospitalized for the duration of antibiotic treatment. Initially, he or she should be thoroughly evaluated and monitored for any complications of endocarditis. Once signs of systemic infection have resolved and blood cultures have cleared with appropriate antibiotic treatment, reliable access for long-term administration of antibiotics should be arranged, such as a peripherally inserted central catheter (PICC) line.

DISPOSITION

Discharge Goals

The patient will require either placement in a subacute facility for administration of intravenous antibiotics or home care if the patient is reliable and not actively using illicit substances.

TABLE 28-2
Antibiotic Regimens for Infective Endocarditis

	Regimen	
Pathogen	Native Valve	Prosthetic Valve
MSSA	Oxacillin or nafcillin 6 weeks	Oxacillin or nafcillin 6 weeks PLUS
	OPTION to add	Rifampin 6 weeks PLUS
	Gentamicin 3–5 days	Gentamicin 2 weeks
MRSA	Vancomycin 6 weeks	Vancomycin 6 weeks PLUS
	OPTION to add	Rifampin 6 weeks PLUS
	Gentamicin 3–5 days	Gentamicin 2 weeks
PCN-sensitive streptococci	Penicillin G or ceftriaxone 4 weeks	Penicillin G 6 weeks PLUS Gentamicin 2 weeks
PCN relatively resistant streptococci	Penicillin G 4 weeks PLUS Gentamicin 2 weeks	Penicillin G 6 weeks PLUS Gentamicin 4 weeks
Enterococcal species	Penicillin G 4–6 weeks PLUS Gentamicin 4–6 weeks	Penicillin G 6 weeks PLUS Gentamicin 6 weeks
HACEK species	Ceftriaxone 4 weeks	Ceftriaxone 6 weeks

HACEK, *Haemophilus, Actinobacillus, Cardiobacterium, Eikenella*, and *Kingella*; MRSA, methicillin-resistant *Staphylococcus aureus*; MSSA, methicillin-sensitive *S. aureus*; PCN, penicillin. (Bonow R. Carabello BA, Kanu C et al. ACC/AHA 2006 guidelines for the management of patients with valvular heart disease: a report of the American College of Cardiology/American Heart Association Task Force on practice guidelines. *Circulation.* 2006:114(5)e84–e231.)

Outpatient Care

The patient should follow up with his or her primary care physician after completing the intravenous antibiotic course. In some cases, a referral to an infectious disease specialist may be warranted, particularly if the specific pathogen was unusual. If there are cardiac or neurologic complications, follow-up with the appropriate specialist should be arranged. Patients with a cardiac history or prosthetic valve should continue with regular cardiology care. Finally, intravenous drug users should be referred to substance abuse treatment facilities and support groups.

WHAT YOU NEED TO REMEMBER

- Left-sided and right-sided endocarditis occur in different demographic groups and have different manifestations and associated complications.
- Multiple blood cultures separated in time and space are critical.
- TTE is specific but not sensitive and TEE may be required in certain cases.
- Complications can occur through direct cardiac extension or valve dysfunction or through embolic events affecting the CNS, lungs, and mesentery.
- Remember to search for patients who meet criteria for surgical intervention.

REFERENCE

1. Hoen B. Epidemiology and antibiotic treatment of infective endocarditis: an update. *Heart.* 2006;92:1694–1700.

SUGGESTED READINGS

Bonow RO, Carabello BA, Kanu C, et al. ACC/AHA 2006 guidelines for the management of patients with valvular heart disease: a report of the American College of Cardiology/American Heart Association Task Force on practice guidelines. *Circulation.* 2006;114(5):e84–e231.

Durack D, Lukes A, Bright DK. New criteria for diagnosis of infective endocarditis: utilization of specific echocardiographic findings. *Am J Med.* 1994;96:200–209.

Haldra S, O'Gara P. Infective endocarditis: diagnosis and management. *Nat Clin Prac Cardiovasc Med.* 2006;3(6):310–317.

Karchmer AW. Infective endocarditis. In: Fauci AS, Braunwald E, Kasper DL, et al., eds. Harrison's *Principles of Internal Medicine,* 16th ed. New York: McGraw-Hill; 2005.

Li, J, Sexton D, Mick N, et al. Proposed modifications to the Duke criteria for the diagnosis of infective endocarditis. *Clin Infect Dis.* 2000;30:633–638.

Mylonakis E, Calderwood S. Infective endocarditis in adults. *N Engl J Med.* 2001; 345:1318–1330.

CHAPTER

29

Sepsis

THE PATIENT ENCOUNTER

A 62-year-old man presents to the emergency department complaining of shortness of breath and cough productive of green sputum. Vital signs reveal a temperature of 102.2°F (39°C), a heart rate of 110 bpm, blood pressure of 80/50 mm Hg, and an oxygen saturation of 80% on room air. He is tachypneic and has crackles posteriorly in the right lower lobe. A chest radiograph reveals a consolidation in the right lower lobe with a small pleural effusion.

OVERVIEW

Definition

Sepsis is a clinical syndrome that complicates severe infection and is characterized by systemic inflammation and widespread tissue injury. There is a continuum of inflammation that ranges from systemic inflammatory response syndrome (SIRS) to septic shock. The different categories along that continuum—SIRS, sepsis, severe sepsis, and septic shock—are important to differentiate as they are associated with escalating levels of mortality.

SIRS is a global inflammatory response to any one of multiple possible clinical insults such as pneumonia, trauma, or pancreatitis. The syndrome is defined by the presence of two or more of the following:

- Temperature >100.4°F (>38°C) or <96.8°F (<36°C)
- Heart rate > 90 bpm
- Respiratory rate >20 breaths per minute *or* $PaCO_2$ <32
- White blood cell count >12,000 cells/mm^3, <4,000 cells/mm^3, or with >10% bands

CLINICAL PEARL

Blood pressure is not a criterion for the definition of SIRS.

Sepsis is the combination of SIRS with infection. Infection is defined as an inflammatory response to the presence of microorganisms or the invasion of a normally sterile host tissue by those organisms. Severe sepsis is sepsis with hypotension, hypoperfusion, or end-organ damage. Clinical manifestations can include acute renal failure, oliguria, a change in mental status, and/or lactic acidosis. Septic shock is severe sepsis with hypotension that persists despite adequate fluid resuscitation. If pressors are required, then the patient has septic shock.

Pathophysiology

Sepsis results from the dysregulation of normal host inflammatory mechanisms. In response to severe infection, cytokines such as tumor necrosis factor-α and interleukin-1 that are normally crucial to local immune responses may produce injury in distant tissues. Specific bacterial substances, such as endotoxin in gram-negative infections, may activate the complement system and cause dysregulation in both normal coagulation and vasodilatory pathways. The ability of tissues to locally extract oxygen may be adversely affected, leading to tissue hypoxia and further cellular injury. The combination of these events leads to a cycle of malignant inflammation and even relative immunosuppression that further results in critical illness and possibly multiorgan dysfunction.

Epidemiology

There are approximately 750,000 cases of sepsis each year in the United States. The incidence of sepsis and sepsis-related deaths continues to increase, although the overall mortality rate is declining. The number of deaths from sepsis is equal to that seen from myocardial infarctions (1,2).

Etiology

Pneumonia is the most common infectious process that results in sepsis. In some studies, up to half of patients with community-acquired pneumonia meet criteria for sepsis on presentation. The most common cause of sepsis is gram-positive bacteremia, followed by gram-negative bacteremia; fungemia is a less common cause.

ACUTE MANAGEMENT AND WORKUP

Recognizing the "golden time" of initial resuscitation in a patient with severe sepsis is the key to improved survival.

The First 15 Minutes

Immediate fluid resuscitation should be initiated as soon as a patient with severe sepsis or septic shock is identified.

Initial Assessment

It is important to consider the diagnosis of sepsis in any patient with evidence of an infection. For example, the patient in our encounter clearly has a pneumonia but also has severe sepsis marked by hypotension and end-organ hypoperfusion. However, the diagnosis may be more subtle at times. A patient with a urinary tract infection, borderline tachycardia, and a low-grade fever may also have sepsis, and early recognition and management before hypotension occurs will improve outcome. Because a number of patients with sepsis will go on to develop acute respiratory distress syndrome (ARDS), it is also important to screen patients with presumed sepsis for signs and symptoms of respiratory failure (see Chapter 17). It is critical to perform a thorough cardiovascular examination because it can sometimes be difficult to distinguish sepsis from other forms of shock.

Admission Criteria and Level of Care Criteria

Patients with recognized sepsis will most likely require intermediate or intensive care unit management. If a patient responds to initial antibiotics and fluid resuscitation, he or she may be able to remain on a regular medicine floor with close observation. However, the need for vasopressors, ventilatory support, or even frequent fluid boluses should prompt urgent referral to the intensive care unit (ICU).

The First Few Hours

The goal of initial resuscitation is to meet certain physiologic criteria within the first 6 hours. Patients should be treated with aggressive adjustments in cardiac preload, afterload, and contractility to balance oxygen delivery with oxygen demand in order to prevent cardiovascular collapse.

During the first 6 hours of resuscitation, the goals should include all of the following:

- Central venous pressure (CVP) 8 to 12 mm Hg
- Mean arterial pressure ≥65 mm Hg
- Urine output ≥0.5 mL/kg/hr
- Central venous or mixed venous-oxygen saturation ≥70%

In patients undergoing mechanical ventilation, a higher target CVP of 12 to 15 mm Hg should be considered due to the increased intrathoracic pressure from positive-pressure ventilation.

In a single-center study that evaluated the initial resuscitation in sepsis, the group that received "early goal-directed therapy" using these physiologic parameters had a 30.5% in-hospital mortality as opposed to a mortality of 46.5% in the control group. One life can be saved for every seven patients treated with early goal-directed therapy (3).

Every patient is different, but in general, septic patients will require about 5 to 6 L of intravenous fluids in the first 6 hours. Do not be afraid to "overresuscitate" your patient, especially early on. A patient with a history of systolic heart failure who has severe sepsis will likely need aggressive fluid resuscitation despite having a low ejection fraction.

History

In taking the patient history, you should focus on identifying the likely source of sepsis and seek to identify risk factors that may affect outcome. A history of chemotherapy, neutropenia, immunosuppressive medications, or human immunodeficiency virus may help identify a patient at risk for opportunistic infections and help guide the choice of empiric antibiotics. A history of recent hospitalization may identify a patient at risk for nosocomial infection. Indwelling catheters and lines also pose a risk of infection and the duration of such devices should be elicited. Finally, a review of any previous infections may help to guide initial antibiotic therapy.

Physical Examination

In general, the exam should focus on assessing volume status, searching for evidence of end-organ dysfunction, and localizing the source of the infection. The jugular venous pressure (JVP) exam is critical. A flat JVP is consistent with a patient who is volume depleted, vasodilated, or both. An elevated JVP in the setting of hypotension would not be consistent with sepsis and might suggest either cardiogenic shock or obstructive shock from a pulmonary embolism or pericardial effusion. Examination of the peripheral pulses and extremities may provide information about cardiac output and systemic vascular resistance. You might expect to feel brisk pulses and warm extremities in a patient with sepsis, which reflects a high cardiac output and peripheral vasodilation. However, sepsis may result in a low cardiac output state and may even be characterized by vasoconstriction early on.

The pulmonary examination should focus on identifying patients with pneumonia or patients who may be developing respiratory failure. A mental status exam is helpful in identifying patients with altered mental status that may be caused by the infection itself or that may result from hypoperfusion of the brain.

Labs and Tests to Consider

There are a number of diagnostic tests that can aid in the diagnosis and management of sepsis.

Key Diagnostic Labs and Tests

Cultures should always be obtained prior to the initiation of antibiotics. At least two blood cultures should be obtained, of which at least one should be percutaneous. If the patient has an indwelling vascular device, then a blood culture should be drawn from each port of the device. If the clinical situation warrants, cultures from urine, cerebrospinal fluid, wounds, respiratory cultures, or other body fluids should be obtained before or while antibiotic therapy is being initiated.

Other laboratory tests may provide information about end-organ dysfunction; for example, serum creatinine and blood urea nitrogen should be measured to look for acute renal failure, liver function tests should be sent to assess for hepatic dysfunction, and coagulation studies should be performed to assess for disseminated intravascular coagulation. A serum bicarbonate and arterial blood gas should be obtained to look for metabolic acidosis and to assess ventilatory reserve. A serum lactate may be useful to assess for end-organ hypoperfusion, although a normal level is not necessarily reassuring.

Imaging

Diagnostic studies should be performed as promptly as possible to determine the source of infection and the likely causative organism. This need should be balanced against the risk of transporting a sick patient to an imaging device where monitoring and access to the patient can be difficult. If possible, a bed-side imaging technique may be done until the image of choice can be obtained.

Treatment

In addition to aggressive volume resuscitation, there are a number of treatments that have been shown to affect outcome in patients with sepsis.

Antibiotics

The time to initiation of appropriate antimicrobial therapy is one of the strongest predictors of mortality in patients with septic shock. The goal is to have intravenous antibiotic therapy initiated within the first hour of recognition of severe sepsis, once appropriate cultures have been obtained. Empiric antibiotic therapy should include one or more drugs that have activity against likely pathogens (bacterial or fungal) and that penetrate the presumed source of sepsis. The initial choice of antibiotics is complex and takes into account a patient's history of drug allergies, underlying disease, hospital and community susceptibility patterns, and the overall clinical picture. Neutropenic or other immunosuppressed patients present a special challenge. Empiric antibiotic therapy is usually broadened and should be continued until neutropenia resolves.

Source Control

In every patient with severe sepsis, a search for a potential source of infection that is amenable to source control should be undertaken. In the case of the patient from our encounter, the possibility of empyema should be considered as a complicating feature of his pneumonia. When possible, the least invasive means of source control should be chosen. For example, a computed tomography–guided drainage of an abdominal abscess is preferable to an open surgical procedure. Indwelling catheters or devices should be removed as soon as possible if they are thought likely to be the source of infection.

Vasopressors

Patients who are not responding to appropriate fluid challenges and in whom hypoperfusion and hypotension persist require vasopressor therapy

TABLE 29-1

Vasopressors in Septic Shock

Agent	Receptors	Effects	Potential Disadvantages
Norepine-phrine	α_1 and β_1	Vasoconstriction Increased cardiac output	Due to the increased mean arterial pressure, a reflex bradycardia usually occurs and the β_1 effects are cancelled out
Dopamine	Dopaminergic, α_1, and β_1	Renal vasodilation Increased heart rate Vasoconstriction	Possible tachyarrhythmias
Epine-phrine	α_1, β_1, and B_2	Increased heart rate Increased inotropy Vasoconstriction	Decreased splanchnic, coronary blood flow
Phenyle-phrine	Purely α_1	Vasoconstriction	Less tachycardia due to no β_1 effects
Arginine Vasopressin	V_1 and V_2	Vasoconstriction Increases vasculature responsiveness to catecholamines	Be careful in patients with coronary heart disease

(Table 29-1). Vasopressors should be viewed as second-line therapy for septic patients who have failed intravenous fluids; however, not infrequently, vasopressor therapy may be required transiently to sustain life and maintain perfusion while a fluid challenge is in progress and hypovolemia is being corrected.

First-line agents for septic shock include norepinephrine or dopamine, ideally through a central venous catheter. This is based on a recommendation from the Surviving Sepsis Campaign (4), and no large controlled trials have been performed comparing one agent to another. Phenylephrine, a pure α-adrenergic agonist, may be particularly useful when tachyarrhythmias preclude the use of agents with β-adrenergic activity. Epinephrine, in animal studies, causes impairment in splanchnic circulation and is typically not used as a first-line agent in septic shock. Arginine vasopressin may be considered in patients with refractory shock who are on high doses of norepinephrine, do not have coexisting heart disease, and have been adequately resuscitated with fluids.

Activated Protein C

Microcirculatory dysfunction plays a large role in the pathogenesis of sepsis. As a result, a recombinant form of the naturally occurring anticoagulant, activated protein C, has been studied as an adjunctive treatment. Activated protein C is recommended for patients at high risk of death. This group includes those with an APACHE II score greater than or equal to 25, sepsis-induced multiple organ failure, septic shock, or sepsis-induced ARDS. Its administration must be carefully weighed, as there is an increased risk of serious bleeding events.

Glycemic Control

The management of hyperglycemia is likely critical in patients with sepsis. There have been several trials comparing "aggressive" glycemic control to more "liberal" glycemic control in intensive care unit patients. Although a mortality benefit in sepsis has not been demonstrated, it is possible that tighter control might improve outcomes, although the risk of severe hypoglycemia must be carefully weighed.

Corticosteroids

There have been several trials on the use of "stress-dose" corticosteroids in patients with sepsis and laboratory evidence of adrenal insufficiency. The results have been mixed but suggest that patients with relative adrenal insufficiency and refractory hypotension may be able to come off vasopressors sooner if given supplemental steroids. However, there is certainly an increased risk of complications such as infection, hyperglycemia, and neuromuscular weakness. The jury is still out on the use of corticosteroids in patients with sepsis.

Other Therapies

Prophylaxis of deep vein thrombosis (DVT) and stress ulcers is key to management of patients with severe sepsis. No single study has been done that looks at patients with severe sepsis or septic shock; however, numerous trials have been performed that have shown the benefit of DVT prophylaxis in an ICU setting. Not infrequently, septic patients will have a contraindication to either low-molecular-weight heparin or low-dose unfractionated heparin (recent intracerebral hemorrhage, active bleeding, severe coagulopathy, or thrombocytopenia); these patients should receive compression stockings and an intermittent compression device.

EXTENDED IN-HOSPITAL MANAGEMENT

The specific long-term management of patients with sepsis will depend in large part on the source of their infection. A few circumstances warrant specific mention.

Patients with severe sepsis and septic shock frequently require mechanical ventilation and develop ARDS. Patients with ARDS benefit from specific ventilatory strategies centered around the delivery of low tidal volumes. The specifics of these ventilatory strategies are beyond the scope of this text but their use in an ARDS network landmark study reduced mortality from 39.8% to 31.0%. As a result of the lung protective strategy, patients may develop a respiratory acidosis. This "permissive hypercapnia," if severe, may be treated with a sodium bicarbonate infusion in selected patients (5).

Patients with sepsis oftentimes are bedbound for extended periods of time. They are also frequently on either sedative infusions or neuromuscular blocking agents, especially when they require mechanical ventilation for ARDS or respiratory failure. As a result, early and aggressive physical and occupational therapy, even while the patient is still in the intensive care unit, is an important part of patient care and should be initiated once a patient is hemodynamically stable. This will likely help to decrease thromboembolic and pressure ulcer complications, and may reduce the incidence of critical illness polyneuropathy and myopathy.

The patient's nutritional status is likely also important for successful long-term outcomes. There is currently debate regarding the right time to initiate feeding in critically ill patients (i.e., early feeding or delayed feeding), but it is clear that improving overall nutritional status will help improve long-term outcomes.

DISPOSITION

Discharge Goals

Discharge criteria are largely dependent on the underlying etiology of sepsis. However, it is clear that patients must be hemodynamically stable and recovering from end-organ dysfunction before they are ready to be released from the hospital. A short inpatient stay in a rehabilitation unit is fairly common following the resolution of sepsis.

Outpatient Care

Patients will likely require close follow-up with their primary care physician following an admission for sepsis.

WHAT YOU NEED TO REMEMBER

- There is a "golden time" of initial resuscitation in patients with severe sepsis; early recognition and management are critical to the long-term outcome.
- Patients may be septic with a "normal" blood pressure.
- Early antibiotics and source control are important determinants of the outcome.
- Aggressive fluid resuscitation is an important part of initial management.
- Patients with sepsis are at high risk for ARDS and respiratory failure.
- DVT and stress ulcer prophylaxis, as well as aggressive physical and occupational therapy, should be part of routine sepsis management.

REFERENCES

1. Russell JA. Management of sepsis. *N Engl J Med.* 2006;355(16):1699–1713.
2. Stanchina ML, Levy MM. Vasoactive drug use in septic shock. *Semin Respir Crit Care Med.* 2004;25(6):673–681.
3. Rivers E, Nguyen B, Havstad S, et al. Early goal-directed therapy in the treatment of severe sepsis and septic shock. *N Engl J Med.* 2001;345(19):1368–1377.
4. Dellinger RP, Levy MM, Carlet JM, et al. Surviving Sepsis Campaign: International Guidelines for Surviving Sepsis and Septic Shock: 2008. *Crit Care Med.* 2008;36(1).
5. Ventilation with lower tidal volumes as compared with traditional tidal volumes for acute lung injury and the acute respiratory distress syndrome. The Acute Respiratory Distress Syndrome Network. *N Engl J Med.* 2000;342(18):1301–1308.

SUGGESTED READINGS

Bernard GR, Vincent JL, Laterre PF, et al. Efficacy and safety of recombinant human activated protein C for severe sepsis. *N Engl J Med.* 2001;344(10):699–709.
Landry DW, Oliver JA. The pathogenesis of vasodilatory shock. *N Engl J Med.* 2001;345:588–595.

HIV/AIDS in Hospitalized Patients

Definition

With the advent of highly active antiretroviral therapy (HAART) in the mid-1990s, the morbidity and mortality associated with human immunodeficiency virus (HIV)-1 infection in the United States has declined substantially, and hospitalization rates are estimated to have decreased by one quarter to one third. Despite this, studies suggest that nearly one in every four patients with HIV/acquired immunodeficiency syndrome (AIDS) has had at least one hospitalization in the past year. Because these patients have a unique set of risk factors, it is important to have a sound approach to the management of HIV/AIDS patients in the hospital setting.

Pathophysiology

Causes of hospitalization in HIV/AIDS patients can broadly be grouped into three categories: (a) AIDS related (Table 30-1), (b) non–AIDS related, and (c) antiretroviral medication related (Table 30-2). AIDS-related hospitalizations are a consequence of immune deficiency and tend to occur when the CD4 count is <200 cells/mm^3. Non–AIDS-related hospitalizations can be due to myriad causes and can generally be approached diagnostically, as one would approach a patient who is HIV negative. It is important to understand how to appropriately administer antiretroviral medications to HIV/AIDS patients while they are hospitalized to ensure proper prophylaxis before discharge and to recognize potential drug–drug interactions before starting any new medications.

Epidemiology

Although the face of the HIV epidemic has changed considerably with the advent of HAART, AIDS-defining illness continues to be the primary reason for hospitalization in approximately 20% of hospitalizations for HIV/AIDS patients.

Etiology

The most common AIDS-defining illness in several series is *Pneumocystis* pneumonia followed by candidal esophagitis. Non–AIDS-related admissions span a variety of causes, but gastrointestinal disease, vascular disease, and renal disease appear to be among the most common. Though not a cause of admission, medication errors are common among hospitalized HIV patients.

TABLE 30-1

HIV and AIDS-related Causes of Hospitalization Organized by CD4 Count

CD4 Cell Count	HIV- and AIDS-related Disease
Any CD4 Count	HIV nephropathy
200–500	Bacterial pneumonia Pulmonary tuberculosis Herpes zoster Oropharyngeal candidiasis Cryptosporidiosis Kaposi sarcoma Oral hairy leukoplakia
<200	*Pneumocystis* pneumonia Disseminated histoplasmosis/coccidiomycosis Miliary or extrapulmonary tuberculosis Progressive multifocal leukoencephalopathy
<100	Disseminated herpes simplex Toxoplasmosis Cryptococcosis Microsporidiosis Candidal esophagitis
<50	Disseminated cytomegalovirus Disseminated *Mycobacterial avium* complex

TABLE 30-2

Antiretroviral Medication Complications

Lactic acidosis/hepatic steatosis
Abacavir hypersensitivity (and other hypersensitivity reactions)
Immune reconstitution inflammatory syndrome
Drug eruptions—most common Bactrim, NNRTIs, some PIs
Pancreatitis–associated with PI-related hypertriglyceridemia

NNRTI, nonnucleoside reverse transcriptase inhibitors; PI, protease inhibitor.

Such errors may have more significance for HIV-infected patients because inappropriate medication administration may allow for the development of drug resistance and limit future treatment options.

HOSPITALIZATION FOR COMMON AIDS-DEFINING ILLNESSES

The pathology that you will encounter in HIV patients is incredibly broad. In the sections that follow, we will explore the evaluation and management of three of the most common hospital presentations in patients with HIV: (a) *Pneumocystis* pneumonia, (b) esophagitis, and (c) cryptococcal meningitis.

Pneumocystis Pneumonia

The most common causes of pneumonia in the AIDS patient are bacterial pneumonia, *Pneumocystis jiroveci* pneumonia (PCP), and idiopathic pneumonia (see Chapter 25).

Clinical Presentation

Key features of the history should include the patient's last CD4 count, whether he or she is on prophylaxis for PCP, and the tempo of symptom onset. Bacterial pneumonia is likely to present as it would in an HIV-negative patient—with fever and purulent cough for up to 1 week. PCP, on the other hand, has a more insidious onset with symptoms of nonproductive cough, fever, and dyspnea often being present for weeks before presentation. HIV/AIDS patients are at increased risk for PCP once the CD4 count falls below 200 cells/mm^3. This risk is markedly reduced if the patient is on appropriate prophylaxis, most commonly trimethoprim/sulfamethoxazole.

Physical Examination

The physical examination may be notable for fever, tachypnea, tachycardia, and rales. Dyspnea is a key feature of PCP and an oxygen saturation should always be obtained to assess whether the patient is hypoxemic (oxygen saturation <92% to 93%) on room air either at rest or with exertion. While it does not secure the diagnosis, a lactate dehydrogenase >500 mg/dL is suggestive in the right clinical context.

Diagnosis

The diagnosis of PCP is made from an induced sputum (when a saline solution is inhaled to provoke expectoration of sputum from the lower airways) or bronchoalveolar lavage. Usually the induced sputum is obtained first because it is a noninvasive test. If the induced sputum is negative and there is high clinical suspicion for PCP, then a bronchoscopy should be performed because of the low sensitivity of induced sputum (about 56%).

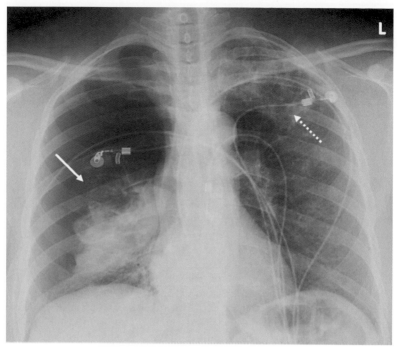

FIGURE 30-1: Chest radiograph in an HIV patient with *Pneumocystis* pneumonia demonstrating a right-sided pneumothorax (*solid arrow*) as well as left upper lobe infiltrate with cystic changes (*dashed arrow*). (*Courtesy of Brian T. Garibaldi, MD, Division of Pulmonary and Critical Care Medicine, The Johns Hopkins Hospitals.*)

Key Diagnostic Tests

The chest radiograph is a key diagnostic test that may help to distinguish bacterial from *Pneumocystis* pneumonia. In bacterial pneumonia, an infiltrate often appears as a dense consolidation, while in PCP, the infiltrates may be interstitial, atypical, or not present at all, particularly early in the disease course. Pneumothoraces may also be present with PCP (Fig. 30-1).

Treatment

Treatment should begin once the clinical diagnosis is suspected because the mortality rate is 100% in untreated disease! The treatment of choice is high-dose trimethoprim/sulfamethoxazole for 21 days. Steroids should be added to the regimen if the patient has severe disease with hypoxia (defined as a PaO_2 <70 or an alveolar-arterial gradient >35). Watch for toxicity from treatment (rash, gastrointestinal intolerance, hyperkalemia).

Response to therapy may not be seen until 5 to 7 days, especially for more severe disease. In addition, some patients have a paradoxical worsening in their clinical status several days into treatment. This is a result of the immune response to the *Pneumocystis*-infected pneumocytes.

It is important that the patient have appropriate follow-up with his or her HIV provider upon discharge to ensure completion of therapy and continua-

---

 WHAT YOU NEED TO REMEMBER

- PCP and bacterial pneumonia are common causes of hospitalization for HIV/AIDS patients.
- The CD4 count, the presence or absence of PCP prophylaxis, and the tempo of symptom onset may help to distinguish between these common causes.
- Untreated PCP has 100% mortality, so treatment should begin once the diagnosis is suspected.

---

tion of appropriate prophylaxis. The patient should understand that he or she will need to be on PCP prophylaxis after completion of the treatment course.

Esophagitis

Esophagitis is a common AIDS-defining illness that may require inpatient management. Candidal esophagitis is the most common cause, but cytomegalovirus (CMV) and herpes simplex virus (HSV) are other important causes.

Clinical Presentation

Esophagitis is unlikely to present fulminantly, but volume depletion may be present in patients who have not been able to tolerate oral intake. Odynophagia (painful swallowing), dysphagia (difficulty swallowing), heartburn, and chest pain are common presenting symptoms. Dysphagia may be more prominent with candidal esophagitis, whereas fever and odynophagia is more common in patients with CMV esophagitis. The patient's CD4 count is generally <100 cells/mm^3 with candidal disease and <50 cells/mm^3 with CMV disease.

Physical Examination

Depending on the severity of presentation, the patient may have signs of dehydration with dry mucous membranes. Close attention should be paid to the patient's blood pressure, pulse, and orthostatic vital signs in order to assess for hemodynamic stability. Thrush or angular cheilosis is commonly seen with candidal esophagitis, whereas CMV and HSV tend to cause esophageal ulcers. Oral ulcers are often visible when HSV is the causative agent.

Diagnosis

Because *Candida* is responsible for more than half of the cases of esophagitis in patients with HIV/AIDS, patients are often treated empirically for candidal esophagitis, especially if clinical clues are more suggestive of candidal disease. Further workup will be necessary if the patient does not improve with empiric treatment or the patient's presentation is more consistent with another etiology.

Key Diagnostic Tests

In such cases, the diagnosis is typically made via direct visualization with endoscopy and biopsy. With candidal disease, pseudomembranous plaques may be seen. With CMV and HSV, classic viral changes are seen on biopsy.

Treatment

The first-line treatment for candidal esophagitis is fluconazole. If the patient has poor tolerance of oral intake, it can be given intravenously for a duration of 14 to 21 days. Acyclovir and ganciclovir are the treatments of choice for HSV and CMV esophagitis, respectively.

The patient should be tolerating oral intake by the time of discharge.

 WHAT YOU NEED TO REMEMBER

- *Candida* is the most common cause of esophagitis in HIV/AIDS patients.
- Severe odynophagia and fever should raise the possibility of CMV esophagitis.
- If the patient does not respond to empiric treatment for *Candida*, further workup with endoscopy and biopsy is warranted to rule out less common causes.

Cryptococcal Meningitis

Although cryptococcal meningitis, like other AIDS-defining illnesses, is becoming less common in the post-HAART era, appropriate recognition and management of this disease process are critical to patient survival. Prompt recognition of the signs and symptoms of meningitis and elevated intracranial pressure (ICP) are vital in the management of these patients (see Chapter 26).

Clinical Presentation

Unlike other, more common causes of infectious meningitis, patients with cryptococcal meningitis tend to have a subacute presentation with headache as a primary feature. It is important to ascertain the patient's most recent CD4 count as patients with cryptococcal meningitis typically present with a CD4 count <100 cells/mm^3. A high index of suspicion for this disease should be present in the face of unusual symptoms, such as a change in behavior or personality or unexplained fevers. *Cryptococcus* enters the host through the lungs, so patients with cryptococcal meningitis may also have manifestations of lung or skin disease.

Physical Examination

Examination should identify any signs of elevated intracranial pressure, such as altered mental status and papilledema. A detailed neurologic exam should be performed to assess for focal deficits. Other signs of meningitis should be explored, although classic signs of meningeal inflammation are often not seen. The skin should be examined for vesicular or papular eruptions that might represent cutaneous disease. In addition, auscultation and percussion of the lungs should be performed to assess for any abnormalities consistent with pneumonitis.

Diagnosis

A patient with HIV and a headache likely warrants a lumbar puncture (LP). Likewise, a patient with HIV and an unexplained fever should have an LP. Lumbar puncture is critical to making the diagnosis of cryptococcal meningitis and can potentially help relieve symptoms of intracranial hypertension.

Key Diagnostic Tests

Because elevated ICP may be caused by a mass or other space-occupying lesion in addition to infection (meningitis, encephalitis, or abscess), a prompt noncontrast head computed tomography (CT) scan can help to assess for these possibilities. If no mass or space-occupying lesion is present and the head CT scan does not show signs of intracranial hypertension, lumbar puncture should be obtained and an opening pressure recorded.

In addition to the standard workup for meningitis, the cerebrospinal fluid (CSF) should be analyzed for cryptococcal antigen as well as for other pathogens that are rarely seen in immunocompetent hosts (i.e., CMV, varicella zoster virus, Ebstein Barr virus, JC virus, etc.). Serum cryptococcal antigen can also be obtained and is positive in nearly all patients with cryptococcal meningitis.

Treatment

The goal of treatment is to eradicate infection and to control intracranial hypertension. Treatment begins with a 2-week induction phase with amphotericin B and flucytosine followed by 8 weeks of maintenance therapy with fluconazole.

Serial LPs, lumbar drain, or ventriculoperitoneal shunt may be necessary to control intracranial pressure in severe cases. Inappropriate or ineffective management of this complication is a common but potentially fatal mistake. In general, if your patient develops a worsening headache or worsening neurologic status, a repeat LP with likely removal of excess CSF is in order.

Patients often need to stay in the hospital or another inpatient facility for the induction phase of treatment. They should show clinical improvement, with no new neurologic symptoms or evidence of elevated ICP before discharge. Close follow-up should be scheduled with the patient's HIV provider as the patient will need to be maintained on prophylactic therapy with fluconazole until the CD4 count is >100 to 200 cells/mm^3 for 6 consecutive months.

WHAT YOU NEED TO REMEMBER

- Cryptococcal meningitis has a subacute presentation with headache as a primary symptom.
- Elevated intracranial pressure is a common feature of disease that can prove fatal if not managed appropriately.

MANAGEMENT OF ANTIRETROVIRAL MEDICATIONS IN HOSPITALIZED HIV/AIDS PATIENTS

Regardless of the cause of admission to the hospital, HIV/AIDS patients on antiretroviral medications are at risk for medication errors. As many as 25% of patients may be exposed to entirely preventable mistakes, the most common of which include inappropriate dosage or frequency and initiating medications contraindicated for use with HAART. Inappropriate administration of antiretroviral medications can put patients at risk for the development of drug resistance, especially if the patient continues this dosing regimen after discharge and if he or she is on medications that have a low genetic barrier for resistance.

For those patients who meet criteria for treatment, the initiation of antiretroviral medications is rarely done emergently in the hospital without the consultation of an HIV specialist. This is important because patients should have an established relationship with a care provider and should have sufficient counseling about the medication regimen, the potential side effects, and the importance of adherence for preventing drug resistance. Recent data do support, however, that early initiation of HAART (within 2 weeks) of the first opportunistic infection is associated with a better outcome.

When a patient with HIV is admitted to the hospital, a detailed history should include a complete medication list. If the patient is unsure of his or her medications, the medication list can be confirmed with the HIV provider and/or the patient's pharmacy. It is not uncommon for patients to develop metabolic derangements or other lab abnormalities while admitted to the hospital. Most of the reverse transcriptase inhibitors need to be dose-adjusted in renal failure, and most of the protease inhibitors given in combination with ritonavir need to be dose-adjusted in hepatic failure.

CLINICAL PEARL

One of the protease inhibitors, atazanavir, often causes an indirect hyperbilirubinemia. This is a known side effect that is not always recognized by non-HIV providers, and should not prompt discontinuation of the drug.

Unless the patient is suffering from a medication-related toxicity, antiretroviral medications should be continued while the patient is hospitalized. It is wise to look up the names and dosages of all medications to avoid errors. If the underlying reason for admission precludes the patient's ability to take antiretroviral medications (such as poor oral tolerance or absorption), it is reasonable to discontinue HAART. It is generally recommended to discontinue all medications at once. Exceptions occur with efavirenz- and nevirapine-based regimens. These nonnucleoside reverse transcriptase inhibitors (NNRTIs) have a long half-life, and if the entire HAART regimen is discontinued at once, the patient will effectively be on monotherapy until these medications are metabolized. In this setting, there is increased risk for development of resistance that would compromise nearly an entire class of medications (NNRTIs).

Before adding a new medication to the patient's regimen, be sure to investigate for drug–drug interactions. All of the protease inhibitors (PIs) are inhibitors of the cytochrome P450 enzymes and thus are associated with many interactions. Statins are among the most commonly prescribed medications in the United States and many are metabolized by P450 enzymes. Simvastatin and lovastatin, for example, are contraindicated for use with protease inhibitors. Similarly, rifampin is contraindicated for use with PIs. In addition, oral contraception may be unsafe for use in combination with protease inhibitors, and other forms of contraception should be considered. Proton pump inhibitors should not be used in combination with the PI atazanavir. Warfarin may have unpredictable interactions with PIs, so coagulation factors should be followed closely until a stable dose is attained.

The goals of antiretroviral medication management at discharge are to ensure proper dosing, to avoid the addition of contraindicated drugs, and to minimize potential drug–drug interactions. In addition, all HIV/AIDS patients should be discharged on appropriate prophylaxis based on his or her CD4 count (Table 30-3). In general, vaccinations should be reserved for patients with a CD4 count $>200/mm^3$ and care must be taken to avoid live-attenuated vaccines except in specific circumstances.

TABLE 30-3

Prophylaxis Against Opportunistic Infections

Opportunistic Infection	CD4 Risk Category	Prophylactic Regimen
Pneumocystis (*jiroveci*) pneumonia	<200	Bactrim or dapsone or aerosolized pentamidine
Toxoplasma gondii	<100	Bactrim or dapsone or atovaquone
Mycobacterium avium complex	<50	Azithromycin

 WHAT YOU NEED TO REMEMBER

- Medication errors are common among hospitalized HIV/AIDS patients and most commonly involve improper dosage and drug–drug interactions.
- Antiretroviral medication drug interactions are common with protease inhibitors and high vigilance should be maintained to avoid potentially dangerous drug interactions.

SUGGESTED READINGS

Bartlett J. Pneumonia in the patient with HIV infection. *Infect Dis Clin N Am.* 1998;12(3):807–820.

Bartlett J, Gallant J. *Medical Management of HIV Infection.* Baltimore, MD: Johns Hopkins Medicine Health Publishing Business Group; 2007.

Betz M, Gebo K, Barber E, et al., for the HIV Research Network. Patterns of diagnoses in hospital admissions in a multistate cohort of HIV-positive adults in 2001. *Med Care.* 2005;43(9):s3–14.

Gardner L, Klein R, Szczech L. Rates and risk factors for condition-specific hospitalizations in HIV-infected and uninfected women. *JAIDS.* 2001;34(3):320–330.

Rastegar D, Knight A, Monolakis J. Antiretroviral medication errors among hospitalized patients with HIV infection. *Clin Infect Dis.* 2006;43:933–938.

Saag M, Graybill R, Larsen R, et al., for the Mycoses Study Group Cryptococcal Subproject. Practice guidelines for the management of cryptococcal disease. *Clin Infect Dis.* 2000;30:710–718.

Approach to the Gastrointestinal Evaluation

The gastrointestinal evaluation can be among the most challenging in internal medicine, in part because the abdomen contains a number of different organ systems whose pathology can present with a wide range of signs and symptoms. This chapter will attempt to provide a framework to approach patients with complaints referable to the abdomen.

Physiology of the Gastrointestinal System

As with any disease process, knowledge of normal physiology greatly enhances recognition and understanding of pathology. However, given the breadth of organs found in the abdomen, it would not be practical to review each one in great detail here. Where indicated, we will review the physiology of specific organs in the chapters that follow.

PATIENT EVALUATION

Because there are many conditions that can produce symptoms referable to the abdomen, a good clinical history can often secure the diagnosis or at least narrow the differential diagnosis. A thorough physical examination and directed laboratory and imaging studies can then guide further management.

History

It is important to focus on the onset, timing, duration, and character of symptoms. It is also particularly relevant to identify specific exacerbating or relieving factors. For example, right upper quadrant pain made worse after eating fatty meals points to gallbladder pathology, while midepigastric pain relieved by eating might suggest a duodenal ulcer.

Pain, in particular, is an important historical concept to review. Pain is an incredibly complex phenomenon that is made even more complicated by the overlap of visceral and somatic innervation in the abdomen. In general, visceral pain is poorly localized and is usually perceived in the midline because most structures are bilaterally innervated. Notable exceptions to this rule include the gallbladder and the ascending and descending colons. Structures that have unilateral innervation (i.e., the ureters) or somatic innervation (i.e., the peritoneum) are more readily localizable. The evolution of a patient's pain with these particular distinctions may provide insight into the pathophysiology of his or her disease. Acute appendicitis provides a great example. Initial distension of the appendix causes visceral pain that is perceived in the midepigastrium. As the inflammation progresses to involve the peritoneum, the pain becomes sharper and localized to the right lower quadrant. "Referred pain" further complicates the issue and is likely caused by crosstalk between visceral and somatic pain fibers as they enter the spinal cord. Perhaps the best example is right-sided scapular pain in the setting of cholecystitis.

When investigating pain or any abdominal symptom, it is sometimes helpful to divide the abdomen into discrete sections in order to help narrow your differential diagnosis. For example, right upper quadrant pain is usually referable to the biliary tree but can also be caused by liver capsular stretch from such processes as right-sided heart failure. Remember that abdominal symptoms can also be caused by processes outside the abdomen, such as a right lower lobe pneumonia that causes right upper quadrant pain or myocardial ischemia that causes midepigastric pain.

Physical Examination

As always, observation is a critical component to your physical examination. For example, patients with an acute abdomen will often lie as still as possible. They may breathe rapidly and shallowly, and may attempt to limit their speech to avoid uncomfortable motion of their abdominal wall. This is in marked contrast to a patient with nephrolithiasis, who will most likely be in constant motion in an attempt to find a comfortable position. As you talk with your patient, look for signs of chronic illness, such as temporal wasting, cachexia, and muscle wasting. Look carefully at the color of his or her skin and eyes to assess for jaundice. A thorough nail examination can be quite useful. For example, "half-and-half" nails (proximal pallor and distal redness) are suggestive of chronic kidney disease, while Muehrcke lines (double, parallel transverse white lines) oftentimes signify hypoalbuminemia from either protein wasting or liver disease.

CLINICAL PEARL

As you approach the bedside, it is sometimes helpful to be a little indirect in your physical examination maneuvers. For example, if you're concerned that someone has an acute abdomen, you can assess for rebound tenderness by "accidentally" knocking into the bed and carefully observing your patient's response.

When you're ready to assess the abdomen, the patient should be placed completely flat, arms by his or her side with the knees slightly bent to relax the abdominal muscles. First, inspect for asymmetry, which might suggest masses or organomegaly. Look for signs of chronic liver disease, such as spider angiomata. Abnormally dilated veins might be consistent with portal hypertension (flow radiating from the navel, also called *caput medusae*), inferior vena cava obstruction (flow is superior), or superior vena cava obstruction (flow is inferior). Obvious distention with a noticeable periumbilical hernia might suggest tense ascites. Periumbilical ecchymosis (Cullen sign) and flank ecchymosis (Grey-Turner sign) can be markers of intra-abdominal hemorrhage from conditions such as acute pancreatitis. Be sure to note the locations and size of any scars.

The abdominal exam is the one examination in which using your stethoscope first is sometimes advantageous. You can assess for the presence or absence of bowel sounds but you can also be sneaky and use the stethoscope to assess for rebound tenderness and guarding. Remember that you need to listen for a full minute to say for sure that someone has hypoactive or absent bowel sounds.

Percussion can help to identify masses, ascites, dilated loops of bowel, and both hepatomegaly and splenomegaly. Both light and deep palpation (usually done by dividing the abdomen into quadrants) can further characterize the above conditions, and they provide additional information, such as the contour of the liver edge (i.e., nodularity suggestive of cirrhosis). Palpation can also help to identify specific pathology, such as acute cholecystitis with a positive Murphy sign (worsening right upper quadrant tenderness with cessation of respiratory effort on inspiration).

When the liver, kidneys, or spleen is markedly enlarged, it can be difficult to know which one is the culprit organ. If you can get above the mass, then it is likely to be in the kidney. Percussion can also be useful—the spleen and liver are always dull to percussion in comparison to the kidneys because the kidneys are retroperitoneal and have air-filled loops of bowel anterior to them. Serial examinations are incredibly useful in charting a patient's clinical course and may provide the key piece of information that determines whether a patient requires an emergent intervention.

Key Diagnostic Evaluations

There are a number of labs that can be helpful in the evaluation of a patient with abdominal complaints. A comprehensive panel provides information about renal function, liver function, acid–base status, and even nutritional status. A complete blood count provides information about chronic illness, infection, anemia, and thrombocytopenia. We will review the significance of each of these components in the chapters that follow.

One lab test deserves particular mention in this section: lactate. Elevated lactate levels can be the result of increased lactate production from anaerobic metabolism/ischemia or from decreased liver lactate clearance. As a result, following serial lactate levels can provide information about the severity and duration of intra-abdominal processes such as bowel ischemia, but they must be interpreted in the appropriate clinical context.

Imaging

There are a number of radiology modalities that can provide useful information in the evaluation of a patient with a gastrointestinal complaint. Plain radiography can show evidence of obstruction or perforation. Abdominal ultrasound can identify cholecystitis and gallstones and provide information about the liver parenchyma and vasculature. Abdominal computed tomography scanning and magnetic resonance imaging can better characterize specific abnormalities and can provide important information about vasculature, including the abdominal aorta. Where appropriate, we will discuss these modalities in more detail in the chapters that follow.

 WHAT YOU NEED TO REMEMBER

- Because the abdomen contains a number of different organ systems, obtaining a thorough history is critical in the evaluation of a patient with an abdominal complaint.
- Abdominal pain may be visceral, somatic, or both. Referred pain to other areas of the body may also result from intra-abdominal processes.
- As always, observation is a key part of your physical examination and may provide critical insight into your patient's underlying disease process.
- Use your stethoscope to listen for bowel sounds and also to palpate for tenderness, rebound, and guarding.
- Imaging studies are important diagnostic tools that should be guided by the patient's history and your physical exam.

SUGGESTED READINGS

Bickley LS, ed. *Bates' Guide to Physical Examination and History Taking*. 9th ed. Philadelphia: Lippincott Williams & Wilkins; 2007.

Feldman M, Friedman LS, Brandt LJ, eds. *Sleisenger & Fordtran's Gastrointestinal and Liver Disease*. 8th ed. Philadelphia: Saunders Elsevier; 2006.

Silen W. Abdominal pain. In: Kasper DL, Braunwald E, Hauser S, et al., eds. *Harrison's Principles of Internal Medicine*. New York: McGraw-Hill; 2005.

Acute Pancreatitis

A 35-year-old woman presents to the emergency department with a 2-day history of nausea, vomiting, and severe midepigastric pain that radiates to her back. She normally drinks a pint of vodka daily and has recently been drinking even more than usual. She is tachycardic, hyperglycemic, and found to have an elevated white blood cell count.

OVERVIEW

Definition

Pancreatitis is an inflammatory process that results from autodigestion of the pancreas parenchyma by the enzymes it synthesizes. Pancreatitis can be divided into both acute and chronic types based on the duration and character of symptoms. This chapter will focus on the evaluation and management of patients with acute pancreatitis.

Pathophysiology

Acute pancreatitis results from the malfunction of normal gland physiology, which includes both endocrine (2%) and exocrine (98%) function. Pancreatic enzymes are produced by acinar cells as inactive proenzymes that are then activated in the duodenum by a cascade of reactions. The presence of activated pancreatic enzymes within pancreatic tissue leads to autodigestion and initiates a vicious cycle of gland destruction. The pancreas goes to extreme measures to protect itself against premature activation and autolysis. Such defense mechanisms include the secretion of the enzymes in the proenzyme form as well as production of a pancreatic secretory trypsin inhibitor protein to bind and inactivate trypsin. When these defense mechanisms fail or are overwhelmed by an inflammatory insult, acute pancreatitis occurs.

Epidemiology

Acute pancreatitis accounts for more than 200,000 hospital admissions yearly in the United States, and its incidence has significantly risen in the past 20 years (1). This rise may be explained by improved diagnostic abilities, continued or increased alcohol consumption, increased rates of gallstones, more evaluations using endoscopic retrograde cholangiopancreatography (ERCP), and higher rates of prescriptions for medications that cause pancreatitis.

Etiology

The most frequent causes of pancreatitis arise as complications from biliary tree pathology, specifically cholelithiasis, choledocholithiasis, biliary sludge, and microlithiasis. Biliary pancreatitis has the highest mortality rate, likely due to the fact that it afflicts an older population and carries with it a greater incidence of infectious-related complications, including bacteremia, cholangitis, pancreatic abscess formation, and infected necrosis.

The second most common cause is alcohol abuse. A dose-response relationship between the amount of alcohol consumed and the risk of alcoholic pancreatitis likely exists. Additional risk factors include tobacco abuse, race, diet, drinking pattern, genetic variations in metabolizing enzymes, and mutations of specific pancreas-related proteins. Pancreatitis from alcohol presents more commonly in younger women drinkers.

In addition to biliary and alcohol-related pancreatitis, many other sources trigger pancreatitis, including hypertriglyceridemia, hypercalcemia, toxins, various medications, infections, postsurgical changes, ischemia, autoimmunity, malignancy, and trauma.

ACUTE MANAGEMENT AND WORKUP

Patients with pancreatitis can manifest signs of severe systemic inflammation. As a result, the initial assessment should focus on confirming the diagnosis of pancreatitis as well as identifying patients at risk for decompensation.

The First 15 Minutes

The cardinal symptom of acute pancreatitis is epigastric abdominal pain that increases in severity over hours with radiation to the back. Patients usually experience associated nausea and vomiting. In the right clinical scenario, such as our patient in the encounter who describes classic symptoms in the presence of a clear precipitant, the diagnosis of pancreatitis can be made from this initial history alone. However, when first evaluating a patient, it is important to entertain other potential causes of severe abdominal pain, such as abdominal aortic dissection or aneurysm rupture; myocardial infarction; bowel ischemia, obstruction, or perforation; nephrolithiasis; pyelonephritis; peptic ulcer disease; and acute cholecystitis.

Initial Assessment

After screening for common risk factors for pancreatitis, such as drinking, a history of biliary problems, and medications, a focused abdominal examination provides useful information. Pancreatitis may cause severe midepigastric tenderness to palpation with voluntary guarding. However, in the absence of severe complications of pancreatitis, such as hemorrhage or necrosis, pancreatitis itself will not produce marked peritoneal signs. Such findings should prompt immediate surgical consultation and rapid abdominal imaging to identify their source.

It is also important to be vigilant for signs of either the systemic inflammatory response syndrome (SIRS) or sepsis because patients with pancreatitis are at risk of developing uncontrolled systemic inflammation. Pancreatitis is also a common nonpulmonary cause of acute lung injury and acute respiratory distress syndrome (ARDS), so an initial cardiopulmonary examination helps to identify patients who may be developing respiratory failure.

During this initial assessment, intravenous fluids for likely volume depletion as well as intravenous pain medications should be initiated while awaiting the results of diagnostic tests.

Admission Criteria and Level of Care

Patients with evidence of SIRS, worsening oxygen requirements, or hemodynamic instability should be managed in an intensive care unit. Sinus tachycardia that does not resolve with initial fluid resuscitation in the emergency department is a warning sign that may warrant an intermediate level of care in the absence of other concerning signs and symptoms.

The First Few Hours

Once the diagnosis of pancreatitis has been established, the remainder of your evaluation should focus on identifying the cause of the acute episode as well as screening for comorbid conditions that can complicate management.

History

The time course of abdominal pain can sometimes provide helpful clues as to the etiology of pancreatitis. Subacute worsening pain, especially when associated with fatty meals, might indicate underlying gallstones as the etiology of the pancreatitis. Pain that begins shortly after alcohol consumption or illicit drug use should strongly point to those substances as the inciting cause. Pay close attention to any recently added medications that may be temporally associated with the onset of symptoms. Some of the more commonly implicated medications include nonsteroidal anti-inflammatory drugs, furosemide, hydrochlorothiazide, corticosteroids, azathioprine, and sulfonamides.

Recurrent bouts of pancreatitis may point to either occult substance abuse issues, structural abnormalities, or even genetic causes of pancreatitis. It is helpful to screen for signs and symptoms of chronic pancreatitis, such as steatorrhea and pancreatic endocrine insufficiency, because even patients without a prior known history may have had subclinical pancreatitis in the past.

Physical Examination

Fever, tachycardia, and tachypnea are common responses to the inflammatory nature of pancreatitis. In general, the abdominal exam is the most abnormal part of the exam in milder cases in which inflammation remains local and not systemic. The abdomen is often quiet with diminished bowel sounds due to the paralytic nature of peritoneal irritation with associated tenderness localizing to the epigastrium. The more acute the abdomen is on examination, the more aggressive you should be about staging severity and considering radiologic imaging to rule out complications or other diagnoses.

Two signs remarkable for pronounced inflammatory disease and serious complications include the Grey-Turner and Cullen signs. The Grey-Turner sign is a reddish-brown discoloration of the flanks concerning for retroperitoneal blood dissecting down tissue planes. The Cullen sign is a bluish discoloration around the umbilicus that indicates hemoperitoneum, often from rupture of the splenic artery.

Icterus and jaundice may suggest biliary pathology, while a ruddy complexion with a scent of alcohol on the breath could suggest alcohol abuse. Xanthomas would raise the possibility of dyslipidemia or hypertriglyceridemia, and a purpuric rash may indicate a vasculitis. Finally, cachexia and wasting could place human immunodeficiency virus or malignancy higher on the differential list.

Labs and Tests to Consider

Pancreatitis is largely a clinical diagnosis, but laboratory enzyme measurements, specifically elevation of amylase and lipase, provide useful information.

Key Diagnostic Labs and Tests

Elevated amylase levels generally indicate pancreas destruction, although other intra-abdominal inflammatory conditions and salivary pathology also produce increases in serum amylase. Amylase typically rises within 12 hours of damage to the pancreas and may return to normal within 3 to 5 days. In approximately 30% of cases, amylase levels may be normal due to late presentation or pancreatic insufficiency from chronic exocrine damage. Marked elevations of amylase may reach 95% specificity, especially with levels over 1,000 IU/L.

Serum lipase remains elevated for much longer than amylase, approximately 8 to 14 days, and can be more helpful in patients who present farther along in their illness course. Other intra-abdominal inflammatory conditions and renal insufficiency also cause a rise in lipase as do certain common medications, such as furosemide, but, in general, lipase is a very specific marker, especially when elevated above 600 IU/L.

Initial presenting labs should include not only amylase and lipase, but also a complete metabolic panel, complete blood count, serum volatile screen (i.e., alcohol level), toxicology screen, and triglyceride level.

Imaging

Radiography is not required to make the diagnosis of acute pancreatitis. However, radiologic modalities are often utilized to help rule out other entities when the diagnosis is in question, to help determine the cause of pancreatitis, to assist in severity staging, and to determine if associated complications exist.

Computed tomography (CT) is the most commonly utilized radiologic test in the evaluation of acute pancreatitis. CT may help determine the underlying cause by identifying choledocholithiasis or biliary ductal dilatation from mechanical obstructions like malignancies or other anatomic distortions. It can also identify associated complications such as fluid collections, pseudocysts, abscesses, necrosis, or vascular compromise. CT can also provide prognostic information when it is used to calculate a severity index based on the detection and quantification of pancreatic necrosis. Perhaps equally important, CT can help to identify alternative etiologies for a patient's abdominal complaints.

There is some debate over which patients benefit most from CT scanning. In mild cases in which the patient is clinically improving, CT is not likely to provide useful information. Furthermore, CT scanning provides the most information when done with intravenous contrast to enhance any changes or edema within the pancreas; some studies indicate that contrast may exacerbate disease severity by impairing oxygenation of the pancreatic parenchyma. Most clinicians agree that patients with moderate to severe pancreatitis warrant CT imaging.

Magnetic resonance imaging (MRI) with gadolinium is comparable to CT for acute pancreatitis. However, cost, expertise, length of the study, claustrophobia, and potential toxicities of gadolinium limit MRI in comparison to CT.

The usefulness of transabdominal ultrasound in acute pancreatitis is limited. However, it can be used to evaluate biliary dilatation as well as the presence of cholelithiasis or biliary sludge.

Treatment

Understanding the precipitating cause of pancreatitis is essential to the appropriate treatment. The avoidance of toxins, suspected medications, and alcohol, as in the patient from our encounter, is paramount.

Supportive Management

Supportive management, specifically hemodynamic resuscitation with intravenous fluids, is probably the most important aspect of the treatment of acute pancreatitis. Volume resuscitation and expansion may prevent hypotension and subsequent ischemic consequences, such as bowel hypoperfusion, lactic acidosis, and acute liver or renal failure, all of which would worsen the prognosis.

Pain Control

Pain control frequently requires high-dose narcotics and occasionally patient-controlled analgesic devices. Historically, meperidine was the narcotic of choice because it does not cause sphincter activation like other opiates. However, such effects do not appear to be clinically significant and the less favorable side effect profile of meperidine makes it a second-line agent in most instances. Nausea and vomiting may require the liberal use of intravenous antiemetics.

Nutritional Support

Nutrition continues to be a prominent issue in patients with acute pancreatitis. The classic teaching is bowel rest because stimulation of the pancreas increases enzyme production and worsens the cycle of autodigestion. However, improved nutrition during times of systemic inflammation may reduce morbidity and improve prognosis. At first glance, parenteral nutrition would seem to provide the best of both worlds, but in some studies, enteral feeding via nasogastric or nasojejunal feeding tubes has been found to be superior to parenteral nutrition. Currently, there is no consensus about the appropriate timing of feeding, but typically, physicians order some period of bowel rest followed by the initiation of a clear liquid diet once the patient is hemodynamically stable and pain-free. The diet is then slowly advanced to a low-fat diet as symptoms allow.

Surgical Management

The timely identification of biliary pathology is crucial because early interventional procedures, such as ERCP and endoscopic sphincterotomy, reduce the number of biliary sepsis complications by relieving any obstruction. In patients with gallstone pancreatitis who subsequently pass the stone but have persistent cholelithiasis, cholecystectomy should be performed. The optimal surgical timing of the intervention is debatable; some opt for cholecystectomy during the hospitalization, while others prefer sphincterotomy and discharge with cholecystectomy 6 weeks later.

EXTENDED IN-HOSPITAL MANAGEMENT

As mentioned previously, pancreatitis can produce signs of profound systemic inflammation, so it is important to be vigilant and search for ongoing inflammation throughout a patient's hospital stay. There are several clinical scoring systems that help to identify patients most likely to have a difficult course. Perhaps the most commonly used is the Ranson criteria (Table 32-1).

A score of 1 to 3 indicates mild pancreatitis, while scores >3 suggest severe pancreatitis; such patients likely require more intensive monitoring. One disadvantage of the Ranson score is that it cannot be fully calculated until 48 hours. As a result, some clinicians prefer using the APACHE-II score, a validated objective scoring system of illness severity that is commonly used in the intensive care unit.

Severe pancreatitis often reflects the presence of significant glandular necrosis. The morbidity and mortality rises as the amount of necrosis increases. The necrotic tissue provides a rich media for infection, especially

TABLE 32-1
Ranson's Criteria for Acute Pancreatitis

On Admission	At 48 Hours
WBC count >16,000 cells/mm^3	PaO$_2$ <60 mm Hg
LDH >350 IU/L	Hematocrit decrease >10%
AST >250 U/L	Base deficit >4 mEq/L
Age >55	Fluid sequestration >6 L
Glucose >200 mg/dL	Calcium <8 mg/dL
	BUN increase >5 mg/dL

AST, aspartate aminotransferase; BUN, blood urea nitrogen; LDH, lactate dehydrogenase; WBC, white blood cell.
Ranson JHC, Rifkind KM, Roses DF, et al. Prognostic signs and the role of operative management in acute pancreatitis. *Surg Gynecol Obstet.* 1974;139:69.

from local bowel inflammation and bacterial translocation. Therefore, preventing infection remains a primary objective, as sterile necrosis has only a 10% mortality rate while infected necrosis has upwards of a 30% to 90% mortality rate. Prophylactic antibiotics should likely be given to patients with severe clinical symptoms and radiographic evidence of more than 30% necrosis. Empiric antibiotics should include gram-negative and anaerobic coverage; imipenem-cilastatin is probably the most effective of all antibiotics studied.

In addition to monitoring for the complications of uncontrolled systemic inflammation, such as ARDS and SIRS, there are a number of local intra-abdominal problems that may arise following a bout of acute pancreatitis. Pseudocysts are the most common complication, occurring in 7% to 25% of cases. Typically, the development of such cysts occurs between 4 and 6 weeks from the onset of pancreatitis. They can usually be managed conservatively but it is sometimes difficult to distinguish a pseudocyst from an abscess or a pancreatic tumor.

Multiple vascular catastrophes may arise as a result of the significant inflammation associated with pancreatitis. Such consequences may include arterial erosion or a pseudoaneurysm that leads to hemoperitoneum. Portal vein and especially splenic vein thromboses are also common, particularly when the inducing trigger is alcohol.

CLINICAL PEARL

A small number of patients with acute pancreatitis may progress to develop either portal hypertension or isolated gastric varices from portal and splenic vein thromboses.

Another common complication of acute pancreatitis is the progression to chronic pancreatitis. Chronic pancreatitis is characterized by the loss of both exocrine and endocrine pancreatic function. Common sequelae include diabetes (usually requiring insulin), fat and therefore vitamin malabsorption, chronic pain, and malodorous steatorrhea. Treatment includes nutritional support, pancreatic enzyme supplementation, and pain control.

It is also important to follow patients for complications related to their other medical comorbidities. For example, a patient who presents with alcoholic pancreatitis may be at higher risk for alcohol withdrawal and will require close observation and possible treatment early on in his or her hospital course (see Chapter 48).

DISPOSITION

Discharge Goals

A patient with pancreatitis is ready for discharge when he or she is able to tolerate oral intake and is able to have his or her pain controlled on oral medications. In rare cases, patients may be sent home on parenteral nutrition, but this is usually reserved for patients who have had recurrent episodes of pancreatitis that have severely limited their nutritional status. It is important to have a plan in place to help prevent recurrent pancreatitis whenever possible. For example, surgical follow-up for patients with gallstone pancreatitis and aggressive substance abuse counseling in patients with alcoholic pancreatitis should be arranged prior to discharge.

Outpatient Care

Patients should follow up with their primary care physician within a few weeks of discharge and should be encouraged to keep appointments with substance abuse counselors, gastroenterologists, and surgical specialists as appropriate.

WHAT YOU NEED TO REMEMBER

- Acute pancreatitis is a common cause of abdominal pain, nausea, and vomiting.
- Biliary pathology and alcohol use are the most common causes in the United States.
- Pancreatitis may be accompanied by severe systemic inflammation, resulting in either SIRS or ARDS.
- Pancreatitis is a clinical diagnosis, but laboratory testing and imaging may provide useful information.

- The timing and type of nutritional supplementation in acute pancreatitis are controversial.
- Antibiotics are only indicated in the case of significant pancreatic necrosis or worsening systemic manifestations.

REFERENCE

1. Carroll JK, Herrick B, Gipson T, et al. Acute pancreatitis: diagnosis, prognosis, and treatment. *Am Fam Physician.* 2007;75:1513–1520.

SUGGESTED READINGS

Attasaranya S, Abdel Aziz AM, Lehman GA. Endoscopic management of acute and chronic pancreatitis. *Surg Clin N Am.* 2007;87:1379–1402.

Baron T, Morgan D. Acute necrotizing pancreatitis. *N Engl J Med.* 1999;340: 1412–1417.

Frossard J, Steer ML, Pastor CM. Acute pancreatitis. *Lancet.* 2008;371:143–152.

Matull W, Pereira SP, O'Donohue JW. Biochemical markers of acute pancreatitis. *J Clin Pathol.* 2006;59:340–344.

O'Keefe S, Sharma S. Nutrition support in severe acute pancreatitis. Gastroenterol Clin N Am. 2007;36:297–312.

Yadav D. Alcohol-associated pancreatitis. *Gastroenterol Clin N Am.* 2007;36:219–238.

New-onset Jaundice

THE PATIENT ENCOUNTER

A 56-year-old previously healthy woman presents with a 2-week history of jaundice and fatigue. In the emergency room, she is found to be lethargic and deeply jaundiced. Laboratory results reveal a total bilirubin of 55 mg/dL, a direct bilirubin of 35 mg/dL, an alkaline phosphatase of 2,800 IU/L, an alanine aminotransferase of 135 IU/L, and an aspartate aminotransferase of 230 IU/L. A significant leukocytosis with a left shift is discovered. A right upper quadrant ultrasound shows marked intrahepatic and extrahepatic biliary ductal dilatation with a mass in the left hepatic lobe.

OVERVIEW

Definition

Jaundice, also known as *icterus*, is the yellow discoloration of the skin, sclera, and mucous membranes caused by elevated levels of bilirubin in the blood. The word *jaundice* is derived from the French word *jaune*, which means yellow. Typically, jaundice is detected when the serum bilirubin concentration is >2.5 mg/dL. There are a variety of conditions, ranging from benign to serious, that may result in jaundice. This chapter will focus on the diagnostic approach and management of patients who present with new-onset jaundice.

Pathophysiology

There are three basic phases of bilirubin production and metabolism, a disruption in any of which may lead to jaundice (Fig. 33-1). In the prehepatic phase, bilirubin is formed from the metabolism of heme, the majority of which comes from the breakdown of red blood cells. This unconjugated bilirubin is transported to the liver and is taken into hepatocytes, where it is conjugated with glucuronic acid to become water soluble. In the posthepatic phase, conjugated bilirubin is excreted from the liver as aqueous bile into the biliary and cystic ducts to be stored in the gallbladder or to enter the duodenum via the ampulla of Vater.

Epidemiology

There are a number of processes that may lead to jaundice. As a result, it is difficult to estimate the numbers of patients that present to the hospital with new-onset jaundice.

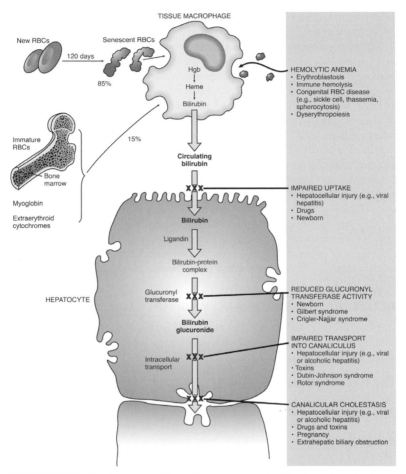

FIGURE 33-1: Mechanisms of jaundice at the level of the hepatocyte. Jaundice results from overproduction of bilirubin (hemolytic anemia) or defects in its hepatic metabolism. The locations of specific blocks in the metabolic pathway of bilirubin in the hepatocyte are illustrated. (From Rubin E, Farber JL. *Pathology*, 3rd ed. Philadelphia: Lippincott Williams & Wilkins; 1999, with permission.)

Etiology

It is clinically useful to think about the causes of jaundice in terms of disorders that result in predominately unconjugated versus conjugated hyperbilirubinemia.

The most common causes of unconjugated hyperbilirubinemia are overproduction of bilirubin, as in the case of hemolysis, and defective conjugation, which occurs in hereditary conditions such as Gilbert syndrome. They generally result in mild elevations in bilirubin, usually no greater than 5 mg/dL.

Conjugated hyperbilirubinemia reflects either the presence of hepatocellular disease or biliary obstruction. Among the most common causes of hepatocellular injury are viruses (hepatitis A through E, Ebstein-Barr virus, herpes simplex virus, and varicella zoster virus), drugs and toxins such as alcohol and acetaminophen, and autoimmune hepatitis. Other causes include nonalcoholic steatohepatitis; sepsis; low perfusion states, such as heart failure; and hereditary disorders, such as Wilson disease and hemochromatosis. The most common cause of biliary obstruction in the United States (also referred to as extrahepatic cholestasis) is cholelithiasis. Gallstones may become impacted in the common bile duct, which leads to jaundice, resulting in a condition known as choledocholithiasis. Malignancies, including cholangiocarcinoma, pancreatic cancer, and ampullary cancer, are less common but serious conditions that may result in obstructive jaundice. Strictures after biliary surgery, acute and chronic pancreatitis, infections in patients with acquired immunodeficiency syndrome, and primary sclerosing cholangitis are also other possibilities.

ACUTE MANAGEMENT AND WORKUP

It is important to make the distinction quickly about whether a patient with jaundice is "sick" or "not sick" as jaundice may represent a medical emergency in certain situations.

The First 15 Minutes

Recognizing several common clinical scenarios will help you initially evaluate a patient with new-onset jaundice.

Initial Assessment

The presence of fever and/or chills, right upper quadrant (RUQ) pain, and jaundice make up the Charcot triad, which is used to clinically diagnosis ascending cholangitis. Cholangitis results from biliary infection from partial or complete obstruction of the biliary tree. It may rapidly progress from local biliary infection to the systemic inflammatory response syndrome or sepsis. It is also critical that you assess the patient's mental status. The presence of mental status changes and hypotension in addition to the clinical findings of the Charcot's triad constitutes the Reynolds pentad, which, although rare, represents a severe form of cholangitis. In such cases, an intensive care unit (ICU) consult should be obtained immediately. While the patient from the encounter does not have fever or pain, her lethargy and leukocytosis in the setting of biliary obstruction (from a likely malignancy) should raise concern about the possibility of cholangitis.

> ### CLINICAL PEARL
> *Two factors that suggest moderate to severe cholangitis are the lack of response to initial medical treatment and the onset of organ dysfunction, including hypotension and disturbance of consciousness.*

Admission Criteria and Level of Care Criteria

Patients who appear to be sick, with signs of fever, abdominal pain, hypotension, or other worrisome clinical or laboratory features, need to be admitted to the hospital for further diagnostic workup and management of their jaundice. Patients who appear to be septic require closer observation in an intermediate care or intensive care unit.

The First Few Hours

Once the patient is stable, you can begin to gather more information to aid in the diagnosis and management of his or her jaundice.

History

Eliciting a good history often can provide you with much of the information you need to make a diagnosis. Important information to specifically ask about includes the use of alcohol; medications, including herbal medications; risk factors for hepatitis; a history of gallstones; a history of prior surgeries, including gallbladder surgery; human immunodeficiency virus status; travel history; prior medical history, such as hemolytic anemia or inflammatory bowel disease; and a family history of liver disease.

The details of a patient's clinical presentation may also provide you with important clues to the etiology. An older patient with recent weight loss, fatigue, pruritus, or light-colored stools likely has pancreatic or biliary tract cancer. Flulike symptoms, such as anorexia, malaise, and myalgias, may indicate a viral hepatitis.

> ### CLINICAL PEARL
> *Painless jaundice in an older patient represents malignancy until proven otherwise.*

Physical Examination

As mentioned previously, the presence of fever, tachycardia, tachypnea, or hypotension should be noted, as this will help you determine the level of care a patient needs.

The physical exam should also be directed at detecting signs of chronic liver failure or cirrhosis such as ascites, bruising, spider angiomata, gynecomastia, splenomegaly, and asterixis. A careful abdominal exam should be performed to assess for RUQ tenderness and liver span. Specific findings may point to certain diseases, such as a Kayser-Fleischer ring in Wilson disease or xanthomas in primary biliary cirrhosis. A careful cardiac exam should also be performed to assess for signs of heart failure that can lead to hepatic congestion and possibly hyperbilirubinemia.

Labs and Tests to Consider

Initial laboratory testing should include measurement of both total and conjugated (direct) bilirubin concentrations, alkaline phosphatase (AP), aminotransferases, prothrombin time (PT), albumin, and a complete blood count with differential. Evidence of systemic hypoperfusion, including blood urea nitrogen and creatinine to assess for acute renal failure and bicarbonate to assess for metabolic acidosis, is also important. Blood cultures should be sent in all patients in whom cholangitis is suspected.

Key Diagnostic Labs and Tests

An increase in serum AP and bilirubin out of proportion to aspartate aminotransferase (AST) and alanine aminotransferase (ALT) generally indicates biliary obstruction or intrahepatic cholestasis, while a predominant increase in aminotransferases reflects hepatocellular injury. Isolated hyperbilirubinemia suggests hemolysis or the presence of an inherited disorder of bilirubin metabolism, such as Gilbert or Crigler-Najjar syndrome.

If the clinical picture is most consistent with hepatocellular injury, screening tests to determine the cause should include serologic tests for viral hepatitis; autoimmune markers such as antinuclear, smooth muscle, and liver/kidney microsomal antibodies; a serum toxicology screen, including measurement of alcohol and acetaminophen levels; and measurement of serum ceruloplasmin, iron, transferrin, ferritin, and α_1-antitrypsin activity. An AST:ALT ratio >2:1 is characteristic of alcoholic hepatitis. Massively elevated aminotransferases (>1,000 U/L) indicate severe hepatitis usually due to viral causes, acetaminophen toxicity, or ischemia. Hypoalbuminemia and an elevated international normalized ratio are other markers of impaired liver synthetic function.

Imaging

Ultrasonography is generally the first recommended test to evaluate cholestasis as it is widely available, noninvasive, and relatively inexpensive. It is an excellent modality for detecting biliary ductal dilatation and obstruction. It can also detect cholelithiasis. Endoscopic ultrasound (EUS) allows for better visualization of the common bile duct and extrahepatic bile ducts as the transducer is placed directly into the duodenum, avoiding intestinal gas. Computed tomography scanning provides more detailed information about the liver as well as extrahepatic disease. Further imaging may be performed by a gastroenterologist or interventional radiologist, including endoscopic retrograde cholangiopancreatography (ERCP) or percutaneous transhepatic cholangiography. ERCP allows direct visualization of the biliary tree and pancreatic ducts. Its advantage is that it permits therapeutic interventions such as sphincterotomy with or without stent placement, stone extraction to relieve obstruction, and tissue diagnosis via biopsy or brushings if masses or strictures are detected. Magnetic resonance cholangiopancreatography (MPCP) is an alternative to diagnostic ERCP.

Treatment

The underlying cause of jaundice as determined by the history, the physical exam, and diagnostic testing directs subsequent therapy. If ultrasound is indicative of obstruction, ERCP may be needed for decompression of the biliary tree and possible diagnosis. Patients with evidence of ascending cholangitis should receive prompt supportive therapy with broad-spectrum antibiotics to cover common enteric microbes, which include gram-negative rods such as *Escherichia coli*, *Klebsiella*, and *Proteus*, and anaerobes such as *Bacteroides* and *Enterococcus*. Urgent biliary drainage, via ERCP or percutaneous drainage, is necessary in severe cases because an obstructed biliary system behaves essentially like an abscess that will respond poorly to antibiotics alone. The patient from our encounter will likely require empiric antibiotics for possible cholangitis, endoscopic or percutaneous decompression of her biliary system, and further diagnostic testing to confirm the suspicion that her hepatic mass is malignant.

EXTENDED IN-HOSPITAL MANAGEMENT

Patients with obstructive jaundice may develop cholangitis during their hospital stay and require admission to the ICU. Prompt diagnosis is critical for appropriate management.

Patients in whom a new diagnosis of pancreatic or biliary malignancy is established should be evaluated by a surgeon to determine whether their cancer is considered resectable. If their disease is deemed inoperable, as is often the case, a palliative care approach can be taken with possible referral to hospice care, depending on the patient's wishes.

DISPOSITION

Discharge Goals

Patients are ready to be discharged once the appropriate diagnostic and therapeutic workup for their jaundice has been performed and the necessary follow-up has been arranged. They should be afebrile and tolerating oral intake well, particularly if they need to continue taking oral antibiotics at home.

Outpatient Care

Communication with the patient's outpatient primary care physician should occur during his or her hospital stay, with the results of any diagnostic workup communicated promptly. Appropriate follow-up should be scheduled as necessary.

WHAT YOU NEED TO REMEMBER

- A careful history and physical exam are the first steps in evaluating a patient with jaundice.
- Screening laboratory tests may reveal a pattern of hepatocellular injury with a predominant elevation in AST and ALT versus a cholestatic pattern with a predominant elevation in AP.
- RUQ ultrasound is the initial test of choice when biliary obstruction is suspected.
- The most common cause of biliary obstruction is gallstones.
- Malignancy should always be considered in older patients who present with painless jaundice.
- The prompt diagnosis and management of ascending cholangitis, including the administration of early broad-spectrum antibiotics, referral to an ICU, and urgent biliary decompression in severe cases, can be life saving.

SUGGESTED READINGS

Bansal V, Schuchert VD. Jaundice in the intensive care unit. *Surg Clin N Am.* 2006;86:1495–1502.

Roche SP, Kobos R. Jaundice in the adult patient. *Am Fam Physician.* 2004; 69:299–304.

Rogoveanu I, Gheonea DI, Saftoiu A, et al. The role of imaging methods in identifying the causes of extrahepatic cholestasis. *J Gastrointest Liver Dis.* 2006;15(3): 265–271.

Vuppalanchi R, Liangpunsakul S, Chalasani N. Etiology of new-onset jaundice: how often is it caused by idiosyncratic drug-induced liver injury in the United States? *Am J Gastroenterol.* 2007;102:558–562.

Wada K, Takada T, Kawarada Y, et al. Diagnostic criteria and severity assessment of acute cholangitis: Tokyo guidelines. *J Hepatobiliary Pancreat Surg.* 2007;14:52–58.

Acute Hepatitis

THE PATIENT ENCOUNTER

A 22-year-old man is brought to the emergency department by his family with complaints of a 1-day history of yellow discoloration of his eyes, general malaise, and dull right upper quadrant pain. He is alert and oriented to person and place only, and has mild asterixis. He is tachycardic with no stigmata of liver disease. His comprehensive metabolic panel is significant for a severe elevation in his transaminases with a normal prothrombin time.

OVERVIEW

Definition

Acute hepatitis is a nonspecific term that includes all disorders that are characterized by a histologic inflammatory response of the liver that lasts no longer than 6 months. This chapter will focus on the approach to and management of inpatients that present with acute hepatic injury.

Pathophysiology

There are many potential causes of hepatic injury, including drug reactions, infections, and toxins, as well as metabolic, circulatory, and neoplastic insults. The pathophysiology of these diseases may differ, but in each case, one of five potential morphologic patterns is likely present at the cellular level: inflammation, degeneration, necrosis, regeneration, and/or fibrosis. A discussion of the pathophysiology of each of these injury patterns is beyond the scope of this chapter.

Epidemiology

The prevalence and incidence of acute hepatitis is difficult to determine because there are so many potential causes.

Etiology

The liver usually manifests disease in one of three patterns: cholestatic, hepatocellular, or mixed. In general, cholestasis is characterized by elevated levels of direct bilirubin and alkaline phosphatase, while hepatocellular injury is characterized by an elevation in the level of aspartate aminotransferase (AST) and alanine aminotransferase (ALT). The differential diagnosis

TABLE 34-1
Cholestatic Liver Disease

Obstructive	Intrahepatic
Choledocholithiasis	Primary biliary cirrhosis
Biliary stricture	Medications
Malignancy	Sepsis
Extrinsic compression	Cholestasis of pregnancy
Sclerosing cholangitis	Dubin-Johnson syndrome

for the underlying cause of liver injury is greatly informed by the predominant pattern seen on liver function testing.

Tables 34-1 and 34-2 list the most common causes of abnormal liver chemistries.

ACUTE MANAGEMENT AND WORKUP

The acute management and workup of acute hepatitis are largely dependent on the underlying cause of liver injury.

The First 15 Minutes

In the first 15 minutes of evaluating a patient with suspected acute hepatitis, it is very important to ensure that the patient is clinically stable before taking time to review his or her history.

Initial Assessment

After establishing stability, beneficial information can be gained by quickly reviewing the patient's vital signs and most recent laboratory values (complete blood count, comprehensive metabolic panel, and coagulation studies) if available. This initial review may suggest infection, metabolic derangement, liver dysfunction, and/or coagulopathy that may require immediate attention.

Your goal should be to obtain a focused history of the risk factors associated with liver disease; the recent use of prescription, over-the-counter, herbal, and illicit drugs; and a focused physical examination. Remember that while the patient may present with laboratory values consistent with an acute hepatitis, an extrahepatic diagnosis could be the underlying cause for the liver dysfunction. Liver injury in the setting of hypotension or passive liver congestion with decompensated congestive heart failure can each contribute to elevated liver tests.

TABLE 34-2
Hepatocellular Injury

Hepatocellular Injury	Infiltrating Disorders
Acute viral hepatitis	Malignancy
Chronic viral hepatitis	Hepatocellular carcinoma
Alcoholic liver disease	Lymphoma
Nonalcoholic fatty liver disease	Leukemia
Toxins	Metastatic disease
Hereditary liver disease	Granulomatous disease
Wilson disease	Tuberculosis
Hemochromatosis	Sarcoidosis
α_1-Antitrypsin deficiency	Histoplasmosis
Congestive/ischemic liver disease	Medications
Congestive heart failure	
Constrictive pericarditis	
Hypotension	
Budd-Chiari syndrome	
Veno-occlusive disease	
Inferior vena cava occlusion	

Care should be taken to establish the onset of signs and symptoms. While evaluating for common diseases that may cause elevations in liver chemistry tests, also keep in mind that there are many idiosyncratic drug reactions and potential side effects of commonly prescribed therapies and medications (e.g., blood product transfusions, nonsteroidal anti-inflammatory drugs, HMG-Co A reductase inhibitors, azole antifungals, and some antibiotics) that may cause these abnormalities.

A brief but focused examination should evaluate for the presence of encephalopathy as manifested by confusion, delirium, and possibly aster-ixis, as is the case in the patient from the encounter. You should look carefully for signs of jaundice, including scleral icterus and the color of the frenulum of the tongue. Attempt to palpate the liver. A large nodular liver might indicate cirrhosis, although end-stage cirrhotic livers may be too small to palpate, especially if the underlying cause is alcohol use. A pulsatile, tender liver might point to right-sided heart failure and subsequent congestive hepatopathy. A positive Murphy sign may indicate an acute cholecystitis. Splenomegaly is a reliable predictor of portal hypertension in patients with known liver disease. While less reliable, other stigmata of chronic liver disease might indicate cirrhosis, such as palmar erythema, spider angiomata, gynecomastia, and caput medusae. Patients with acute liver failure will often not have any signs of chronic liver disease because these signs develop over months to years.

It is important to do a thorough cardiovascular and pulmonary examination because patients with liver disease may have underappreciated cardiopulmonary disease or may have a lower afterload because of gut bacterial translocation and splanchnic vasodilation. They may also present with systemic inflammation or infection.

Admission Criteria and Level of Care Criteria

Acute liver failure (ALF) is defined as the onset of hepatic encephalopathy and coagulopathy (prothrombin time [PT] >15 seconds or international normalized ratio [INR] >1.5) within 26 weeks of acute liver injury in a patient without preexisting liver disease. Although this is a rare complication of many causes of acute hepatitis, ALF carries a very high mortality rate and should prompt immediate admission and evaluation by a hepatologist because liver transplantation may be indicated. Patients with acute liver failure are often severely ill on presentation. In general, you should have a very low threshold to call the intensive care unit to help evaluate such patients.

Any patient with elevated liver enzymes and a suspected toxic ingestion should be admitted for observation and possible treatment, depending on the ingestion. If the patient is clinically stable and has mild elevations in the transaminases without signs of worsening liver injury, altered mental status, or coagulopathy, an outpatient workup may be reasonable.

The First Few Hours

The history is tremendously important in identifying an underlying etiology of liver diseases in the early stages of liver injury. If vascular compromise, coagulopathy, or encephalopathy is suspected, you must take prompt action to initiate potentially therapeutic strategies.

History

It is important to identify patient risk factors for chronic liver disease, including blood transfusions, body fluid exposures, intravenous drug use, alcohol consumption, and recent toxic ingestions. Reviewing the patient's medical history for the diagnoses of right-sided congestive heart failure, recent episodes of hypotension, and pancreatitis may help in clarifying the etiology of the liver injury. The patient's social history could be very helpful in identifying risk factors for infectious hepatitis, alcoholic hepatitis, and infectious etiologies that may be associated with travel. In addition, the patient should be asked about genetically inherited diseases such as hereditary hemochromatosis, Wilson disease, and α_1-antitrypsin deficiency. Signs and symptoms of infection should be actively sought because ascending cholangitis, cholecystitis, and hepatic abscess can all present with elevated liver enzymes.

Physical Examination

In addition to the physical exam findings already discussed, there are certain signs to look for in patients with acute liver enzyme abnormalities. Fetor hepaticus is a characteristic breath odor that is often present in patients with hepatic encephalopathy. A respiratory alkalosis may also be seen with encephalopathy. You should look carefully for the stigmata of chronic alcohol use, such as muddy sclerae, lacrimal gland hypertrophy, and parotid swelling. However, remember that the physical examination may be unrevealing in patients with acute liver function test abnormalities.

Labs and Tests to Consider

On initial laboratory evaluation, you should order a complete blood count, basic metabolic panel, albumin, total bilirubin, direct bilirubin, AST, ALT, alkaline phosphatase, γ-glutamyl transferase, PT, INR, and urinalysis (urinary bilirubin, β-human chorionic gonadotropin). These tests will help to characterize the liver injury as predominantly cholestatic, hepatocellular, or mixed and will likely help to guide further testing.

Key Diagnostic Labs and Tests

In addition to the aforementioned tests, all patients with predominantly hepatocellular injury on initial laboratory testing should be screened for viral hepatitis. In most patients, this includes testing for hepatitis A, B, and C. Testing for hepatitis D should only be in done in patients with known hepatitis B (because hepatitis D requires coinfection with hepatitis B). Likewise, testing for hepatitis E should only be done in individuals with recent travel to endemic areas. All patients should have a serum volatile toxicology screen performed, mostly to evaluate for alcohol use, but also to screen for unsuspected ingestions. A serum acetaminophen level should be drawn in all patients, and an attempt made to document the time of last ingestion, since this will greatly impact treatment options as well as help in determining prognosis.

In the appropriate clinical context, serologic testing for autoimmune hepatitis should be performed including antinuclear antibody, anti–smooth muscle antibody, and anti–LKM-1 antibody.

CLINICAL PEARL

Acetaminophen hepatotoxicity is unfortunately very common and should be suspected in all patients who present with fulminant hepatic failure or acute hepatitis.

Imaging

Imaging of the liver can be of benefit in the initial evaluation of an acute elevation in the transaminases. Ultrasound (US), computed tomography (CT), and magnetic resonance imaging (MRI) all have roles in the evaluation of potential liver disease. However, the decision about which modality to use depends on the clinical scenario. A right upper quadrant ultrasound is a good option for the initial evaluation of a patient with suspected cholestasis. In addition to imaging the intra- and extrahepatic bile ducts, US with Doppler can also aid in the evaluation of liver vasculature, providing evidence of vascular occlusion such as portal vein thrombosis or hepatic vein thrombosis (i.e., Budd-Chiari syndrome). CT imaging with intravenous contrast can also provide a valuable look at the biliary system and vasculature but may also highlight liver masses or abscesses that could be potential causes of liver enzyme elevation. Magnetic resonance cholangiopancreatography (MRCP) may provide a more detailed look at the biliary system and may be indicated in cases in which the biliary system appears to be dilated on CT or ultrasound.

Further Testing

In cases of acute liver failure, or if the hepatic inflammation progresses despite a thorough workup, a liver biopsy may be indicated to search for the underling cause of hepatic dysfunction.

Treatment

Acute hepatitis is often self-limiting. Treatment is determined by the underlying cause. If hepatocellular damage is identified to be secondary to toxic ingestions or secondary to a specific drug, withdrawal of the offending agent is the treatment. In the case of known or suspected ingestions, a specific antidote, such as *N*-acetylcysteine in the case of acetaminophen ingestion, may be available to help prevent further hepatic injury (1,2). The patient in our encounter should be tested for acetaminophen levels and should have his treatment tailored based on the results and the clinical suspicion of ingestion. It is important to contact your local poison control center if you are able to identify a known ingestion because they are often able to provide specific instructions regarding the treatment and monitoring of at-risk patients.

If a hepatitis virus is found to be the cause of injury, acute therapy may be warranted, as in the case of acute hepatitis A.

EXTENDED IN-HOSPITAL MANAGEMENT

The extended hospital course of a patient with acute hepatitis will depend on the underlying etiology. Patients with acute liver failure require close monitoring until they either progress to liver transplantation or recover from their acute injury. Other patients require varying levels of inpatient monitoring.

If diagnostic studies reveal no evidence of hepatitis A or hepatitis B exposure, the patient should be screened for potential vaccination. In addition, alcohol cessation should be discussed with all patients with liver disease.

DISPOSITION

Discharge Goals

The discharge goals for a patient with acute hepatitis depend on the underlying etiology of the hepatitis and her or his overall clinical course.

Outpatient Care

After discharge, close follow-up with a primary care provider is important to continue to monitor the patient's liver chemistry tests. In the cases of acute hepatitis B and C, continual follow-up is necessary to document potential clearance of the virus or its continued course as chronic hepatitis. Depending on the underlying etiology of hepatitis, specialty care by a gastroenterologist or hepatologist may be warranted.

 WHAT YOU NEED TO REMEMBER

- Acute hepatitis is a nonspecific term that includes all disorders that are characterized by a histologic inflammatory response that lasts no longer than 6 months.
- There can be many causes of acute hepatitis; close attention paid to the patient's history and physical examination may give clues to the underlying etiology.
- A patient with acute liver injury should be admitted to the hospital when accompanied by signs of hepatocellular insufficiency or encephalopathy, or when the transaminases continue to rise without a known etiology.
- If the diagnoses of ALF is made, consideration of liver transplantation is urgent in all patients
- Acute hepatitis is usually self-limiting. The treatment of acute hepatitis is directly related to the diagnosis. If hepatocellular damage is identified to be secondary to toxic ingestions or to a specific drug, withdrawal of the offending agent is the treatment.

REFERENCES

1. Larson AM. Acetaminophen hepatotoxicity. *Clin Liver Dis.* 2007;11(3):525–548.
2. Lee WM. Etiologies of acute liver failure. *Semin Liver Dis.* 2008;28(2):142–152.

SUGGESTED READINGS

Ahmed A, Keeffe E. Liver chemistry and function tests. In: Feldman M, Friedman LS, Brandt LJ, eds. *Sleisenger & Fordtran's Gastrointestinal and Liver Disease.* 8th ed. Philadelphia: Saunders Elsevier; 2006.

Green RM, Flamm S. AGA technical review on the evaluation of liver chemistry tests. *Gastroenterology.* 2002;123(4):1367–1384.

Larson AM. Acetaminophen hepatotoxicity. *Clin Liver Dis.* 2007;11(3):525–548.

Lee WM. Etiologies of acute liver failure. *Semin Liver Dis.* 2008;28(2):142–152.

Stravitz RT, Kramer AH, Davern T, et al.; Acute Liver Failure Study Group. Intensive care of patients with acute liver failure: recommendations of the U.S. Acute Liver Failure Study Group. *Crit Care Med.* 2007;35(11):2498–2508.

Surveillance for acute viral hepatitis—United States, 2006. *MMWR Surveill Summ.* 2008;57(2):1–24.

Chronic Liver Disease and Portal Hypertension

THE PATIENT ENCOUNTER

A 55-year-old man with hepatitis C and cirrhosis is brought to the emergency department for a 1-week history of jaundice, increasing abdominal girth, and somnolence. His temperature is 38.1°C (100.6°F), his pulse rate is 100 bpm and regular, and his blood pressure is 110/70 mmHg. Spider angiomata, asterixis, and mild muscle wasting are noted. An abdominal examination shows a tender, distended abdomen with significant ascites, splenomegaly, and a nonpalpable liver. A bedside paracentesis is remarkable for a white blood cell count of 750 (83% polymorphonuclear cells), a serum albumin–to–ascites gradient of 2.4 g/dL, and a total protein of 0.8 g/dL.

OVERVIEW

Definition

The term *chronic liver disease* refers to any liver disease that results in the gradual destruction of liver tissue over time, frequently leading to cirrhosis and portal hypertension. This chapter will focus on the approach to and management of inpatients with cirrhosis and portal hypertension.

Pathophysiology

Cirrhosis is a chronic, degenerative disease in which normal liver cells are damaged and then replaced by scar tissue. This fibrous scar tissue causes vascular channels to become irregular and tortuous with accompanying increases in hepatic resistance and obstruction to portal venous flow. When portal vein pressure exceeds the pressure in the inferior vena cava, portal hypertension occurs. Portal hypertension remains one of the most serious sequelae of chronic liver disease and can lead to severe gastrointestinal bleeding, as well as to metabolic, renal, and circulatory complications.

As the pressure in the portal system begins to increase, dilation of veins at the portal-caval anastomoses begins to develop. The most frequently affected area is the gastroesophageal junction, with the distal 2 to 5 cm of esophagus being the most common site. These "varices" are at risk for serious bleeding as portal pressures elevate over time.

Increased pressures in the portal system also cause local production of vasoactive substances, such as nitric oxide, which causes splanchnic arterial vasodilatation and a decrease in effective arterial blood volume. Activation of the renal-angiotensin system ensues, leading to increased sodium and fluid retention. Additionally, this combination of portal hypertension and splanchnic vasodilatation causes increases in intestinal and liver capillary pressure and permeability, leading to the accumulation and retention of fluid in the abdominal cavity (ascites). Translocation of intestinal bacteria can subsequently infect ascitic fluid, causing spontaneous bacterial peritonitis (SBP). At advanced stages of cirrhosis, free water excretion becomes impaired and maximal renal vasoconstriction occurs, leading to a dilutional hyponatremia and development of the hepatorenal syndrome. Lastly, overall poor hepatic function leads to the impaired production of glucose and clotting proteins, and to the accumulation of bilirubin and unmetabolized ammonia, which leads to hypoglycemia, coagulopathy, jaundice, and hepatic encephalopathy.

Epidemiology

Cirrhosis was the twelfth leading cause of death in the United States in 2000, accounting for more than 25,000 deaths (1). Approximately 25% to 35% of cirrhotic patients will experience variceal hemorrhage (2). Hepatic encephalopathy may be present in 50% to 70% of all patients with cirrhosis (3).

Etiology

The causes of cirrhosis include a broad differential diagnosis of infectious, autoimmune, inherited, metabolic, toxic, and acquired origins. The most common causes in the United States are alcoholic liver disease and chronic hepatitis C infection. Additionally, while portal hypertension is often a result of cirrhosis, there are many other nonhepatic causes of portal hypertension (Table 35-1).

ACUTE MANAGEMENT AND WORKUP

Cirrhosis spans a wide clinical spectrum, from a presentation that is completely asymptomatic to severe hepatic dysfunction. Your initial evaluation needs to focus on identifying the degree of hepatic impairment, the correction of the ongoing insult, the prevention of further complications, and the appropriate evaluation and need for emergent liver transplantation.

The First 15 Minutes

When evaluating a patient, it is imperative to determine whether his or her liver disease is no longer compensated. The term *decompensated cirrhosis* is often used to denote the development of ascites, jaundice, gastrointestinal bleeding, electrolyte derangements, or hepatic encephalopathy. The patient in our vignette likely has decompensated cirrhosis because of his ascites and apparent encephalopathy.

TABLE 35-1
Causes of Portal Hypertension

Sinusoidal

Cirrhosis

Acute hepatitis

Extensive malignancy (hepatocellular carcinoma, metastatic disease, etc.)

Postsinusoidal

Right-sided heart failure including constriction and tricuspid regurgitation

Budd-Chiari syndrome, veno-occlusive disease

Presinusoidal

Portal or splenic vein thrombosis

Schistosomiasis

Initial Assessment

Hemodynamic function and mental status should be immediately determined upon meeting a patient with cirrhosis. Tachycardia (heart rate >100) and hypotension (systolic blood pressure <90 mm Hg) may indicate circulatory collapse from gastrointestinal hemorrhage or septic shock. An obtunded or confused patient may have hepatic encephalopathy, cerebral hemorrhage from a coagulopathy, or severe electrolyte derangements (e.g., hyponatremia, hypoglycemia). Basic labs, such as a complete blood count, comprehensive metabolic panel, coagulation studies, and a fingerstick glucose, should be obtained immediately to verify any of these abnormalities. A febrile patient may herald an underlying infection (e.g., SBP) that may progress to sepsis. Impaired respiratory status may indicate the presence of a hepatic hydrothorax, a condition in which ascitic fluid enters the pleural space through tiny defects in the diaphragm.

CLINICAL PEARL

Cirrhotic patients with ascites have massive volume redistribution that leads to a low blood pressure. A hemodynamically "stable" patient will often have hyperdynamic pulses and low systolic blood pressures in the range of 100 to 110 mm Hg.

Admission Criteria and Level of Care Criteria

Patients who have cirrhosis and are admitted to an intensive care unit often have a poor prognosis, with a median survival of 1 month. While there are no standardized criteria, admission to a higher level of care is usually based on the presence of the aforementioned complications and the need for managing a severe metabolic, circulatory, or neurologic impairment. For example, patients with high-grade hepatic encephalopathy are at risk for increased intracranial pressure and cerebral edema if ammonia accumulates too quickly in the blood. Although this is not as frequent as in acute liver failure/fulminant hepatic failure, these patients may require monitoring for increasing intracranial pressure.

The First Few Hours

After being placed in the appropriate level of care, patients with cirrhosis and new or worsening decompensation require evaluation for a precipitating cause.

History

Information should initially be gathered regarding the etiology of liver disease, whether a previous diagnosis of cirrhosis has been made (and how), and the duration of the patient's liver disease and/or cirrhosis. A previous history of complications should also be obtained to help gauge the severity of the patient's disease.

A patient's medication list, dietary regimen, and compliance history should also be obtained. Common causes of hepatic encephalopathy include a decrease in dose or discontinuation of medications such as lactulose, usually because of gastrointestinal side effects (i.e., frequent, loose stools). Taking medications such as sedative-hypnotics and narcotics is a common cause as well. Increases in diuretics can precipitate encephalopathy as well as inducing renal failure. Conversely, decreased diuretics can lead to increased fluid retention and worsening ascites. Increases in protein and sodium intake can also contribute to hepatic encephalopathy and worsening ascites, respectively.

A thorough review of systems should always be performed to help determine other factors that may have contributed to decompensation.

Physical Examination

The physical exam can provide a great deal of information about the severity and duration of cirrhosis and should focus on identifying stigmata of chronic liver disease and portal hypertension. The skin may reveal evidence of jaundice, spider angiomata/telangiectasias, or palmar erythema. Jaundice is usually detectable when bilirubin in the blood reaches 2.0 to 2.5 mg/dL and is most evident beneath the frenulum and in the sclerae. Vascular spiders may be present on the trunk, face, or upper extremities. Although their presence is not specific for cirrhosis and can be found in a number of other medical conditions (e.g., pregnancy, malnutrition), the number and size of these vascular lesions have been shown to correlate with the severity of chronic liver disease.

The abdominal exam should look to identify the presence of ascites, liver size, splenomegaly, or caput medusae (distended and engorged umbilical veins). Dullness in the flanks with tympany in the central abdomen is classic for ascites. "Shifting dullness" is often present, as confirmed by performing percussion with the patient on his or her back and then rolling the patient to one side. If ascites is present, the level where dullness begins will rise as the fluid pools on the dependent side. A fluid wave may also be appreciated in the presence of ascites. Tenderness on examination may be due to infection, but may also result simply from distention.

An enlarged liver may be palpated with a firm or nodular edge in chronic liver disease. However, the liver may begin to shrink in size and may not be felt in late stages of the disease. The presence of abdominal tenderness (rebound, involuntary/voluntary guarding) may suggest SBP, although its absence is not helpful in ruling out this diagnosis. As mentioned earlier, a thorough neurologic examination should be performed to identify the presence and/or severity of hepatic encephalopathy. Asterixis (flapping tremor) will be detected in early stages of encephalopathy. This is best demonstrated by having the patient extend the arms and dorsiflex the hands. In an obtunded patient, a gag or cough reflex should be assessed to determine if the patient can protect his or her airway. Examination of the pupils should also be performed to evaluate for any severe neurological insult (e.g., herniation). In addition to the findings mentioned above, other common physical exam findings in chronic liver disease and portal hypertension include the following:

- Clubbing and hypertrophic osteoarthropathies
- Cruveilhier-Baumgarten murmur—an abdominal venous hum in patients with portal hypertension
- Dupuytren contracture
- Fetor hepaticus—a sweet, pungent breath odor
- Gynecomastia
- Muehrcke nails—paired horizontal white bands separated by normal color
- Terry nails—proximal two thirds of nail plate appears white, whereas the distal one third is red
- Testicular atrophy

Labs and Tests to Consider

Routine blood work, including a complete blood count, comprehensive metabolic panel, and coagulation studies, should always be obtained to evaluate the extent of liver disease as well as to assess renal and circulatory function.

Key Diagnostic Labs and Tests

Elevated transaminases reflect damaged hepatocytes following hepatocellular injury or death. Patients with cirrhosis often have normal or only slightly elevated serum aspartate aminotransferase (AST) and alanine aminotransferase (ALT) levels, especially in those with long-standing disease. However, AST and ALT levels will be higher in cirrhotic patients with continuing inflammation or necrosis. Levels that are >10 to 15 times the upper limit of normal often indicate another acute process.

Impaired hepatic synthetic function is reflected by hyperbilirubinemia, hypoalbuminemia, and an elevated prothrombin time. Low platelet levels may be a marker of hypersplenism due to portal hypertension and splenic sequestration. Additionally, decreased levels of thrombopoietin from hepatic injury will contribute to thrombocytopenia.

Renal and circulatory dysfunction is usually reflected by hyponatremia and an elevated creatinine level from excessive renal vasoconstriction and impaired free-water excretion. A 24-hour urine sodium and protein collection may help determine the degree of renal impairment. If the hepatorenal syndrome is suspected, a workup to exclude other causes of renal failure should be performed in order to make a diagnosis. The diagnostic criteria for the hepatorenal syndrome include the following (4):

- Serum creatinine >1.5 mg/dL or 24-hour creatinine clearance <40 mL/minute
- Absence of shock, bacterial infection, fluid loss, or nephrotoxic drugs
- Absence of sustained improvement of renal function after a trial of plasma expanders (i.e., albumin)
- Absence of proteinuria (<500 mg/day) or hematuria (<50 red blood cells per high-powered field)
- Absence of obstructive uropathy or parenchymal renal disease by renal ultrasound
- Urinary sodium concentration <10 mmol/L

Other labs include fingerstick or serum glucose to evaluate for hypoglycemia from impaired hepatic gluconeogenesis, serum α-fetoprotein level to evaluate for hepatocellular carcinoma, and serum ammonia to aid in assessing hepatic encephalopathy.

CLINICAL PEARL

Plasma ammonia levels are usually elevated in patients with hepatic encephalopathy, but the degree of elevation does not correlate with the severity of encephalopathy; levels may be normal in up to 10% of patients with encephalopathy.

In almost all cirrhotic patients with ascites admitted to the hospital, a diagnostic paracentesis should be performed to rule out SBP. SBP is defined by an ascitic fluid polymorphonuclear cell (PMN) count >250 or a positive ascitic fluid culture with a single organism. The three most common organisms are *Escherichia coli, Klebsiella pneumoniae,* and *Pneumococcus.* The yield of a culture being positive in a patient with SBP (PMNs >250) increases from 50% to 80% with bedside inoculation of the culture bottles during the paracentesis. If the diagnosis of portal hypertension is in doubt, a serum albumin–to–ascites gradient >1.1 g/dL will confirm the presence of portal hypertension. A total protein >2.5 g/dL may further distinguish cardiac cirrhosis (congestive heart failure leading to portal hypertension) from hepatic cirrhosis.

Upper endoscopy should be routinely performed in patients with portal hypertension to evaluate for the presence of gastric and esophageal varices.

A liver biopsy is the gold standard for diagnosing cirrhosis but is not usually indicated in patients admitted to the hospital with previously known disease. However, based on the clinical setting, this may be of use in selected patients, especially in cases in which a diagnosis has not been made yet and/or another cause of liver disease is suspected.

Imaging

Diagnostic imaging in cirrhotic patients can be useful to evaluate the progression and extent of cirrhosis and/or to identify a new process responsible for acute hepatic decompensation. Abdominal ultrasound, computed tomography (CT), and magnetic resonance imaging (MRI) are commonly used to evaluate the liver, spleen, portal/hepatic vasculature, and abdominal cavity for the presence of ascites. Advanced cirrhosis often reveals liver surface irregularities/nodularities and increased areas of echogenicity. The use of duplex imaging with abdominal ultrasound can further evaluate for the patency of the hepatic and portal vasculature when obstruction is suspected (e.g., Budd-Chiari syndrome, portal vein thrombosis, veno-occlusive disease) and to evaluate for the presence of venous collateralization. CT may be indicated for evaluating the hepatic parenchyma further and to look for evidence of mass lesions (e.g., hepatocellular carcinoma). MRI can provide higher-resolution images if previous tests are equivocal. Additionally, magnetic resonance angiography is more sensitive than duplex ultrasound in detecting vascular abnormalities.

Treatment

The treatment of hospitalized patients with chronic liver disease will depend in part on their reason for admission.

Variceal Hemorrhage

Therapy for variceal hemorrhage should first be aimed at achieving hemodynamic stability with aggressive volume repletion via normal saline and/or blood. If present, a coagulopathy should be corrected using fresh frozen plasma with or without platelets. Octreotide and antibiotics (usually a third-generation cephalosporin) should be started to reduce splanchnic blood flow/portal pressures and for SBP prophylaxis, respectively. A continuous infusion of a proton pump inhibitor should also be started if variceal bleeding is suspected. A gastrointestinal consult should be obtained for upper endoscopy to evaluate for gastric and esophageal varices and to rule out other causes of bleeding. Endoscopic band ligation or sclerotherapy may be performed on bleeding esophageal varices. Gastric varices, however, are often located deeper in the submucosa and band ligation and sclerotherapy are usually ineffective. In the case of recurrent gastric variceal bleeding or refractory esophageal bleeding, portosystemic shunting by transhepatic portosystemic shunting (TIPS) or surgical shunting may be warranted. In all patients with known varices, prophylaxis should be addressed. Primary prophylaxis with a nonselective beta-blocker with or without the addition of a nitrate is typically initiated in patients with cirrhosis and known large varices. However, secondary prophylaxis should be instituted in all patients after an initial episode due to the high risk of recurrent variceal bleeding. The goal should be to titrate up the beta-blocker for a heart rate of approximately 55 bpm or to reduce the patient's baseline blood pressure by 25%.

Ascites

In mild ascites from portal hypertension, a reduction in dietary sodium intake is usually sufficient to reduce fluid accumulation. Unfortunately, most patients do not present until they have moderate ascites, so the initiation of diuretics in combination with sodium restriction is usually necessary. An aldosterone antagonist, such as spironolactone, is the first-line therapy, in part due to the presence of hyperaldosteronism in most patients with portal hypertension. Limitations to spironolactone include its side effects (gynecomastia, hyperkalemia), a lack of effectiveness in treating lower extremity edema, and an inability to use the medication in renal impairment due to an increased risk of severe hyperkalemia. Often, dual therapy that combines furosemide (a loop diuretic) and spironolactone is necessary when ascites is present with lower extremity edema. Furosemide causes hypokalemia; when combined at a ratio of 100 mg of Aldactone to every 40 mg of furosemide, potassium often remains within normal limits, as one agent wastes potassium while the other spares it. High doses of both may be required (400 mg of spironolactone and 160 mg of furosemide daily). Even at lower doses, occasionally patients become significantly intravascularly volume depleted, resulting in hypotension and hyponatremia. Such "refractory" ascites requires either regularly scheduled large-volume paracentesis with intravenous albumin after the procedure or the placement of a shunt that bypasses the liver (i.e., a transjugular intrahepatic portosystemic shunt).

A patient with ascites from portal hypertension may also develop a recurrent large, right-sided pleural effusion termed a hepatic hydrothorax. Management of hepatic hydrothorax is usually conservative but may involve recurrent thoracentesis for symptomatic relief. A chest tube should be avoided because the high-output drainage will make it difficult to remove the tube, exposing the patient to possible infection and potentially excessive protein loss.

Spontaneous Bacterial Peritonitis

Spontaneous bacterial peritonitis presents with complaints ranging from abdominal pain and fever, as in the case of our patient encounter, to altered mental status, to simply nausea and vomiting in a patient with ascites. Treatment should be started immediately if the paracentesis cell count has >250 PMNs or if the clinical suspicion is high before the results of the paracentesis are available. Usually, a third-generation cephalosporin such as ceftriaxone or cefotaxime is the treatment of choice. Culture-negative SBP is more prevalent than culture-positive SBP. However, morbidity and mortality appear to be the same for both conditions. If SBP is diagnosed, intravenous albumin is also given at day 0 and day 2 as this volume expansion has been shown to reduce the likelihood of developing hepatorenal syndrome. While being treated with antibiotics for SBP, large-volume paracenteses should likely be avoided as they may increase the likelihood of developing hepatorenal syndrome. Patients with a prior episode of SBP should be on lifelong prophylaxis. Patients with an active gastrointestinal bleed should receive 7 days of prophylaxis, while patients with a low total ascitic fluid protein (<1.0 g/dL) should be on prophylaxis while in the hospital. Fluoroquinolones are usually the drugs of choice for prophylaxis.

Hepatorenal Syndrome

Patients who develop hepatorenal syndrome have an extremely poor prognosis with a median survival of <1 month without therapy. Treatment is with vasoconstricting agents (vasopressin analogs or α-adrenergic drugs) along with albumin for 5 to 15 days. Octreotide alone does not work and, if used, is only beneficial in combination with midodrine. The treatment of hepatorenal syndrome increases the likelihood of survival to undergo orthotopic liver transplant, and improving the patient's renal function before transplant reduces posttransplant morbidity and mortality. In patients whose renal function does not improve after use of vasoconstrictors, hemodialysis may be warranted.

Hepatic Encephalopathy

Hepatic encephalopathy in patients with chronic liver disease is often due to clinically apparent precipitating events, and treatment should focus on identifying and correcting the underlying cause. Gastrointestinal bleeding and SBP should be treated as outlined previously. Metabolic disturbances (hyponatremia, hypokalemia) as a consequence of diuretic therapy should be corrected by electrolyte and fluid replacement in combination with medication readjustment. Sedative-hypnotic and narcotic medications should be discontinued. All patients experiencing hepatic encephalopathy should be prescribed lactulose, a nondigestible disaccharide and osmotic cathartic. Lactulose acts to decrease the absorption of ammonia. It should be titrated to result in two to three soft stools per day. Antibiotics against urease-producing bacteria, such as metronidazole and rifaximin, can also be used in combination with lactulose to decrease colonic production of ammonia. Refractory hepatic encephalopathy as a complication of TIPS may require implantation of a reducing stent to decrease blood flow through the TIPS.

Liver Transplantation

Patients with end-stage cirrhosis and severe hepatic decompensation may ultimately require orthotopic liver transplantation for definitive treatment. The nature and severity of liver disease should be categorized using standard techniques such as the Child-Pugh score or model for end-stage liver disease (MELD):

$$MELD = 3.78 \times \log[\text{serum bilirubin (mg/dL)}] + 11.2 \times \log[\text{INR}] + 9.57 \times \log[\text{serum Cr (mg/dL)}] + 6.43 \ (5)$$

Indications for transplantation are a MELD score ≥26, recurrent or severe hepatic encephalopathy, refractory ascites, SBP, and recurrent variceal bleeding. Unfortunately, not all patients will be eligible for transplant. Active substance abuse, extrahepatic malignancy, advanced human immunodeficiency virus, ongoing bloodstream infections, and the presence of severe comorbidities are contraindications to transplantation.

EXTENDED IN-HOSPITAL MANAGEMENT

The hospital course for a patient admitted with decompensated cirrhosis depends largely on the precipitating event. A patient who develops hepatorenal syndrome due to SBP may have a prolonged stay, whereas a patient who has hepatic encephalopathy because of medication noncompliance may be ready for discharge in several days after resuming lactulose. Patients who have changes to diuretic therapy or who undergo large-volume fluid removal (e.g., paracentesis, thoracentesis) should be watched closely for electrolyte, renal, and circulatory changes. Patients who undergo an upper endoscopy for variceal bleeding often require at least 48 to 72 hours of postprocedure observation to ensure that rebleeding does not occur. Most patients who require admission to an intensive care unit often have an extended hospital course and may oftentimes undergo transplantation if clinically indicated.

DISPOSITION

Discharge Goals

A patient is ready for discharge when the cause for decompensation has been identified and treated and all renal, circulatory, and electrolyte parameters are stable and/or have returned to baseline. Not all patients admitted to the hospital will make a recovery well enough for discharge and oftentimes may stay until transplantation can occur.

Outpatient Care

Patients should follow up with their primary care physician in 1 to 2 weeks as well as a hepatologist within 1 to 2 weeks. Patients with refractory ascites and recurrent hepatic hydrothorax may require more frequent visits with scheduled large-volume paracentesis and therapeutic thoracentesis as needed. All patients should continue to undergo routine screening for hepatocellular carcinoma with serum α-fetoprotein and hepatic imaging every 6 to 12 months.

 WHAT YOU NEED TO REMEMBER

- Alcohol-related liver disease and chronic hepatitis C are the most common causes of cirrhosis in the United States.
- Cirrhosis spans a wide clinical spectrum, from a presentation that is completely asymptomatic to severe hepatic dysfunction with jaundice, ascites, encephalopathy, variceal hemorrhage, coagulopathy, metabolic derangements, and renal failure.
- Patients with cirrhosis and new or worsening decompensation require evaluation for a precipitating cause, such as infection, electrolyte abnormalities, or gastrointestinal bleeding.
- All patients with cirrhosis should undergo upper endoscopy to evaluate for the presence of esophageal and gastric varices and, as appropriate, should be started on prophylaxis against variceal bleeding.
- Hepatic encephalopathy is often caused by metabolic disturbances from diuretic use, the use of sedative-hypnotics and narcotics, noncompliance with medications (lactulose), gastrointestinal bleeding, and SBP.
- SBP is an independent risk factor for developing hepatorenal syndrome and requires early diagnosis and prompt administration of antibiotics and albumin.
- The severity of liver disease should be categorized using either the Child-Pugh classification or the MELD score for appropriate evaluation and listing for orthotopic liver transplantation.

REFERENCES

1. Ginès P, Cárdenas A, Arroyo V, et al. Management of cirrhosis and ascites. *N Engl J Med.* 2004;350(16):1646–1654.
2. Sharara AI, Rockey DC. Gastroesophageal variceal hemorrhage. *N Engl J Med.* 2002;346(11):860–862.
3. Riordan SM, William R. Treatment of hepatic encephalopathy. *N Engl J Med.* 1997;337(7):473–479.
4. Paoli A, Merkel C. Pathogenesis and management of hepatorenal syndrome in patients with cirrhosis. *J Hepatol.* 2008;48:S93–S103.
5. Kamath PS, Wiesner RH, Malinchoc M, et al. A model to predict survival in patients with end-stage liver disease. *Hepatology.* 2001;33:464–470.

SUGGESTED READINGS

Green RM, Flamm S. AGA technical review on the evaluation of liver chemistry tests. *Gastroenterology.* 2002;123(4):1367–1384.
Karnath B. Stigmata of chronic liver disease. *Hospital Physician.* 2003;39(7):14–20.

Acute Gastrointestinal Bleeding

A 63-year-old man presents to the emergency department complaining of three episodes of bright red blood and clots passed rectally over the preceding 4 hours. He experienced an episode of dizziness when standing after the last bowel movement. He denies hematemesis and abdominal pain. The rectal exam is remarkable for gross blood.

OVERVIEW

Definition

Acute gastrointestinal (GI) bleeding is acute blood loss from the gastrointestinal tract (from the esophagus to the anus), which can result in hemodynamic instability. Hematemesis (frequently described as bright red or "coffee-ground") and melena (black, tarry stools) suggest an upper GI source defined as proximal to the ligament of Treitz. Hematochezia (bright red blood passed rectally) suggests a lower GI source or a very brisk upper GI bleed. The appearance of the stool, although suggestive, does not definitively localize the source of the GI bleed.

Pathophysiology

The pathophysiology of a GI bleed depends on its underlying etiology.

Epidemiology

Acute GI bleeding results in approximately 300,000 hospital admissions annually with an estimated cost of more than $900 million. Overall, the incidence of upper GI bleeds is approximately 100 cases per 100,000, while lower GI bleeds are less common, with an average of 20 to 27 cases per 100,000 (1).

Etiology

There are multiple causes of GI bleeding, and the differential is guided by distinguishing between upper and lower GI bleeds (Table 36-1). Although the patient's presentation can aid in distinguishing the source of the bleeding, it is important to note that brisk upper GI bleeds can cause hematochezia—indeed, 11% of suspected lower GI bleeds are ultimately found to have an upper GI source. It is also important to note that only a

TABLE 36-1

Causes of Acute Gastrointestinal (GI) Hemorrhage

Upper GI	Lower GI
Peptic ulcer disease (stomach or duodenum)[a]	Colonic diverticulosis[a]
Gastric erosions	Colorectal malignancy
Esophageal varices	Ischemic colitis
Mallory-Weiss tears	Acute colitis, unknown cause
Erosive esophagitis	Hemorrhoids/anal fissure
Angiodysplasia (Dieulafoy lesion)	Postpolypectomy hemorrhage
Neoplasm	Colonic angiodysplasia
Other (nosebleed, lung source with aspiration)	Neoplasm
	Crohn disease
	Other (menstrual bleeding)

[a]Most common.

small amount of blood will cause a heme-occult–positive stool, and this result may remain positive for up to a week postbleed.

ACUTE MANAGEMENT AND WORKUP

The acute management and workup will focus on hemodynamic stability as well as localization of the bleeding source.

The First 15 Minutes

When approaching any patient with GI bleeding, the assessment must first begin with determining the hemodynamic stability of the patient. Symptoms of orthostasis, as observed in our patient encounter, suggest a significant amount of blood loss. Postural changes greater than 10 mm Hg in systolic blood pressure or an increase of more than 10 bpm in pulse may indicate an acute blood loss of more than 800 mL (15% of total circulatory blood volume). Marked tachycardia, tachypnea, hypotension, or a change in mental status can suggest an acute blood loss of more than 1,500 mL (30% of total circulatory blood volume). If the patient has continued active bleeding, attention must be paid to frequent checks of the vital signs to ensure expeditious care and triage. New or worsening sinus tachycardia may be a sign that the bleeding has resumed or has increased in severity.

Initial Assessment

In an actively bleeding patient or a patient with vital signs suggestive of significant blood loss, prompt resuscitation is critical. This includes establishing intravenous access with a minimum of two large-bore (14- to 18-gauge) intravenous catheters to allow rapid delivery of crystalloid fluids to the patient. These patients may also require central venous access with a large-bore catheter (i.e., a Cordis), which allows for very rapid infusion of blood products. Initial blood work should include a complete blood count, electrolytes, and a coagulation profile. The blood bank should be notified immediately so that cross-matching can be initiated (nonmatched blood can be used in an emergency). In ordering initial blood products, attention should also be directed toward coagulopathy and thrombocytopenia. Further assessment with nasogastric (NG) tube placement and NG lavage should be performed in patients with suspected upper GI bleeding. Finally, attention must be directed to the patient's ability to protect his or her airway.

CLINICAL PEARL

Patients with extensive suspected lower GI blood loss should undergo NG lavage since the absence of hematemesis does not reliably exclude a brisk upper GI bleed.

Admission Criteria and Level of Care Criteria

The proper triage of a patient with gastrointestinal bleeding must take into account hemodynamic instability, continued bleeding, and response to initial resuscitation efforts. Retrospective studies have shown that patients with GI bleeding who are at higher risk for adverse outcomes during hospitalization include those with greater comorbidities, a lower serum albumin level, and a higher prothrombin time. In such patients, a higher level of care may be warranted. Intensive care is appropriate for any patient who is hemodynamically unstable or unresponsive to initial resuscitation fluids. For a hemodynamically stable patient with GI bleeding, a cardiac monitor is not immediately indicated unless the patient has shown ischemic changes related to the blood loss. Closer monitoring is always preferred for a patient with GI bleeding to permit early detection of clinical deterioration should bleeding resume.

The First Few Hours

Once the patient is hemodynamically stable, you can begin to explore the etiology of the bleeding in more detail.

History

The patient's history can provide much insight into the source of the bleeding and should include the following: (a) the nature and duration of bleeding, including changes in stool color, the frequency of bleeding, and the cessation of bleeding; (b) associated symptoms, including fever, weight loss, nausea, vomiting, abdominal pain, and tenesmus; (c) a past medical history, especially of prior episodes of bleeding (i.e., diverticulosis), prior abdominal surgeries (particularly aortic), liver disease, peptic ulcer disease, inflammatory bowel disease, radiation therapy, and any age-appropriate cancer screenings; (d) current medications, with particular attention paid to use of aspirin, nonsteroidal anti-inflammatory drugs (NSAIDs), and oral anticoagulation medications; (e) a social history, including alcohol and drug use, recent travel, and animal exposures; and (f) a family history of gastrointestinal malignancy or inflammatory bowel disease.

Physical Examination

The physical exam should begin with a review of vital signs, specifically pulse and blood pressure, including supine and upright measurements to assess for orthostatic hypotension. An examination of the conjunctivae and sublingual tissue for pallor can suggest anemia. The cardiac exam may reveal tachycardia and a hyperdynamic precordium. A murmur of aortic stenosis may suggest angiodysplasia as a source of GI bleeding (i.e., Heyde syndrome). The abdominal examination should be focused on identifying localizable tenderness, masses, hepatosplenomegaly, and the stigmata of chronic liver disease. Finally, the rectal exam must be performed in all cases to look for gross blood, evidence of hemorrhoids, fissures, and masses.

Labs and Tests to Consider

A number of laboratory and imaging studies may help you to determine the severity and location of the bleeding as well as to direct interventions aimed at preventing further blood loss.

Key Diagnostic Labs and Tests

A complete blood count is a critical first test. If possible, the patient's hemoglobin level should be compared to baseline values to establish a range and trend. Remember that active blood loss may not be immediately reflected in the hemoglobin level, since it takes time for the hemoglobin to equilibrate after acute blood loss. In addition, the hemoglobin level may fall after appropriate fluid resuscitation. If you suspect that a decreased hemoglobin level is due to hemodilution, be sure to evaluate for a trend in the other cell lines.

CLINICAL PEARL

Do not be reassured by a "normal" hemoglobin level in a patient who is actively bleeding, since it may take several hours for equilibration of the hemoglobin level to occur.

The complete blood cell count also provides the platelet count, which should be kept above 50 in an actively bleeding patient. The mean corpuscular volume can provide further diagnostic clues. For example, microcytosis suggests iron deficiency anemia from chronic blood loss as might be seen in a patient with colon cancer. Macrocytic anemia may suggest chronic alcohol use, which should raise the suspicion for liver disease. In the acute setting, the patient's hemoglobin level should be checked every 4 to 6 hours while the patient is bleeding.

Particularly in patients with underlying liver disease, a coagulopathy may be present at the time of the bleeding. Fresh frozen plasma (FFP) and vitamin K should be administered to achieve an international normalized ratio of <1.5 times normal.

Lastly, a ratio of blood urea nitrogen to creatinine >35 can suggest GI tract absorption of blood proteins, which suggests a more proximal source of bleeding. In all patients with GI tract bleeding, it is critical to ensure that a blood typing and cross-match is sent at the time of admission and kept active throughout the hospital stay. In a patient with continued bleeding, it is reasonable to have 2 to 3 units of packed red blood cells on hold in the blood bank, as well as FFP or platelets as necessary.

Finally, an electrocardiogram should be obtained on admission to look for ischemic changes that may indicate the need for more aggressive transfusion goals.

Imaging

The decision about when to pursue abdominal imaging for gastrointestinal bleeding is entirely dependent on the hemodynamic stability of the patient, as well as on the suspected cause of the bleeding. Abdominal computed tomography scanning (with oral and intravenous contrast) may demonstrate bowel wall thickening, evidence of diverticulosis, and intra-abdominal free air.

If the patient continues to have active bleeding, the ^{99m}Tc-pertechnetate labeled red blood cell (RBC) nuclear medicine scan can detect the source with variable reliability. Nuclear medicine scans have come to be the primary imaging modality in the radiologic evaluation of gastrointestinal bleeding. In general, a tagged RBC scan will yield a positive test with bleeding rates as low as 0.1 to 0.4 mL/minute, while angiography requires extravasation of approximately 1.0 to 1.5 mL/minute. Angiography does offer the benefit of immediate intervention by embolization. It should be noted that once the nuclear scan is begun, if the patient should bleed again within 24 hours, the patient can be returned to the radiology suite for further imaging, which is an added benefit to the tagged RBC scan.

Treatment

After the initial stabilization of the patient, the treatment of GI tract bleeding depends on whether the bleeding localizes to the upper or to the lower GI tract. Up to 80% of GI bleeding will spontaneously resolve, but it is not possible to predict which patients will stop bleeding without intervention. In general, consultation with gastroenterology should be sought early to guide further care of the patient.

The medical management of upper GI bleeding includes intravenous proton pump inhibitors. The data for the continuous infusion of proton pump inhibitors versus twice-daily administration remains inconclusive; the practice is often institution based, although most clinicians would probably use a continuous infusion in the case of a suspected variceal bleed. In the case of a variceal bleed, an octreotide infusion can lower the portal pressures and should also be considered (octreotide 50-μg intravenous bolus, then 50 μg/hour infusion).

After consultation with gastroenterology, an upper endoscopy may be performed for acute GI bleeding; in general, this is most successful if the bleeding has stopped. Direct visualization of the bleeding source permits endoscopic banding, thermal coagulation, the injection of vasoconstrictors, and/or sclerotherapy. For lower GI bleeds, if the bleeding has lessened and the patient is hemodynamically stable, the decision is likely to be made to administer a bowel preparation to ease the colonoscopy and endoscopic intervention. Bowel preparation has not been shown to worsen or reactivate bleeding.

Other considerations include the following: (a) ensuring that the patient takes nothing by mouth; (b) possibly withholding antihypertensive medications in the setting of severe bleeds; (c) withholding the administration of aspirin, NSAIDs, and oral anticoagulant medications (TED stockings and spontaneous compression devices should be used for deep venous thrombosis prevention); and (d) volume resuscitation, usually through intermittent boluses of intravenous fluids or blood products.

The patient in the encounter likely has a lower GI bleed from diverticulosis. He requires aggressive fluid resuscitation, and depending on his hemodynamic response may need a tagged RBC scan or angiography to localize the bleed. An NG lavage should likely be performed initially to exclude the possibility of a brisk upper GI bleed. If the NG lavage is negative and the bleeding stops spontaneously, he should be considered for colonoscopy to confirm the suspected diagnosis and look for other potential sources of lower GI bleeding.

EXTENDED IN-HOSPITAL MANAGEMENT

After stabilization of the patient and further diagnostic interventions to localize and potentially control the source of bleeding, consideration should be given to secondary prevention. For example, if an ulcer is found on an upper endoscopy, NSAID and aspirin use may need to be stopped. Patients with alcoholic gastritis or alcoholic liver disease will need aggressive lifestyle modification and substance abuse treatment. Remember to follow up on any biopsies that were taken at the time of the endoscopy since the results will help to substantiate a diagnosis of ischemic colitis or inflammatory bowel disease. In patients with peptic ulcer disease, the pathology should be examined for *Helicobacter pylori* or evidence of dysplasia. Lastly, if the patient has had significant bleeding, iron supplementation can be considered at discharge.

DISPOSITION

Discharge Goals

Patients with acute gastrointestinal bleeding are ready for discharge once their bleeding has stopped and their hemoglobin level is stable. If a source of bleeding cannot be localized, further diagnostic testing, such as a capsule endoscopy, or follow-up with a gastroenterologist should be arranged prior to discharge.

Outpatient Care

After a GI bleed, patients should follow up with their primary care physician within 1 to 2 weeks to make sure that their blood counts are stable. In cases in which a specific etiology has been identified (or even in cases in which the cause is not apparent), patients may need to follow up with a gastroenterologist, a hepatologist, or sometimes even a surgeon in order to explore further diagnostic and treatment options.

WHAT YOU NEED TO REMEMBER

- The most common causes of upper GI bleeding include peptic ulcer disease and gastric erosions; the most common causes of lower GI bleeding include diverticulosis and angiodysplasia.
- *Prepare for the worst.* Appropriately triage the patient; secure vascular access; aggressively provide fluid resuscitation; obtain a blood typing

and cross-match early, with a request for blood products to be on hold; and have a low threshold to call gastroenterology, surgery, and interventional radiology consults.

- Nasogastric lavage helps localize the source of the bleeding and provides useful information on the briskness of a bleed to guide management.
- Aggressive fluid resuscitation, the early initiation of proton pump inhibitors (plus octreotide in the setting of variceal bleeds), and the correction of any underlying coagulopathy are essential components of bleeding management.

REFERENCES

1. Chung P, Kim K. Epidemiology of acute gastrointestinal bleeding. In: Kim K, ed. *Acute Gastrointestinal Bleeding: Diagnosis and Treatment.* Totowa, New Jersey: Humana Press; 2003.

SUGGESTED READINGS

Gralnek IM, Barkum AN, Bardou M. Management of acute bleeding from a peptic ulcer. N Engl J Med. 2008;359(9):928–937.

Lau JY, Leung WK, Wu JC, et al. Omeprazole before endoscopy in patients with gastrointestinal bleeding. N Engl J Med. 2007;356(16):1631–1640.

Luk GD, Bynum TE, Hendrix TR. Gastric aspiration in localization of gastrointestinal hemorrhage. JAMA. 1979;241(6):576–578.

Zuccaro G Jr. Management of the adult patient with acute lower gastrointestinal bleeding. American College of Gastroenterology. Practice Parameters Committee. Am J Gastroenterol. 1998;93(8):1202–1208.

Approach to the Renal Evaluation

The majority of medical patients with renal dysfunction that you will encounter will present without specific urologic complaints. That is, most patients with renal dysfunction will be identified on the basis of an elevated serum creatinine level seen on a basic metabolic panel that was performed for another reason. In this context, many times renal dysfunction will be identified without the classic "symptoms and signs of kidney failure" as the initial presenting features.

While a patient's renal dysfunction may not be apparent in the initial history, a good review of systems and a thorough physical examination (often repeated after the discovery of an elevated creatinine level) will provide insight into the chronicity and etiology of the renal dysfunction. In contrast, some patients with renal dysfunction present quite strikingly with classic symptoms and signs of acute renal failure, including uremia, pyelonephritis, nephrolithiasis, and nephritic/nephrotic syndromes. In most instances, a thorough history and physical examination, coupled with a urinalysis and evaluation of the urine sediment, will lead to the correct diagnosis.

THE PATHOPHYSIOLOGY OF THE RENAL SYSTEM

The kidneys are fascinating organs that are involved in critical physiologic activities in order to maintain homeostasis in an ever-changing environment. They are responsible for maintaining fluid balance, regulating plasma tonicity and electrolyte balance, and removing the nonvolatile end products of nitrogen metabolism (i.e., maintaining acid–base equilibrium). The kidney has an increasingly apparent role as an endocrine organ, such as activating vitamin D, producing erythropoietin, and regulating the renin-angiotensin system. A fundamental knowledge of these normal physiologic properties will allow you to understand in greater detail the abnormalities that you encounter in patients with renal dysfunction.

Renal Ultrafiltration and Reabsorption

The normal excretory output of urine averages about 1 mL/minute. This volume is determined by the opposing forces of glomerular filtration and tubular reabsorption—the leftover product is excreted in the urine. The normal glomerular filtration rate (GFR) is about 125 mL/minute. Because urine output is normally about 1 mL/minute, you can infer that most of the filtered plasma is reabsorbed. In order to accomplish this, we need a lot of glomeruli and tubules. In fact, humans have between 225,000 and 900,000 nephrons in each kidney. The glomeruli are actually able to "hyperfiltrate" by increasing the tone of the efferent arteriole. In this manner, the injured or aging kidney is able to compensate for a loss of nephrons until about 50% or more of the total nephrons are lost before the serum creatinine level becomes "elevated" on a basic metabolic panel. While hyperfiltration can be beneficial in the short term, prolonged hyperfiltration and glomerular hypertension leads to glomerular hypertrophy and eventual scarring and fibrosis of the remaining kidney. Angiotensin-converting enzyme inhibitors and angiotensin receptor blockers lower glomerular pressure by decreasing the tone of the efferent arteriole, therefore delaying the progression of chronic kidney disease.

Renal Tubules

The kidney is responsible for maintaining acid–base equilibrium by maintaining a buffering system and by excreting noncarbonic nonvolatile acids. The renal tubules are also responsible for resorbing and secreting electrolytes and ultimately concentrating or diluting the urine. Generally, two physiologic concepts are of utmost clinical importance for the student or resident in understanding abnormalities of the renal tubular system: (a) acid–base equilibrium and (b) the renal solute gradient and action of antidiuretic hormone (ADH) on water resorption.

Acid–Base Metabolism

Noncarbonic nonvolatile acids are the result of dietary consumption and waste product metabolism (i.e., the liver). In a normal human under steady-state conditions, these acids amount to 1 mmol/kg/day. These acids use the intracellular (bicarbonate) and extracellular (phosphate, ammonia) buffering systems, which must be regenerated by the kidney. The kidney works to maintain a pH of approximately 7.4 and is able to increase or decrease acid elimination in order to maintain this level. With increases in dietary or metabolic acid production, the normal kidney is able to handle excretion of about 300 to 400 mmol/day of H^+. A damaged or an aging kidney must lose about 75% of total nephrons in order to begin to see clinical and/or laboratory derangements in levels of arterial pH, HCO_3, or $PaCO_2$.

Solute Gradient, Antidiuretic Hormone, and Serum Tonicity

The solute gradient of the kidney increases as one goes farther into the medulla. These solutes are primarily urea and NaCl. The dietary consumption of adequate solute is necessary for adequate dilution of the urine. The ability of the kidney to dilute or concentrate the urine relies on the following two elements: (a) the solute gradient and (b) the presence or absence of ADH (and its effect on the collecting tubules).

The effect of solute intake and ADH on serum tonicity and water balance is best understood first by remembering that the normal maximal free water clearance by the kidney is approximately 15 L/day. This assumes that the solute intake is adequate and that the renal tubules are able to maximally dilute the urine (in the absence of ADH). This means that the normal human can consume about 15 L/day of free water with no change in serum sodium. This can be overwhelmed acutely, as in the recent cases of water toxicity in college students.

Under normal conditions, approximately 600 (mOsm) of solute is taken in per day, which maintains the renal solute gradient. If the average urine concentration is approximately 300 mOsm/L, then the obligate urinary excretion per day to remove the solute is about 2 L. Substances that turn off arginine vasopressin production (e.g., coffee, beer) increase the obligate free water excretion by diluting the urine. In the absence of ADH, the urine osmolality decreases to 50 to 100 mOsm/L and the obligate urinary excretion to excrete the solute is 6 to 12 L.

Patients may have problems with serum tonicity when their solute intake is chronically low. This is frequently seen in two populations: (a) alcoholics who primarily get their nutritional intake from beer and (b) crash dieters who have an excessive intake of water. These clinical scenarios are referred to as beer and water potomania.

If the solute gradient in the kidney is only 200 mOsm (rather than 600 mOsm) and ADH is suppressed (i.e., urine osmolarity is 100 mOsm/L), the patient is only obligated to excrete 2 liters of urine per day. If a patient increases free water (in the form of beer or water) to more than 2 L/day, he or she is unable to excrete this and "owns" this free water. This excess free water will manifest as a decrease in serum sodium. See Chapter 41.

PATIENT EVALUATION

In subsequent chapters within the Nephrology section of this book, other clinical situations that affect total body water, serum osmolality and tonicity, and urine osmolality will be addressed. Of utmost clinical importance in these situations is determination of the patient's volume status. This aspect of the physical examination is most important for interpreting the laboratory abnormalities encountered in patients with renal dysfunction.

History and Physical Examination

Determine the patient's volume status by assessing the jugular venous pressure, checking orthostatic vital signs, and assessing the patient for edema (in the abdomen and presacral and pretibial areas).

When encountering a patient with a new diagnosis of renal failure, you should ask about the quantity and color of the patient's urine output, dysgeusia, or altered mental status (i.e., clouded thinking). You should also elicit the presence or absence of asterixis, rashes, or nail changes that can be helpful in narrowing the differential diagnosis. Costovertebral tenderness can make the diagnosis of pyelonephritis in the correct clinical and laboratory context.

Key Laboratory Evaluations

Key laboratory evaluations include serum creatinine testing, urinalysis, and urine sediment testing. These simple laboratory tests should be performed on the initial evaluation of every patient with renal dysfunction.

Serum Creatinine Testing

The assessment of the serum creatinine level is the test most commonly used as a surrogate for the GFR. In order to measure GFR, one needs a substance that is freely filtered in the glomerulus but is not secreted or reabsorbed. Creatinine is the most commonly used marker, although a small amount is secreted. Creatinine is a product of creatine phosphate, which is found in muscle tissue. This must be kept in mind when looking at the serum creatinine level because patients with more muscle mass will have a higher serum creatinine, and those with less muscle mass will have a lower serum creatinine level. A serum creatinine level of 1 mg/dL may be normal in a man who weighs 60 kg, but is abnormally high in a thin, elderly female. Frequently, it is helpful to have prior values of serum creatinine in order to correctly evaluate its meaning. Equations such as the Cockcroft-Gault and the (MDRD) equation can provide reasonable estimates of a patient's creatinine clearance, but only if the creatinine level is stable.

CLINICAL PEARL

Equations such as the Cockcroft-Gault and MDRD are not useful if the serum creatinine is changing. For example, if the serum creatinine increases from 0.9 mg/dL to 2 mg/dL overnight, the effective GFR is essentially 0.

Urinalysis

Urinalysis is a quick, inexpensive, and easy test that can give a physician valuable information. The presence or absence of white blood cells, red blood cells, bacteria, and specific gravity (SG) (an insight into the urine osmolality) are some of the most helpful data. The SG, coupled with the determination of the patient's volume status, can provide a quick insight into the cause of the renal failure as well as the ability of the kidneys to appropriately concentrate or dilute the urine. For instance, a patient with prerenal azotemia may be orthostatic, have an increased blood urea nitrogen–to–creatinine ratio, and have a high SG (≥ 1.015).

Consider some examples. A patient who drank too many beers would be expected to have a low SG, while a patient with volume depletion or syndrome of inappropriate antidiuretic hormone would be expected to have a high SG (to differentiate between these two diagnoses, you must know the volume status of the patient!). If the patient has no intrinsic renal damage, the urine sodium measure can also be helpful in confirming the patient's volume status. A urine sodium level <20 mEq/L is usually consistent with volume depletion or another effectively low circulating volume state, such as heart failure or cirrhosis.

Urine Sediment Testing

Urine sediment testing is important in evaluating patients with acute renal failure. One of the most gratifying diagnoses to make is a case of glomerulonephritis picked up by looking at the urine sediment under the microscope. As a medical student, you should make a point to look at the urine sediment of every one of your patients with acute renal failure. With persistence, experience, and, initially, a bit of luck, you will pick up a case of glomerulonephritis or acute tubular necrosis that would have otherwise been missed. This is a quick test to perform, and should be done by the admitting medical student or resident. As in the case of blood smears, don't rely on lab technicians to interpret the test because the clinical context will help guide your interpretation. If you don't know what you're looking at, ask an upper level resident or renal fellow to help you out. Most medical wards still have a "student lab" that has a centrifuge, slides, coverslips, and a microscope. Find this lab and use it often.

WHAT YOU NEED TO REMEMBER

- With a good patient history and physical examination, a little knowledge about renal physiology, and inexpensive but key lab tests, you should be able to make the correct diagnosis in most patients with renal failure.
- More extensive laboratory testing and/or renal biopsy is sometimes required when the diagnosis is undetermined.
- A volume status examination is critical in your assessment of a patient with renal dysfunction.

SUGGESTED READINGS

Denker BM, Rose BD. *Renal Pathophysiology: The Essentials*. Philadelphia: Lippincott Williams & Wilkins; 2006.

Acute Renal Failure

A 21-year-old healthy woman in her first trimester of pregnancy has been vomiting several times a day and unable to keep down food or liquid. She is brought in by a neighbor who noticed that she seemed confused today. Initial vital signs reveal a heart rate of 120 bpm. Her mucous membranes are dry. Initial labs reveal a blood urea nitrogen level of 60 mg/dL and a creatinine level of 3.2 mg/dL.

OVERVIEW

Definition

Acute renal failure (ARF) is defined as a rapid decrease in the glomerular filtration rate (GFR). This loss of renal function leads to the retention of urea and nitrogenous waste products and may lead to electrolyte and fluid imbalances. There are a number of definitions for acute renal failure but most focus on either an acute rise in creatinine (i.e., >50% abrupt increase) or a drop in urine output (i.e., <0.5 mL/kg/hour for more than 6 hours). This chapter will develop a framework for approaching patients with acute renal failure.

Pathophysiology

There are many etiologies of acute kidney injury (AKI) or ARF, but the mechanisms through which the injury is mediated are traditionally categorized by the functional and anatomic site of the disturbance (see Table 38-1). *Prerenal* azotemia encompasses those processes in which there is reduced renal perfusion to the glomeruli. Examples of this include true hypovolemia, a state of globally reduced effective circulating volume such as heart failure or cirrhosis, or, more localized to the kidneys, bilateral renal-artery stenosis. *Postrenal* azotemia refers to any process that prevents passage of formed urine from the body, which can happen at any anatomic level from the renal calyces to the urethra. *Intrarenal* causes of acute renal failure include any kidney pathology at the level of the arterioles, the glomeruli, the tubules, or the interstitium.

Epidemiology

In 2004, there were 221,000 hospitalizations in which acute renal failure was listed as the first discharge diagnosis. For patients who are already hospitalized, the incidence of ARF/AKI is significantly higher, approaching 2%

to 3%, and occurs more frequently in the elderly, African Americans, cardiac surgical patients, and patients with pre-existing renal disease, heart failure, and sepsis (1).

Etiology

Table 38-1 provides a list of the more common causes of acute renal failure.

TABLE 38-1
Major Causes of Acute Renal Failure

Type of Renal Failure	Common Causes of Renal Failure
Prerenal failure	• Intravascular hypovolemia (due to GI or renal losses, bleeding, or third spacing) • Poor cardiac output • Bilateral renal artery stenosis (especially with administration of ACE inhibitors) • NSAIDs (in settings of reduced effective circulating volume) • Hepatorenal syndrome • Aortic dissection with involvement of the renal arteries
Postrenal failure	• Ureteral obstruction (nephrolithiasis, papillary necrosis, retroperitoneal fibrosis or cancer) • Urethral obstruction (prostatic hypertrophy, neurogenic bladder, blood clot)
Intrinsic renal failure	• Glomerular: postinfectious glomerulonephritis, rapidly progressive glomerulonephritis • Tubulointerstitial: postischemic or toxic acute tubular necrosis, acute interstitial nephritis due to allergy or systemic infection, intratubular obstruction (e.g., uric acid crystal deposition, myeloma kidney) • Vascular: atheroemboli, vasculitis, malignant hypertension

ACE, angiotensin-converting enzyme; GI, gastrointestinal; NSAIDs, nonsteroidal anti-inflammatory drugs.

ACUTE MANAGEMENT AND WORKUP

The two most important responsibilities in the management of ARF are (a) to determine if the patient has metabolic, electrolyte, respiratory, mental status, or volume derangements that require immediate attention and (b) to determine the etiology of the acute renal failure, especially because readily reversible causes for acute kidney injury can often be identified. In the case of our patient encounter, aggressive volume resuscitation may be the only initial intervention required since her presentation is most consistent with hypovolemia from nausea and vomiting.

The First 15 Minutes

Recall that among the kidneys' responsibilities are the elimination of fluid, potassium, organic acids, and uremic toxins from the body. Hyperkalemia, pulmonary edema with respiratory distress, metabolic acidosis, and uremic encephalopathy in the setting of acute or chronic renal failure are worrisome and require immediate attention.

Initial Assessment

From a respiratory perspective, tachypnea could be a reflection of pulmonary edema or a compensatory response to a developing metabolic acidosis. Kussmaul respirations, or rapid, large tidal volume breaths, may also reflect compensation for a severe acidosis. Assess the patient's blood pressure and heart rate as well as rhythm. Cardiac arrhythmias require immediate attention. Intravascular volume depletion due to dehydration, bleeding, or third spacing may require prompt fluid resuscitation.

On initial laboratory studies, your evaluation should be directed toward the levels of potassium, bicarbonate, blood urea nitrogen (BUN), and creatinine. Hyperkalemia can promote the formation of arrhythmias by destabilizing the cardiac myocyte membrane. Your initial review of the electrocardiogram is critical. The presence of peaked T waves, prolongation of the PR interval, a diminished P-wave amplitude, and, in severe cases, elongation of the QRS complex all portend a potentially fatal arrhythmia and must be dealt with emergently (see Chapter 42). A low serum bicarbonate level on a metabolic panel requires an assessment of arterial blood gas to evaluate for metabolic acidosis. In general, a patient with ARF will demonstrate the presence of a primary metabolic acidosis with respiratory compensation. It is critical to determine whether this compensation is adequate. Finally, an anion gap should be calculated to determine if other factors beyond the accumulation of organic acids are contributing to the acidosis (see Chapter 40).

Urgent hemodialysis should be considered in patients with acute renal failure in several situations as outlined in the pneumonic AEIOU: A, acidosis; E, electrolyte abnormalities (i.e., hyperkalemia); I, intoxication; O, volume overload; and U, uremia (i.e., uremic pericarditis or a profound alteration in mental status). Blood urea nitrogen levels do not always correlate with the presence or degree of encephalopathy; thus, other reversible causes of altered mental status are usually sought in the immediate period, and trials of dialysis for uremic encephalopathy usually are not warranted until other causes are ruled out. The initiation of hemodialysis is a labor-intensive process, so it is important to get a nephrologist involved as early as possible while efforts to temporize the aforementioned processes are initiated.

Admission Criteria and Level of Care Criteria

Patients with ARF usually require in-hospital evaluation. Severe acidosis, altered mental status, respiratory distress, and cardiac instability are triggers for admission to a higher level of care. If a patient is being considered for urgent hemodialysis, he or she should generally be moved to an intermediate or intensive care unit setting. Patients with acute renal failure often require continuous cardiac monitoring, especially if they present with electrolyte or acid–base abnormalities.

The First Few Hours

Following the initial review and management of metabolic, respiratory, and mental status derangements, a combination of history, physical exam, and targeted laboratory and imaging studies can provide valuable clues as to the etiology of the ARF and identify potential reversible causes.

History

The timing of the onset of azotemia can be an important clue to the etiology. For example, the acute onset of anuric renal failure is highly suggestive of either an obstructive cause or a vascular etiology (i.e., aortic dissection that leads to a lack of blood flow to the renal arteries). For patients presenting with a first episode of renal failure, careful questioning about symptoms such as recent nausea, vomiting, diarrheal illness, lightheadedness, flank pain, hematuria, oliguria, dysuria, fevers, arthralgias, and rashes is helpful in establishing both the acuity and the etiology of the process. A review of recent medications (including over-the-counter agents and herbal supplements) is also important. While almost any medication can be responsible for AKI, certain drugs are more frequently cited as precipitants of acute renal failure, including nonsteroidal anti-inflammatory drugs, aminoglycosides, amphotericin B, indinavir, acyclovir, chemotherapeutic medications such as cisplatin or methotrexate, and angiotensin-converting enzyme inhibitors/angiotensin receptor blockers. Ultimately, temporally correlating a new medication with a decreasing GFR is most helpful in establishing a drug as a causal factor, regardless of its being one of the "usual suspects" or not. Attention should also be directed toward recent computed tomography

(CT) scans with intravenous (IV) contrast, since iodinated contrast agents can cause renal failure.

The patient's history also offers important information about comorbid conditions. Preexisting diagnoses, such as congestive heart failure, diabetes mellitus, cirrhosis, renal artery stenosis, underlying chronic kidney disease, human immunodeficiency virus, systemic lupus erythematosus (SLE), multiple myeloma, and other malignancies (especially acute leukemias and lymphomas), as well as benign prostatic hypertrophy can contribute to ARF.

Physical Examination

A number of physical findings can aid in the diagnostic evaluation. First, assess the patient's intravascular volume status. Dry mucous membranes, poor skin turgor, low jugular venous pressure (JVP), and lack of axillary sweat point to hypovolemia. The presence of an elevated JVP, pulmonary edema, additional heart sounds (S_3), peripheral edema, and ascites may reflect severe cardiomyopathy, cirrhosis, or volume overload. A cardiac exam, in addition to revealing the presence of additional hearts sounds, may reveal the triphasic rub of uremic pericarditis.

Physical findings associated with collagen vascular diseases (rashes, joint effusions, focal neurologic deficits), infective endocarditis (Janeway lesions, Osler nodes, new heart murmur), bladder obstruction (distended and painful bladder on abdominal examination), pyelonephritis (pain to percussion in the costovertebral angle), and prostate processes should also be sought when suggested by the clinical history.

Labs and Tests to Consider

There are a number of diagnostic tests that will aid in the evaluation of the patient with acute renal failure.

Key Diagnostic Labs and Tests

The serum creatinine is often used as a surrogate marker for GFR (see Chapter 39). However, estimates of GFR only hold true in the setting of a stable creatinine level. If a patient's creatinine level has increased from 1 to 3 in the span of 24 hours, then his or her GFR is essentially 0. As a result, the serum creatinine only tells part of the story and is oftentimes not helpful in determining the etiology of acute renal failure. The ratio of BUN to creatinine can be suggestive of prerenal disease if >20:1, but is otherwise of limited utility.

A urinalysis (revealing the presence of blood, protein, white and red blood cells, glucose, and infection) as well as microscopic examination of the urine can provide more useful information. For microscopy, a urine sample is obtained and spun via centrifuge. The resulting sediment is resuspended in a very small volume of the original urine (the rest having been poured off) and examined on a microscope slide. An "active" sediment can be very informative. Red blood cell casts suggest glomerulonephritis, white blood cell casts suggest pyelonephritis or interstitial nephritis, and granular casts suggest acute tubular necrosis. A "bland" sediment can also be helpful, taken together with features of the dipstick analysis. For example, 4+ protein with an unremarkable microscopy can be seen in the nephrotic syndrome, while 4+ heme with no red blood cells seen could indicate heme-pigment toxicity from rhabdomyolysis. A bland urine sediment can also be seen in prerenal and postrenal ARF. A quantification of the amount of protein in the urine can also be helpful in distinguishing nephritic from nephrotic causes of AKI. While there may be some overlap between these two types of renal disease processes, in general, excretion in excess of 3 g in 24 hours implies a nephrotic syndrome, while <3 g, especially if red cell casts are seen on microscopy, implies a nephritic syndrome. A spot ratio of urine protein to creatinine is a reasonable first study, because 24-hour urine collections are sometimes difficult to obtain. A ratio >3.5 (mg/mg) is consistent with nephrotic range proteinuria while, a ratio <0.2 (mg/mg) is within normal limits (2). Dipstick proteinuria is not a reliable way to quantify the amount of proteinuria.

CLINICAL PEARL

IV contrast dye may cause a false-positive dipstick protein.

A complete blood count with a differential should be performed. The presence of an elevated white blood cell (WBC) count with neutrophil predominance suggests infection. An elevated WBC count with an elevation in the eosinophils is consistent with an interstitial nephritis (often secondary to medications).

The quantitation of "spot" urine samples for sodium, creatinine, and urea nitrogen should be performed, as this is necessary for calculation of the fractional excretion of sodium and urea; see the formulas below.

Fractional Excretion of Sodium:
> [(Urine sodium × Serum creatinine) /
> (Serum sodium × Urine creatinine)] × 100

Fractional Excretion of Urea:
> [(Urine urea nitrogen × Serum creatinine) /
> (Serum urea nitrogen × Urine creatinine)] × 100

In acute oliguric renal failure, in the absence of diuretics, the fractional excretion of sodium is a well-validated measure for discriminating prerenal

AKI from other forms. A value <1% indicates a prerenal etiology, while a value >2% is suggestive of an intrinsic renal process. However, in nonoliguric ARF and/or in patients who have been exposed to loop diuretics in the previous day, this formula cannot be used. The calculation of the fractional excretion of urea can be helpful in this situation. A value <35% is consistent with a prerenal etiology. Also remember that, over time, prerenal processes such as intravascular volume depletion can progress to acute tubular necrosis, which is an intrinsic renal process. The prerenal processes are best thought of as a spectrum that leads to intrinsic renal disease.

Other tests should be selected based on the history, examination, or urinalysis (UA) findings. For example, if infection is suspected by the history or from the presence of pyuria on the UA, the urine should also be sent for culture. If the patient has a history of hepatitis C or collagen-vascular diseases such as SLE or Sjögren syndrome, serum cryoglobulins and complements should be obtained. ASO titers may be useful if the patient describes tea-colored urine and edema after a pyogenic infection. If hemoptysis or pulmonary hemorrhage occurs concomitantly with hematuria and rapidly progressive renal failure, antiglomerular basement membrane antibodies and antinuclear cytoplasmic antibodies should be part of the initial investigation to assess for Goodpasture syndrome and Wegener granulomatosis, respectively.

Imaging

Obstructive uropathy should be ruled out in all cases in which the cause of the kidney injury is not obvious and/or the injury does not resolve with a fluid challenge. The test may be as simple as a "postvoid residual" in which the individual attempts to urinate and then a urethral straight catheterization (or ultrasound bladder scan) is performed. If a substantial amount of urine (e.g., 900 mL) is collected in this manner, it indicates that an inability to properly void (due to partial bladder obstruction, neurogenic bladder, stone disease, etc.) is causing enough back pressure to the kidneys to injure them. Imaging tests that can demonstrate obstruction, hydroureter, and hydronephrosis include renal ultrasound and noncontrast CT scanning; the latter is more helpful if nephrolithiasis is suspected.

In addition to ruling out obstruction and hydronephrosis, renal ultrasound testing may reveal renal cysts (as in medullary kidney disease) or even perinephric abscesses. The addition of Doppler imaging can be helpful to look for renal artery stenosis or renal vein thrombosis. A CT scan of the abdomen and pelvis without contrast (to avoid nephrotoxicity) can demonstrate nephrolithiasis, abdominal/pelvic tumor or abscess, or obstruction.

A transthoracic echocardiogram can demonstrate new or worsening heart failure from systolic dysfunction, valvular vegetations as found in infective endocarditis, and the presence of a pericardial effusion, as in the case of severe uremia.

Treatment

The treatment of AKI largely depends on the identified etiology. For prerenal ARF due to hypovolemia, as is most likely the case in the patient encounter, the administration of IV isotonic crystalloid is first-line therapy. Relieving an obstructive uropathy depends on the level of obstruction; an indwelling urinary catheter may be needed for urethral obstruction until the root cause is dealt with medically or surgically, whereas a nephrostomy tube or stent may be needed to temporarily bypass a ureteral blockage. Allergic interstitial nephritis usually resolves after withdrawal of the offending agent, although if it continues to progress, most clinicians would advocate a short course of corticosteroids. ARF in the setting of a lupus flare or systemic vasculitis may also warrant high-dose steroids. Cryoglobulinemia may additionally require cyclophosphamide and even plasmapheresis therapy. Conversely, acute tubular necrosis requires no specific treatment other than careful monitoring and the appropriate management of metabolic and fluid volume derangements; it usually resolves within 2 to 3 weeks.

In addition to treating any suspected cause of AKI, during an episode of acute renal failure, it is absolutely critical to avoid additional nephrotoxic medications or substances.

EXTENDED IN-HOSPITAL MANAGEMENT

In most cases, AKI does not require an extended admission. Diagnosing and addressing reversible causes and observing an improvement in renal function is usually sufficient. If the etiology is identified and nonreversible, a decision must be made about whether the patient is likely to require a period of hemodialysis. If, however, the acute renal failure is unexplained or unclear after a thorough, noninvasive evaluation, a renal biopsy should be considered, especially if the renal failure is progressive and/or involves glomerular hematuria or proteinuria. Biopsy specimens are examined under light and electron microscopy and with immunofluorescence techniques that are used to detect various immunoglobulin subclasses as well as their light chains, complement components, and fibrin. A renal biopsy is most helpful in situations in which a potentially treatable cause of ARF is being considered and the results of this test would alter the patient's management (e.g., high-dose steroids for a rapidly progressive glomerulonephritis). A nephrologist should be intimately involved in the decision to biopsy a patient with acute renal failure.

DISPOSITION
Discharge Goals

A patient admitted for acute renal failure is ready for discharge after you establish the etiology of the renal failure and stabilize the patient's renal function.

Outpatient Care

If long-term dialysis is warranted, then dialysis access and outpatient follow-up with a nephrologist and dialysis center should be arranged prior to discharge. Appropriate follow-up should be arranged with the patient's primary care physician as well as with specialists, as appropriate.

WHAT YOU NEED TO REMEMBER

- Acute renal failure or acute kidney injury disproportionately affects the elderly, those with underlying kidney disease, and those who have comorbid conditions such as cirrhosis, heart failure, and diabetes.
- Immediately identify patients who meet criteria for urgent hemodialysis and mechanical ventilation, as these can be life-saving interventions.
- The history, physical exam, and a complete urinalysis with microscopy are the most important tools in determining the cause of acute kidney injury.
- Unless the cause is obvious, obstructive uropathy should always be excluded.

REFERENCES

1. Flowers NT, Croft JB, Division of Adult and Community Health, National Center for Chronic Disease Prevention and Health Promotion. *Morbid Mortal Wkly Rep.* 2008;57(12):309–312.
2. Ginsberg JM, Chang BS, Matarese RA, et al. Use of single voided urine samples to estimate quantitative proteinuria. *N Engl J Med.* 1983;309:1543–1546.

SUGGESTED READINGS

Brady HR, Brenner BM. Acute renal failure. In: Kasper DL, Braunwald E, Hauser S, et al., eds. *Harrison's Principles of Internal Medicine.* 16th ed. New York: McGraw-Hill; 2005.

Carvounis CP, Nisar S, Guro-Razuman S. Significance of the fractional excretion of urea in the differential diagnosis of acute renal failure. *Kidney Int.* 2002;62: 2223–2229.

McCullough PA. Contrast-induced acute kidney injury. *J Am Coll Cardiol.* 2008; 51(15):1419–1428.

Naughton CA. Drug-induced nephrotoxicity. *Am Fam Physician.* 2008;78(6):743–750.

Palevsky PM. Indications and timing of renal replacement therapy in acute kidney injury [Review]. *Crit Care Med.* 2008;36(4 Suppl):S224–228.

Rose BD, Rennke HG. *Renal Pathophysiology – The Essentials.* Philadelphia: Lippincott Williams & Wilkins, 1994.

Chronic Kidney Disease in the Hospitalized Patient

THE PATIENT ENCOUNTER

A 56-year-old Caucasian man with diabetes, hypertension, and chronic kidney disease (baseline serum creatinine level of 2.6 mg/dL and a baseline weight of 80 kg) was brought to the emergency room complaining of dizziness upon standing. He was seen 1 week prior in an urgent care facility for a gout flare. He was found to have a blood pressure of 183/96 mm Hg and was given a prescription for atenolol 100 mg by mouth daily. Today his blood pressure lying flat is 100/60 mm Hg with a pulse of 46 bpm. While standing, his blood pressure drops to 86/40 mm Hg with a pulse of 47.

OVERVIEW

The diagnosis and treatment of specific kidney diseases are covered elsewhere in this book. This chapter will focus on the management of chronic kidney disease in patients admitted to the hospital for other reasons.

Definition

Chronic kidney disease (CKD) is defined as a glomerular filtration rate (GFR) of <60 mL/minute that has persisted for longer than 3 months. Chronic kidney disease can also be diagnosed with a normal GFR if there are structural or functional defects in the kidney. An example is someone who has significant proteinuria but without a change in his or her creatinine level.

Pathophysiology

The pathophysiology of chronic kidney disease will depend on the underlying cause of the renal dysfunction.

Epidemiology

It is estimated that about 13% of Americans over the age of 20 have chronic kidney disease, up from 10% only a decade ago. This increase is likely driven in large part by the rising prevalence of diabetes and hypertension (1). Elderly patients and African Americans are also at higher risk of developing CKD.

Etiology

The most common cause of chronic kidney disease in the United States is diabetes, followed closely by hypertension. These two disorders account for almost 70% of all new cases of CKD. Other causes include infection, obstruction, and autoimmune and infiltrative diseases.

ACUTE MANAGEMENT AND WORKUP

Patients with chronic kidney disease will usually be admitted to the hospital for another complaint. It is important to address a patient's acute medical issues in the context of his or her underlying renal disease.

The First 15 Minutes

When you are called to evaluate a patient in the emergency room and find that his or her creatinine level is elevated, as is the case in our encounter, an important first question is, "Have you ever been told that you have kidney disease?" Because patients rarely have symptoms until the later stages of kidney disease, they may not know or understand that they have chronic kidney disease. Be persistent! Ask when they last had blood tests done. Prior lab data are often the only way to know if the kidney function is stable, worsening, or improving. Remember that a patient may have chronic kidney disease characterized by proteinuria without an abnormal serum creatinine. A urinalysis should always be done in the initial evaluation of chronic kidney disease to check for protein.

> ### CLINICAL PEARL
>
> *The amount of proteinuria can be as important as serum creatinine to prognosis in CKD. A spot (random) urine protein–to–urine creatinine ratio can be used to estimate total daily protein excretion. In general, the more protein in the urine, the worse the prognosis.*

Initial Assessment

Once you have established that your patient has chronic kidney disease, your initial assessment should be focused on the patient's chief complaint.

Admission Criteria and Level of Care Criteria

The decision to admit a patient with chronic kidney disease will usually hinge on two issues: (a) the nature of the patient's chief complaint and (b) the need for hemodialysis. Patients with chronic kidney disease tend to have more comorbidities such as cardiovascular disease and diabetes so the threshold to admit them to the hospital tends to be much lower.

The First Few Hours

The two primary functions of the kidney are to regulate volume status and to clear physiologic toxins (like urea) from the body. Therefore, in addition to focusing on the chief complaint of the patient, you should look carefully for signs and symptoms of volume overload and the buildup of uremic toxins.

History

In addition to trying to discern the duration and severity of your patient's chronic kidney disease, your history should search for clues of worsening renal function. Symptoms of uremia may include mental status changes, nausea and vomiting, itching (pruritus), loss of appetite (anorexia), and restlessness (insomnia). You should ask about symptoms of volume overload, such as orthopnea and paroxysmal nocturnal dyspepsia, as well as the presence and character of any peripheral edema.

Physical Examination

For volume status, pay attention to the lung exam and cardiac exam. Look for edema. Remember that if a patient has been on his or her back, the edema will probably be on his or her back (sacral edema) more than in his or her legs (pedal edema). The physical exam in a patient with kidney disease must always include a weight. Compare admission weight to any previous weight data available. Continue to check daily weights while the patient is in the hospital to follow volume status.

Signs of uremia include a pericardial rub and asterixis (ask patients to hold their hand in front of them like they are stopping traffic—a flapping motion develops within 30 to 60 seconds). Remember that asterixis and edema can also be signs of liver disease. If your patient has any of the aforementioned uremic symptoms, hemodialysis may be indicated.

Labs and Tests to Consider

There are a number of diagnostic studies that can aid in the evaluation of a patient with chronic kidney disease.

Key Diagnostic Labs and Tests

The patient's creatinine level is often used as a marker of kidney function. It is made in fairly constant amounts and is cleared from the body by the kidneys. The elevation of creatinine in the bloodstream is a fairly specific marker of kidney dysfunction. Creatinine is a protein byproduct of creatine in muscle and, therefore, blood levels reflect the amount of muscle a person has, how much protein he or she ingests, and the rate of muscle turnover (i.e., higher in the case of muscle damage). Creatinine production can also vary significantly by sex, age, and race. Therefore, the serum creatinine level can be a clue to kidney dysfunction but does not really tell you how *well* (or not well) the kidney is working.

The GFR tells you how well the kidney is filtering. It can be estimated in a variety of ways, but the most common is the creatinine clearance. This is calculated by measuring the creatinine in a 24-hour collection of urine and a spot sample of creatinine in blood. A 24-hour collection is sometimes not practical to do and will not give you information right away. As a result, there are several formulas that use immediately available data (such as weight, age, race, and serum creatinine) to calculate the GFR. The two that are most commonly used are the Modification of Diet in Renal Disease (MDRD) and the Cockroft-Gault formulas. The Cockroft-Gault equation is [[140 – age (yrs)] × [weight (kg)] / [72 × Cr (mg/dL)]] (× 0.85 for females).

The GFR will tell you what stage of CKD your patient has. Most patients do not have symptoms directly from kidney disease until they reach stage 4 or 5 (Table 39-1).

Imaging

Iodinated contrast is used to enhance certain radiographic studies, such as computed tomography (CT) scans and angiography. This type of contrast can be nephrotoxic. Patients with diabetes and with pre-existing CKD are at highest risk of having acute renal failure from iodinated contrast. It is best to avoid iodinated contrast entirely if the patient has CKD. If a patient must have contrast, there are several proposed methods to help prevent contrast nephropathy. The most important preventive strategy is to make sure that the patient is not volume depleted. Thus, most patients with CKD who can tolerate it receive intravenous (IV) hydration prior to the test. There is no convincing evidence that fluids that contain bicarbonate are more helpful than normal saline alone. Other strategies include using oral N-acetylcysteine dosed twice daily both before and after contrast administration.

TABLE 39-1
The Stages of Chronic Kidney Disease

Stage 1	Normal GFR (>90 mL/min) AND persistent albuminuria
Stage 2	GFR 60–89 AND persistent albuminuria
Stage 3	GFR 30–59
Stage 4	15–29
Stage 5	<15: often called *end-stage renal disease*

GFR, glomerular filtration rate. Adapted with permission from Scrier RW. *Diseases of the Kidney and Urinary Tract*, 8th ed. Philadelphia: Lippincott Williams & Wilkins; 2006

Before ordering a radiographic test on a patient with CKD, ask yourself the following questions: "Is IV contrast required in order to answer the clinical question?" and "Does my hospital have a protocol for pretreating patients with CKD prior to contrast?"

Magnetic resonance imaging (MRI) can also be enhanced with IV contrast. The contrast agent for MRI studies is often gadolinium. Gadolinium is less toxic to the kidney than iodinated contrast. For many years, in patients with CKD, MRI with gadolinium contrast was used as an alternative to CT scans with iodinated contrast. However, we now know that gadolinium contrast is associated with a rare and serious disease called nephrogenic systemic fibrosis (NSF). In this disorder, there is progressive fibrosis of the skin and other organs. We are still learning about this disease, but we do know that people who have a GFR <30 mL/minute have a higher risk of developing NSF. This includes patients on dialysis. Some centers require that any patient with a GFR <30 mL/minute who has received gadolinium contrast have two full sessions of dialysis over the following 2 days in order to help clear the contrast. We do not know yet if this will prevent NSF, so the best way to prevent this disease is to not give these patients gadolinium unless absolutely necessary.

Treatment

Angiotensin-converting enzyme inhibitors/angiotensin receptor blockers (ACE-Is/ARBs) are classes of drugs that are the mainstay of treatment for most kidney diseases that involve proteinuria. They share two effects that you should be aware of in the hospital setting:

- *ACE-Is/ARBs decrease blood flow through the kidney by decreasing constriction of the blood vessels draining the nephron (efferent arterioles).* This is beneficial to the kidney in that it decreases kidney damage in the long term. However, if the patient has a sudden loss of blood pressure (from volume depletion or surgical or traumatic blood loss), ACE-Is/ARBs can prevent the kidney from maintaining a minimum amount of blood flow. Therefore, if the patient is hypotensive or a surgery is planned, these drugs should be temporarily held.
- *ACE-Is/ARBs can also slightly raise the serum potassium level.* If the potassium level in your patient is high, these medicines may have to be temporarily held. Remember to restart these medicines once the patient is better or the surgery is complete.

Most patients in the United States who have Stage 5 CKD (end-stage renal disease) are started on hemodialysis. Other methods of renal replacement therapy are peritoneal dialysis and kidney transplantation. If your patient is on hemodialysis, then it is important to ask the time of his or her last dialysis session. Most people are on a three-times-weekly schedule. Dialysis patients are prescribed a "dry weight"—this is their target weight after volume removal at dialysis. It is common for patients to gain 2 to 4 kg of fluid weight over this "dry weight" by the time of the next dialysis session. Comparing your patient's "dry weight" to his or her current weight will give you a good idea about his or her volume status. It is important to notify the renal team as soon as possible in order to schedule dialysis in the hospital.

EXTENDED IN-HOSPITAL MANAGEMENT

There are a number of longitudinal issues that need to be addressed in patients with CKD. Dietary issues are particularly important. Patients with Stage 4 or 5 CKD may have trouble getting rid of the phosphorus that they take in each day. You may notice that these patients will be on phosphate binders. Calcium salts, like calcium carbonate or calcium acetate, work well as phosphate binders. If patients have high serum calcium, then non–calcium-containing phosphate binders such as sevelamer or lanthanum carbonate may be used. Patients with Stage 4 or 5 CKD in the hospital should be on a potassium- and phosphorus-restricted diet. Protein restriction of at least 0.75 g/kg/day is suggested in Stage 4 and 5 CKD if the patient is not on dialysis, and 1.2 g/kg/day if the patient is on dialysis.

Cardiac disease is the number one cause of death in dialysis patients. Any complaint of chest pain in a dialysis patient should be taken very seriously. The second most common cause of death is infection. Hemodialysis requires reliable access to the bloodstream. This can be done with a catheter, an arteriovenous graft (a piece of synthetic material that connects an artery and a vein), or an arteriovenous fistula (a surgical connection between an artery and a vein in which no synthetic material is used). Infection of dialysis catheters is very common, whereas infection of an arteriovenous fistula is very rare. The most common cause of infection associated with hemodialysis catheter use is *Staphylococcus aureus*. Up to 30% of these isolates are methicillin resistant. Thus, for dialysis patients with catheters who present with signs of infection, it is common practice to give them a single dose of vancomycin while blood cultures are pending.

It is important to remember to adjust the dose of medications that are renally cleared in patients with CKD. The patient presented at the beginning of this chapter has a GFR of 36 by the Cockroft-Gault formula and therefore has Stage 3 CKD. Atenolol and nadolol are water-soluble beta-blockers and require dose adjustment in patients with CKD. While 50 to 100 mg once a day is listed as an acceptable starting dose of atenolol in patients without kidney disease, a dose of 25 mg/day would have been a more appropriate starting dose in this patient. Antibiotics are probably the most frequent medications you will prescribe that will require dose adjustments.

DISPOSITION

Discharge Goals

Plans for discharge will, in large part, be dictated by the underlying condition that prompted admission.

Outpatient Care

Patients with CKD should have close follow-up with their primary care physician because tight blood pressure control in hypertensive patients and tight glycemic control in diabetics may reduce the rate of progression of their disease. Patients with Stage 4 and 5 CKD should be referred to a nephrologist for further evaluation and for consideration of elective initiation of dialysis in the future. In patients already on dialysis, arrangements with their routine dialysis center should be made prior to discharge to ensure that they do not miss their regularly scheduled dialysis session.

WHAT YOU NEED TO REMEMBER

- The patient's creatinine level does not tell you how well the kidney is working. Calculate an estimated GFR using the MDRD or Cockroft-Gault formula.
- Make sure all medications are dosed appropriately and that iodinated or gadolinium-based contrast is not used unless absolutely necessary.
- The physical exam and review of symptoms in a patient with kidney disease should focus on the signs and symptoms of volume overload and uremia.
- Understand that patients with CKD and those who are on dialysis are at high risk for cardiac disease, so you must tailor your workup accordingly.
- If a dialysis catheter is present, then line infection should be considered if the patient shows any signs of infection.

REFERENCE

1. Coresh J, Selvin E, Stevens LA, et al. Prevalence of chronic kidney disease in the United States. *JAMA*. 2007;298(17):2038–2047.

SUGGESTED READINGS

Daugirdas JT. *Handbook of Dialysis*. 4th ed. Philadelphia: Lippincott Williams & Wilkins; 2007:513.

Eaton DC, Pooler JP. Clearance. In: *Vander's Renal Physiology*. 6th ed. New York: McGraw-Hill; 2004:37.

Grobner T, Prischi FC. Gadolinium and nephrogenic systemic fibrosis. *Kidney Int.* 2007;72:260–264.

Johnson CA, Levey AS, Coresh J, et al. Clinical practice guidelines for chronic kidney disease in adults: part 1. *Am Fam Physician.* 2004;70(5):869–876.

Katneni R, Hedayati SS. Central venous catheter-related bacteremia in chronic hemodialysis patients: epidemiology and evidence based management. *Nat Clin Pract Nephrol.* 2007;3(5):256–266.

Stevens LA, Coresh J, Greene T, et al. Assessing kidney function - measured and estimated glomerular filtration rate. *N Engl J Med.* 2006;354:2471–2483.

Weisbord SD, Pavelsky PM. Prevention of contrast-induced nephropathy with volume expansion. *Clin J Am Soc Nephrol.* 2008;3:273–280.

Metabolic Acidosis

A 21-year-old man is brought to the emergency room by "friends," who depart before further information can be obtained from them. He is mildly febrile, tachycardic, and normotensive, but delirious—varying between agitated and obtunded. Initial electrolyte panel shows a sodium of 141 mEq/L, chloride of 105 mEq/L, bicarbonate of 10 mEq/L, glucose of 96 mg/dL, blood urea nitrogen of 16 mg/dL, and creatinine of 0.9 mg/dL. He is admitted to the step-down unit with a diagnosis of "rule-out sepsis." An arterial blood gas on room air reveals a pH of 7.20, PCO_2 of 16 mm Hg, PO_2 of 102 mm Hg, and calculated bicarbonate of 10 mEq/L.

OVERVIEW

Definition

Metabolic acidosis can be defined as a primary reduction in serum bicarbonate due to either loss of bicarbonate or addition of hydrogen ion. It is important to note that while the pH is usually low in this context, the definition does not include a pH threshold since in the setting of mixed acid–base disorders the pH can be normal or even elevated although a metabolic acidosis is present. This chapter will provide a basic framework for approaching patients with a metabolic acidosis.

Pathophysiology

The pathophysiology of a metabolic acidosis depends in large part on the underlying cause. In general terms metabolic acidosis can result from an overproduction of acid (i.e., lactic acidosis from sepsis), an inability of the kidney to secrete an acid load (i.e., a distal renal tubular acidosis), or a loss of bicarbonate from either the kidneys or gastrointestinal tract (i.e., large-volume diarrhea or a proximal renal tubular acidosis). The pathophysiology of each type of acidosis is beyond the scope of this chapter.

Epidemiology

Since metabolic acidosis may be caused by a variety of clinical conditions, it is difficult to estimate its incidence or prevalence.

TABLE 40-1
Causes of Metabolic Acidosis

Elevated Anion Gap	Normal Anion Gap
Salicylates	**D**iarrhea
Lactic acidosis	**U**reteral diversion
Uremia (renal failure)	**R**enal tubular acidosis
Methanol ingestion	**H**yperalimentation
Paraldehyde	Carbonic **A**nhydrase inhibitors
Ethanol/ethylene glycol	**M**assive saline infusion
Diabetic ketoacidosis/starvation ketoacidosis	Recovery phase of ketoacidosis
	Toluene toxicity (glue sniffing)
	Ca^{2+} or Mg^{2+} Chloride ingestion

Etiology

There are several etiologies for a primary metabolic acidosis. It is generally helpful to divide the common etiologies into anion gap versus nonanion gap causes (Table 40-1).

ACUTE MANAGEMENT AND WORKUP

Severe metabolic acidosis from any cause may result in altered mental status, cardiac depression, and, ultimately, hemodynamic collapse. A metabolic acidosis may also be a consequence of a serious underlying disorder such as sepsis or decompensated heart failure. As a result, the initial management will in part be guided by the underlying cause of the acidosis but must also include a rapid assessment of mental status, respiratory status, and hemodynamic stability.

The First 15 Minutes

The approach to a metabolic acidosis is guided by the presence or absence of an elevated anion gap. The anion gap is calculated as serum $Na - (Cl + HCO_3)$. The patient in our encounter has an anion gap of 26 [141 (Na) – 105 (Cl) – 10 (HCO_3)]. The normal value for an anion gap is usually 12 $\pm$ 2 mmol/L. This expected anion gap can be thought of as a balance between unmeasured cations and unmeasured anions, and can change under certain conditions. For example, albumin is a polyanionically charged serum protein that constitutes part of the anion gap. If the albumin level is low, the calculated anion gap will be lower than expected. This can be corrected by adding 2.5 mEq/L to the measured anion gap for every 1 g/dL in albumin below 4.0 g/dL. Similarly, we can expect a patient with a profoundly elevated level of serum calcium (an unmeasured cation) to have a lower than expected anion gap.

Once it is determined that a patient has an anion gap or nonanion gap acidosis, it is important to determine his or her acid–base status by measuring an arterial blood gas. The body adjusts quite quickly to a metabolic acidosis by increasing minute ventilation (respiratory rate $\times$ tidal volume) to decrease PCO_2. The Winters formula, below, can aid in confirming that a patient is adequately compensating for his or her metabolic acidosis.

$$\text{Expected } PCO_2 = 1.5 \text{ (serum bicarbonate)} + 8 \pm 2$$

If the PCO_2 is higher than this equation predicts, the patient may be relatively hypoventilating, a sign that he or she may require ventilatory support in the near future. In contrast, a PCO_2 significantly lower than predicted indicates a respiratory alkalosis, which, in the setting of an anion gap acidosis, should raise the possibility of salicylate toxicity. Salicylates directly stimulate central nervous system–induced hyperventilation, in addition to causing a metabolic acidosis from their deleterious effects on oxidative metabolism. Our patient's expected PCO_2 from the encounter is 23 ± 2 [$1.5 \times 10 \, (HCO_3) + 8 \pm 2$], while his measured is 16, suggesting that he has a respiratory alkalosis beyond what would be expected from compensation for his anion gap metabolic acidosis. Salicylate toxicity should be seriously considered as a diagnostic possibility.

Admission Criteria and Level of Care Criteria

In truth, "metabolic acidosis" is rarely an admitting diagnosis or the isolated reason for a hospital admission. There are a number of patients in the outpatient arena with a metabolic acidosis who are clinically well. The reason for admission is most often the underlying cause of the metabolic acidosis (e.g., diabetic ketoacidosis, sepsis with tissue hypoperfusion, uremia, etc.). Sometimes, though, a patient will be "sick" enough for admission due to general appearance, altered mental status, or vital sign abnormalities—and yet the cause may not be readily apparent. In these cases, the metabolic acidosis, and the stepwise approach to identifying its origin, may be the key to determining the diagnosis and plan of care.

The First Few Hours

There are a number of studies that will aid in the diagnosis and management of a metabolic acidosis.

History

After a metabolic acidosis has been established with admission labs, specific questions based on the etiologies listed in Table 40-1 can be asked. For example, is the patient a diabetic? Has he or she experienced symptoms of a recent infection? Has he or she had profound diarrhea? The patient's medication history is especially relevant given that several agents can contribute to an acidosis. It is also important to ask about potential toxic ingestions. Alcohol use is a common cause of ketoacidosis but should also raise your suspicion for possible coingestions, such as methanol or ethylene glycol.

Physical Examination

Besides the initial assessment of a patient's hemodynamic and mental status, important information can be present on physical examination. Does the patient smell of alcohol, or is there a "fruity" odor on his or her breath, which would be indicative of a ketosis? Is the patient febrile, warm, and vasodilated, which suggests possible sepsis? On funduscopic examination, is there optic disc hyperemia suggestive of methanol toxicity?

Because hyperventilation is the main way that the body deals with an acute acidosis, it is important to carefully observe and evaluate a patient's respiratory status. Patients with a metabolic acidosis may be noticeably tachypneic or they may be taking larger than normal breaths (i.e., Kussmaul breathing) in an attempt to blow off the acidosis. Patients with poor respiratory reserve may be unable to maintain or even achieve this increased minute ventilation. Even a young, healthy person will eventually tire if the acidosis is severe enough or prolonged indefinitely. If a patient begins to slow down his or her respiratory rate and becomes more somnolent, respiratory and hemodynamic collapse may be imminent. Patients who appear to be tiring should be considered for ventilatory support before they reach this stage.

Labs and Tests to Consider

There are a number of specific laboratory tests that must be sent in the evaluation of a metabolic acidosis.

KEY DIAGNOSTIC LABS AND TESTS

If an elevated anion gap is present, a serum lactate level should be sent. Mild lactic acidosis can sometimes be seen from tissue hypoperfusion due to a number of factors (including dehydration), but lactic acidosis can also be a harbinger of septic or cardiogenic shock or ischemic bowel. Similarly, determining the level of serum ketones can be useful when faced with a high anion gap, as they can be seen in diabetic, starvation, or alcoholic ketoacidosis. A serum volatile toxicology screen as well as a salicylate level should be checked, especially when the patient is unable to provide a history secondary to poor mental status.

In the appropriate clinical context, or if an elevated anion gap cannot be readily explained, an "osmolal gap" should be calculated as follows:

$$\text{Expected osmolality} = 2(\text{Na}) + (\text{serum glucose} / 18) + (\text{Blood urea nitrogen} / 2.8) + (\text{serum EtOH} / 4.6)$$

$$\text{Osmolal gap} = \text{Serum osmolality} - \text{Expected osmolality}$$

If the osmolar gap is >10 and the anion gap is elevated, suspect methanol, ethylene glycol, or propylene glycol toxicity.

CLINICAL PEARL

Isopropyl alcohol will also cause an elevated osmolal gap but the anion gap will be normal.

In cases of an elevated anion gap, it is important to determine whether a superimposed nongap acidosis or metabolic alkalosis is also present. This can be done by calculating the "delta-delta," a ratio of the deviations from normal values for the serum anion gap and bicarbonate. Use the following formula:

"Delta-delta" = (Elevation in anion gap above normal) / (Decrease in HCO_3 below normal)

If the delta-delta ratio is <1, the metabolic acidosis has both a "gap" and a "nongap" component. If it is >2, there is a mixed metabolic acidosis and alkalosis. For reasons related to lactate's clearance in the kidney, a lactic acidosis often results in a "delta-delta" of about 1.6.

Metabolic acidosis without an anion gap has its own differential diagnosis, although there can be some overlap between gap and nongap etiologies. For example, a normal anion gap can be seen in the recovery phase of a ketoacidosis, as the ketoacids are excreted in the urine. A normal gap may also be seen in chronic renal failure.

In the evaluation of metabolic acidosis with a normal anion gap, it is helpful to evaluate the urine anion gap (UAG) using the following calculation:

$$UAG = (Urine\ Na^+) + (Urine\ K^+) - (Urine\ Cl^-)$$

A positive value for a UAG indicates that NH_4^+ is being underexcreted and that a renal tubular acidosis (RTA) is present. This signifies that the kidney is not excreting enough titratable acid (in the form of NH_4CL) in response to an acidemia. Urine pH can distinguish a type I RTA, which is caused by a defect in the ability of the intercalated cells of the collecting duct to excrete adequate hydrogen ion, from a type II RTA, which is due to failure of the proximal tubule to resorb bicarbonate. In type I RTA, urine pH usually cannot be lowered below 6.0, although this can still occur with a type II RTA. A type IV RTA is in fact not a tubular problem, but occurs due to insufficient aldosterone action at the level of the distal tubule. Whether this is due to resistance to aldosterone's effects or to underproduction of aldosterone (as can happen in adrenal insufficiency, diabetic nephropathy, human immunodeficiency virus–associated nephropathy, angiotensin-converting enzyme inhibition, or nonsteroidal anti-inflammatory drug use), the hallmark of a type IV RTA is an associated hyperkalemia.

In the absence of a positive urine anion gap, the cause of a nongap metabolic acidosis is often evident by history (diarrhea, ureteral diversion, hyperalimentation, etc.).

> ## CLINICAL PEARL
>
> *A low serum anion gap can be caused by lithium toxicity, a paraproteinemia from a condition such as multiple myeloma, or bromide ingestion (rarely seen clinically).*

Treatment

In general, treatment of a metabolic acidosis focuses on addressing the underlying cause. This is especially true for the anion gap acidoses. For example, the administration of bicarbonate to treat lactic acidosis has not been shown to provide clinical benefit. Most authorities would suggest avoiding the use of intravenous bicarbonate in this situation unless the pH is <7.0, at which point refractory hypotension or imminent cardiac arrest is a balancing consideration. It is not general practice to supplement bicarbonate in an anion gap acidosis, with exceptions such as salicylate toxicity, in which forced alkaline diuresis is therapeutic. This might be considered in the patient from our encounter if his salicylate screen is positive. In most cases, the focus should be to "treat the patient, not the pH."

In contrast, bicarbonate supplementation in patients with nongap acidoses is common, although the threshold for initiating treatment in the acute setting varies among practitioners. Traditionally, in a patient with a pH of >7.20 and serum bicarbonate >12 mEq/L who is asymptomatic (i.e., not dyspneic), treatment is deferred. Below these thresholds, bicarbonate supplementation is usually initiated. In patients with chronic kidney disease, there are some data to suggest a goal serum bicarbonate level of closer to 20 mEq/L due to the potential long-term effects of acidosis on bone demineralization and muscle breakdown.

EXTENDED IN-HOSPITAL MANAGEMENT

A patient's extended hospital course will be largely determined by the underlying cause of his or her metabolic acidosis. It is important to follow a patient's acid–base status closely with an evaluation of serial blood gases to make sure that the process is resolving. As in an acute presentation, it is also important to make sure that a patient continues to compensate for his or her acidosis while the workup and management for the underlying condition are under way.

DISPOSITION

Discharge Goals

Patients with an anion gap acidosis should remain in the hospital until their acidosis has resolved and the underlying etiology has been treated. Patients with a nongap acidosis may sometimes be discharged before their bicarbonate level has returned to normal if the underlying cause for their acidosis is improving or if they have been started on bicarbonate therapy with an appropriate response.

Outpatient Care

In large part, outpatient follow-up will be dictated by the patient's underlying medical condition that precipitated the acidosis. Patients with nongap acidoses from renal causes may benefit from outpatient follow-up with a nephrologist.

WHAT YOU NEED TO REMEMBER

- A primary metabolic acidosis must be established by a metabolic panel and an arterial blood gas.
- The differential diagnosis of a metabolic acidosis is shaped by the presence or absence of an anion gap.
- If an elevated anion gap is present, testing for lactic acid and ketones in the blood is almost always indicated. Other tests, such as serum osmolality, volatiles, and salicylates, can be sent based on clinical suspicion or if initial tests are unrevealing.
- The "delta-delta" equation can be used with an anion gap metabolic acidosis to tease out a concurrent metabolic nongap acidosis or alkalosis.
- The Winters equation can determine if compensation for a metabolic acidosis is appropriate, or if a superimposed respiratory acid–base disorder is present.
- A "urine anion gap" can be a helpful adjunct to the history in determining the etiology of a nongap metabolic acidosis.
- Treating the underlying cause of a metabolic acidosis is the most important part of the therapeutic strategy.

SUGGESTED READINGS

Kamel KS, Davids MR, Lin S, et al. Interpretation of electrolyte and acid-base parameters in blood and urine. In: Brenner BM, ed. *Brenner and Rector's The Kidney.* 8th ed. New York: Elsevier-Saunders; 2007.

Delaney KA. Acid-Base Disturbances in the Poisoned Patient. In: Ford MD, Delaney KA, Ling LJ, et al. *Clinical Toxicology.* Philadelphia: WB Saunders; 2001.

Kraut JA, Madias NE. Serum anion gap: its uses and limitations in clinical medicine [Review]. *Clin J Am Soc Nephrol.* 2007;2(1):162–174.

Morris CG, Low J. Metabolic acidosis in the critically ill: part 2. Causes and treatment. *Anaesthesia.* 2008;63(4):396–411.

Hyponatremia

A 42-year-old schizophrenic man is brought to the emergency room with increasing somnolence over the past 48 hours. He has a witnessed seizure in triage. Admission labs are notable for a serum sodium level of 108 mEq/L.

OVERVIEW

Definition

Hyponatremia can be defined as a serum sodium level of <135 mEq/L. Patients may be asymptomatic or develop profound alterations in mental status, in part depending on the absolute sodium level but also based on the rapidity of decrease. This chapter will focus on the acute evaluation and management of patients with hyponatremia.

Pathophysiology

Hyponatremia is a water problem. Serum sodium (and in a more global sense, serum osmolality) is a balance between total body solute and total body water. The kidneys maintain this balance by regulating the secretion of water through the action of antidiuretic hormone (ADH). In response to a water load, the resulting drop in serum osmolality shuts off ADH secretion, resulting in a maximally dilute urine and excretion of free water. Normal kidneys are able to maximally excrete up to 15 liters of free water daily. As a result, hyponatremia is most often a problem of failure to suppress ADH that leads to less than maximally dilute urine, although in cases of low solute intake or excessive free water intake, a person may be able to overwhelm the kidneys' capacity to excrete free water.

Even though the primary goal of the ADH system is to maintain osmolality, ADH will be turned on when the body senses a decrease in total body volume at the carotid body, even if osmolality is low. As a result, elevated ADH levels may be "appropriate" in response to volume depletion, or in conditions of effective volume depletion, such as congestive heart failure or cirrhosis. Elevated ADH levels may also be "inappropriate" as in the case of the syndrome of inappropriate ADH (SIADH). Conditions that impair the ability of the kidneys to dilute urine, regardless of ADH levels, such as diuretic therapy or chronic renal insufficiency, will also make patients more susceptible to developing hyponatremia.

In the aforementioned cases, hyponatremia will result in hypo-osmolality because of the increase in free water relative to plasma solute. However, there are some cases in which plasma osmolality may be elevated in the setting of hyponatremia. Perhaps the best example is hyperglycemia. Glucose is an effective osmole that does not freely diffuse across cellular membranes. As a result, hyperglycemia will raise serum osmolality and, in response, water will move out of cells into the extracellular space and "dilute" the serum sodium concentration. Mannitol will similarly cause a hyperosmolar hyponatremia.

There are few causes of hyponatremia with a normal plasma osmolality. One example is the administration of glycine. Another possibility is "pseudohyponatremia," a lab artifact caused most commonly by hyperlipidemia or paraproteinemia.

Epidemiology

Hyponatremia is the most common electrolyte abnormality encountered in hospitalized patients. It has been estimated that the prevalence of hyponatremia in this group is about 3%, although this is likely a gross underestimate of the problem.

Etiology

Remember that hyponatremia is really a water issue, so it may be most helpful to classify patients based on their volume status (Table 41-1). Patients

TABLE 41-1
Causes of Hyponatremia

ADH Level	Hypovolemic	Euvolemic	Hypervolemic
Elevated ADH	Volume depletion (i.e., vomiting, diarrhea) Diuretic use Cerebral salt wasting	SIADH Hypothyroidism Adrenal insufficiency	Heart failure Cirrhosis Nephrotic syndrome
Suppressed ADH		Psychogenic polydipsia Low solute intake (i.e., beer drinker's potomania)	Chronic renal failure

ADH, antidiuretic hormone.

may be hypovolemic, euvolemic, or hypervolemic. Patients with euvolemic hyponatremia (i.e., SIADH) in actuality have a mild increase in total body volume but have not developed signs of peripheral edema or frank volume overload. Cerebral salt wasting usually results in some degree of volume depletion but may be difficult to distinguish from SIADH. Once the volume status is determined, it may be helpful to think about whether or not ADH is elevated or suppressed.

ACUTE MANAGEMENT AND WORKUP

The assessment of volume status is critical to narrowing the differential diagnosis and initiating treatment.

The First 15 Minutes

The most important decision to make early on is how quickly to correct the sodium level.

Initial Assessment

In patients who have neurologic sequelae from their hyponatremia (i.e., seizures, profound altered mental status), the most important initial management step is to raise their serum sodium level by administering hypertonic saline (either 2% or 3%), regardless of the underlying etiology. This is best done in an intensive care unit (ICU) setting to avoid the dangers of overly rapid correction. The patient in our encounter has a number of potential reasons for severe hyponatremia, but his sodium needs to be raised acutely because of his altered mental status and seizure. In all other patients, take some time to perform a thorough volume status examination. In patients with profound volume depletion, restoration of their volume status with the administration of normal saline will most likely lead to correction of their hyponatremia. Likewise, in patients with hypervolemic hyponatremia, oftentimes diuretic therapy plus fluid restriction will move them closer to a normal sodium level.

Admission Criteria and Level of Care Criteria

Patients with asymptomatic hyponatremia can usually be safely managed on a regular hospital floor. Patients with severe hyponatremia (<115 mEq/L) should likely be admitted to an intensive care unit for frequent lab draws and monitoring. Patients with neurologic symptoms or who receive hypertonic saline require ICU-level care.

The First Few Hours

Once the patient is stable from both a hemodynamic and neurologic perspective, you can begin to determine the etiology of his or her hyponatremia and move toward long-term management.

History

Patients with hyponatremia may be entirely asymptomatic or they may have nonspecific complaints. The goal of the history is to identify risk factors for hyponatremia and, if possible, to determine the duration because such information will impact treatment. It is important to ask patients about a prior history of heart failure or liver disease that may put them at risk for "effective volume depletion." It is helpful to ask about decreased oral intake, vomiting, and diarrhea, which may predispose them to true volume depletion. Vomiting is also a potent stimulus for ADH secretion. A medication history may reveal diuretic use or the use of antipsychotics or mood stabilizers that may predispose to hyponatremia or suggest the possibility of an underlying psychiatric disease. A dietary history may uncover a low-solute diet (such as excessive alcohol use). Be sure to ask about a history of endocrine disorders and screen for symptoms of both hypothyroidism and adrenal insufficiency. A neurologic and neurosurgical history is also important to screen for risk factors of SIADH and cerebral salt wasting.

Physical Examination

The focus of the physical examination is to determine the patient's volume status. Resting tachycardia may be a clue to volume depletion, although it can also be seen in both heart failure and infection. Orthostatic vital signs, dry mucous membranes, and poor skin turgor also suggest volume depletion. An elevated jugular venous pressure coupled with peripheral edema suggests hypervolemia. The physical exam may also uncover stigmata of chronic diseases, such as heart failure, liver disease, or nephrotic syndrome, which predispose to hyponatremia.

Labs and Tests to Consider

There are a number of laboratory tests that can aid in both the diagnosis and treatment of hyponatremia.

Key Diagnostic Labs and Tests

Once it is determined that a patient is hyponatremic, it is important to check a serum osmolality level to confirm that he or she is truly hypo-osmolar. Remember that hyperosmolality suggests the presence of another effective osmole, such as glucose or mannitol, while normal osmolality in most cases suggests "pseudohyponatremia." Next, you can check the urine osmolality level to see if ADH is likely to be elevated or suppressed. In a normal kidney, the absence of ADH should lead to a urine osmolality of <100 mOsm/L. If the ADH is elevated, it could be either "appropriate" or "inappropriate." In the absence of diuretic therapy, urine sodium will help to differentiate between these two possibilities. A low urine sodium (<20 mEq/L) suggests that the patient is effectively volume depleted as the kidneys are attempting to hold onto salt to bolster intravascular volume (i.e., true volume depletion or heart failure, etc.). An elevated urine sodium level suggests the possibility of SIADH. It may also be helpful to check a thyroid-stimulating hormone and free thyroxine as well as a serum cortisol level if these endocrine disorders are clinically suspected.

Imaging

Imaging should be guided by the patient's clinical presentation. For example, a head computed tomography scan should be performed in most patients with altered mental status to assess for intracranial pathology that may predispose to SIADH but, more importantly, to rule out alternative diagnoses. Chest radiography might reveal a pulmonary process (such as small cell lung cancer) that might be the source of elevated ADH levels as well.

Treatment

Symptoms of acute hyponatremia are the result of cerebral edema, as water moves into neurons along an osmotic gradient. After about 24 to 48 hours, the brain adapts to this osmotic gradient by secreting its own effective osmoles to reduce the cerebral edema. As a result, the rate at which the sodium falls will determine a patient's symptoms. This also has implications for treatment. If the time course of a patient's hyponatremia is known—for example, in a patient with postoperative hyponatremia who had a normal serum sodium level before surgery—it may be appropriate to correct the serum sodium relative quickly. However, rapid correction of "chronic" hyponatremia will raise the osmolality of the neurons' environment to abnormally high levels, which will pull too much water out of cells. This can lead to osmotic demyelination (or central pontine myelinolysis [CPM]), an oftentimes irreversible neurologic insult. The only way to prevent osmotic demyelination is to correct a patient's hyponatremia slowly, usually by no more than 10 to 12 mEq/L in a 24-hour period.

Patients with acute neurologic complications, such as seizures, should be considered for therapy with hypertonic saline. The goal is not to correct the patient's serum sodium to normal levels, but to raise the sodium acutely to prevent further neurologic complications. In all other patients, your therapy will be determined by the patient's volume status, likely etiology, and chronicity of the hyponatremia.

Patients with true volume depletion will respond to the administration of normal saline by two mechanisms: (a) normal saline is mildly hypertonic relative to plasma and (b) restoring intravascular volume will remove the impetus for ADH secretion. Patients with SIADH and primary polydipsia will respond to water restriction. If the sodium level needs to be corrected more rapidly in a patient with known SIADH, you need to use a solution with a tonicity higher than that of the urine osmolality to raise the serum sodium level.

> ### CLINICAL PEARL
>
> *If a patient has SIADH and his or her urine osmolality is 400 mOsm/L, the administration of normal saline (308 mOsm/L) will result in a lowering of the serum sodium.*

In the past, demeclocycline and lithium were occasionally used to induce collecting duct injury and to limit the action of ADH in conditions in which ADH was not suppressed. More recently, ADH receptor antagonists, call "vaptans," have become available. Their role in the acute treatment of hyponatremia is an area of active investigation. Patients with heart failure and cirrhosis need aggressive modification of their underlying disease in order to restore correct sodium and water balance.

EXTENDED IN-HOSPITAL MANAGEMENT

The intricacies of fluid management in hyponatremia are beyond the scope of this chapter. Two key points to remember: (a) frequently recheck sodium levels to assess response to treatment and (b) be mindful of overly rapid correction. The symptoms of osmotic demyelination may not become apparent for several days, so it is important to carefully observe patients as their hyponatremia improves.

DISPOSITION

Discharge Goals

A patient is ready for discharge once his or her sodium level is stable and his or her comorbid conditions have been addressed.

Outpatient Care

Patients should follow up with their primary care physician within 2 weeks for a repeat check of their sodium level. Given the poor prognosis of hyponatremia in the setting of heart failure and cirrhosis, such patients should be referred for subspecialty care.

WHAT YOU NEED TO REMEMBER

- Hyponatremia is a water issue.
- Hyponatremia portends a worse prognosis in patients with chronic medical conditions.
- Patients with neurologic sequelae from their hyponatremia require rapid correction with hypertonic saline.
- Do not correct patients too aggressively because they may be at risk for central pontine myelinolysis.
- Volume status is the key to understanding the cause of hyponatremia.

SUGGESTED READINGS

Verbalis J, Berl T. Disorders of water balance. In: Brenner BM, ed. *Brenner and Rector's The Kidney.* 8th ed. New York: Elsevier-Saunders; 2007.

Decaux G, Musch W. Clinical laboratory evaluation of the syndrome of inappropriate secretion of antidiuretic hormone. *Clin J Am Soc Nephrol.* 2008;3(4):1175–1184.

Goldsmith SR. Current treatments and novel pharmacologic treatments for hyponatremia in congestive heart failure [Review]. *Am J Cardiol.* 2005;95(9A):14B–23B.

Lien YH, Shapiro JI. Hyponatremia: clinical diagnosis and management. *Am J Med.* 2007;120(8):653–658.

Palm C, Pistrosch F, Herbrig K, et al. Vasopressin antagonists as aquaretic agents for the treatment of hyponatremia. *Am J Med.* 2006;119(7 Suppl 1):S87–92.

Upadhyay A, Jaber BL. Madias NE. Incidence and prevalence of hyponatremia. *Am J Med.* 2006;119(7):S30–S35.

Hyperkalemia

THE PATIENT ENCOUNTER

A 53-year-old woman with end-stage renal disease presents to the emergency department with shortness of breath after missing her last two hemodialysis sessions. Her initial labs are notable for a potassium level of 7.3, and her electrocardiogram demonstrates peaked T waves.

OVERVIEW

Definition

Hyperkalemia is defined as a serum potassium >5 mEq/L. With rising levels of potassium, patients are at risk for cardiac dysrhythmias and, ultimately, cardiac arrest.

Pathophysiology

The serum concentration of potassium depends on dietary intake, renal excretion, and the balance between intracellular and extracellular potassium. After ingestion of a large potassium load, the majority of potassium is taken up into cells via insulin and B-adrenergic receptors that increase Na-K ATPase activity. This excess potassium is then excreted by the kidneys over the next few hours. Hyperkalemia in normal individuals is rare because the kidneys are able to markedly increase potassium excretion in response to either an increased dietary load or increased cellular release. In most individuals, hyperkalemia will result from impaired tubular function, impaired aldosterone activity, or a combination of these two mechanisms. Metabolic acidosis can also acutely cause a shift of potassium out of cells in exchange for a hydrogen ion, but persistent hyperkalemia would be unlikely unless renal impairment is also present.

The primary consequence of hyperkalemia is altered depolarization of the cardiac myocyte with subsequent changes in the action potential. This can lead to cardiac arrhythmias and, ultimately, cardiac arrest if left untreated.

Epidemiology

Hyperkalemia may occur in up to 10% of hospitalized patients. It is certainly more common in patients with underlying kidney disease and may be responsible for as many as 5% of deaths in patients with end-stage renal disease.

TABLE 42-1
Causes of Hyperkalemia

Increased Cellular Release	Impaired Renal Excretion
Metabolic acidosis	Acute renal failure
Rhabdomyolysis	Severe volume depletion
Insulin deficiency	Hypoaldosteronism (including type IV RTA and adrenal insufficiency)
B-adrenergic blockade	Angiotensin-converting enzyme inhibitors or angiotensin receptor blockers
Exercise	Aldosterone receptor antagonists
Tumor lysis syndrome	Type I RTA

RTA, renal tubular acidosis.

Etiology

It is helpful to divide the causes of hyperkalemia into processes that impair renal excretion (including disorders of aldosterone) and processes that increase potassium release from cells (Table 42-1). Dietary ingestion is rarely the sole cause of persistent hyperkalemia.

ACUTE MANAGEMENT AND WORKUP

The most important part of the initial management is recognizing the presence of hyperkalemia and instituting management to prevent cardiovascular complications.

The First 15 Minutes

The level of potassium elevation does not directly correlate with cardiovascular consequences. As a result, the electrocardiogram (ECG) is the most valuable tool in assessing the severity of a patient's hyperkalemia.

Initial Assessment

ECG changes proceed in a relatively predictable pattern. Mild hyperkalemia can result in peaked T waves, best seen across the precordial leads. Moderate hyperkalemia can progress to PR and QRS prolongation, as well as decreased P-wave amplitude. Severe hyperkalemia can lead to absence of P waves, conduction system defects, further widening of the QRS complex, and ultimately sine wave pattern, ventricular fibrillation, or asystole. These patterns are so characteristic that an ECG alone might prompt treatment for hyperkalemia in an unstable patient even before initial lab results are back.

Your initial assessment should include a focused history to identify risk factors for hyperkalemia (i.e., medications, dialysis history), as well as a cardiac and pulmonary examination to better characterize a patient's hemodynamic stability.

Admission Criteria and Level of Care Criteria

Patients with mild hyperkalemia, no ECG changes, and reliable follow-up can usually be managed as outpatients, especially if the cause of their hyperkalemia has been identified and addressed (i.e., stopping the culprit medication). Patients with mild ECG changes should be admitted to a telemetry bed. Patients with moderate to severe hyperkalemia, as in our encounter, will oftentimes require emergent hemodialysis and should be admitted to the intensive care unit until cardiac stability is ensured.

The First Few Hours

Once the patient is stabilized, use the patient history and your physical examination to search for the cause of his or her hyperkalemia.

History

Medications are a fairly frequent cause, so be sure to ask about common culprits such as angiotensin-converting enzyme inhibitors, angiotensin II receptor blockers, aldosterone antagonists, trimethoprim/sulfamethoxazole, and nonsteroidal anti-inflammatory drugs. Heparin, even at deep vein thrombosis prophylaxis dosing, has been shown to cause a transient hypoaldosteronism. Be sure to ask your patients about a history of prior renal disease or endocrine problems that may predispose to hypoaldosteronism, such as Addison disease or diabetes. In addition to the cardiac manifestations already described, patients may complain of muscle weakness and fatigue.

Physical Examination

The physical examination in hyperkalemia may be unremarkable. Pay careful attention to the cardiovascular system, but search for stigmata of chronic kidney disease or other conditions associated with hyperkalemia, such as diabetes.

Labs and Tests to Consider

A basic metabolic panel will provide information about the degree of hyperkalemia and will also provide clues to the etiology.

Key Diagnostic Labs and Tests

A low serum bicarbonate level might point to metabolic acidosis as the cause, whereas a low serum sodium level might implicate adrenal insufficiency. You will also gain valuable information about the patient's renal function from a basic metabolic panel. Pseudohyperkalemia can result from either hemolysis of the sample or release of potassium from markedly elevated white blood cells or platelets. If there is no apparent cause for the patient's hyperkalemia and his or her ECG is unremarkable, it is reasonable to send another sample to reassess.

One potential useful test is the transtubular potassium gradient (TTKG), which is a measurement of aldosterone activity. TTKG = [Urine K ÷ (Urine osmolality / Plasma osmolality)] ÷ Plasma K. In the setting of hyperkalemia, a low TTKG (<5 to 7) suggests that there is not enough aldosterone present to excrete sufficient potassium. The diagnosis can then be confirmed by measuring serum aldosterone levels.

Treatment

In patients with mild hyperkalemia and no ECG changes, therapy may be as simple as stopping implicated medicines. More definitive treatment can be described as therapies that stabilize the cardiac myocyte, that transiently shift potassium back into cells, and that eliminate potassium from the body. Remember that the first two types of treatments are bridges to either more definitive removal of potassium or recovery of tubular function.

Intravenous calcium, in the form of calcium gluconate or calcium chloride, will raise the action potential threshold and reduce myocyte excitability. Calcium should be given immediately to any patient with ECG changes that may be due to hyperkalemia.

CLINICAL PEARL

One ampule (amp) of calcium chloride contains three times the elemental calcium as 1 amp of calcium gluconate, but it should be administered through a central venous catheter because it is caustic to peripheral veins.

Insulin stimulates the uptake of potassium by several tissues, including the liver and skeletal muscle. Ten units should be given intravenously (with the coadministration of dextrose to prevent hypoglycemia) to any patient with ECG changes. Insulin should decrease potassium by up to 1 mEq/L and the effects may last up to 4 to 6 hours.

β-Agonists such as albuterol can also drive potassium into cells, but must be used at much higher doses than for acute asthma (i.e., 10 to 20 mg as opposed to 2.5 mg). Potassium may decrease by as much as 1 mEq/L and the effects last up to 6 hours as well.

Sodium bicarbonate only has a role in patients who are profoundly acidotic and should not routinely be used in the treatment of hyperkalemia.

Intravenous diuretics, particularly loop diuretics, are potent stimulators of potassium excretion but require intact tubular function to work. Fludrocortisone does not have a role in the acute setting but may help in the long term in patients with documented hypoaldosteronism.

Sodium polystyrene sulfonate is a sodium/potassium exchange resin that functions in the colon to increase fecal excretion of potassium. It can be dosed orally or rectally and can decrease potassium by up to 1 mEq/L. Patients must have an intact colon and should not have an ileus or bowel obstruction if dosed orally.

Finally, dialysis can be performed in patients with pre-existing end-stage renal disease, as the patient from our encounter, or in patients with acute renal failure. It can take several hours to initiate emergent dialysis, so you should contact the renal fellow and the intensive care unit early in patients with severe hyperkalemia who may or may not respond to your initial therapies.

EXTENDED IN-HOSPITAL MANAGEMENT

The extended hospital course will be determined in large part by the cause of the patient's hyperkalemia.

DISPOSITION

Discharge Goals

Patients are ready for discharge once the cause of their hyperkalemia has been addressed and they have demonstrated that their serum potassium level is stable, either in the setting of improving renal function, medication changes, the initiation of dialysis, or scheduled doses of sodium polystyrene sulfonate.

Outpatient Care

Patients should follow up with their primary care physician within 2 weeks to have their potassium level checked. Be sure to notify the patient's primary physician about any medications that may have contributed to the hyperkalemia. Patients with new or pre-existing renal disease should be scheduled to see a nephrologist for further evaluation and management.

WHAT YOU NEED TO REMEMBER

- Hyperkalemia can be a cardiac emergency.
- The ECG is critical in determining the clinical significance of hyperkalemia.
- Intravenous calcium is the most important initial medication to stabilize the cardiac myocyte.
- Many treatments only cause transient intracellular shifting of potassium— be mindful of rebound hyperkalemia.
- Dietary intake is a rare cause of hyperkalemia in the absence of renal dysfunction or hypoaldosteronism.

SUGGESTED READINGS

Mount DB, Zandi-Nejad K. Disorders of potassium. In: Brenner BM, ed. *Brenner and Rector's The Kidney*. 8th ed. New York: Elsevier-Saunders; 2007.

Halperin ML, Kamel KS. Potassium. *Lancet*. 1998;352(9122):135–140.

Sood MM, Sood AR, Richardson R. Emergency management and commonly encountered outpatient scenarios in patients with hyperkalemia. *Mayo Clin Proc*. 2007; 82(12): 1553–1561.

Diabetic Ketoacidosis and Hyperosmolar Nonketotic Coma

THE PATIENT ENCOUNTER

A 38-year-old man with a history of type 1 diabetes mellitus presents to the emergency department complaining of excessive thirst and generalized weakness. The patient is taking large, deep breaths; he appears drowsy; and his oropharynx appears dry. His lab data are significant for a glucose level of 345 mg/dL and a serum bicarbonate level of 8 mEq/L with an anion gap of 25. An arterial blood gas shows a serum pH of 7.17 with a PCO_2 of 18 mm Hg. His plasma and urine are positive for ketones.

OVERVIEW

Definition

Diabetic ketoacidosis (DKA) and hyperglycemic hyperosmolar state (HHS) are the most serious acute complications of diabetes. They are extreme manifestations of the impaired carbohydrate regulation that occurs in diabetic patients. DKA is a state of absolute or severe insulin deficiency that consists of the biochemical triad of hyperglycemia, ketonemia, and acidemia. HHS occurs as a result of relative insulin deficiency and usually presents with severe hyperosmolarity and hyperglycemia with variable, but usually mild, degrees of ketosis and acidosis. Although DKA is classically seen in patients with type 1 diabetes and HHS affects patients with type 2 diabetes, presentations may vary. For example, HHS can present with variable degrees of ketosis and acidosis, while DKA is being seen with increasing frequency in patients with type 2 diabetes.

Pathophysiology

Understanding the pathophysiology of DKA will help you understand the pathophysiology of HHS. The phrase "starvation in the midst of plenty" is a fundamental concept in the pathophysiology of DKA. Recall that insulin is the key hormone for the transport of glucose from the blood into cells—in particular, liver, muscle, and fat cells. In states of insulin deficiency, although there is an abundance of glucose in the blood, cells sense an environment of starvation because glucose is unable to enter them. In fact, glucagon and other counterregulatory hormones are released due to the body's perceived "fasting" state, and patients may even complain of excess hunger (polyphagia) and weight loss in the setting of hyperglycemia. Cells therefore transition their biochemical pathways from glucose breakdown for the production and storage of energy (e.g., Krebs cycle and lipogenesis) to glucose synthesis and lipid breakdown (gluconeogenesis, lipolysis). The overwhelming lipid breakdown produces excess acetyl-CoA in the liver, which gets shunted into the production of ketone bodies: acetoacetatic acid and β-hydroxybutyratic acid. Ketone bodies are transported to nonhepatic cells to be converted back to acetyl-CoA, the starting metabolite for the Krebs cycle.

Ketogenesis is an important adaptive mechanism in DKA. Normally, the brain can only utilize glucose for its source of energy, but in the setting of starvation, it makes cellular changes to use ketone bodies for fuel. Acetoacetatic acid and β-hydroxybutyratic acid are both weak acids that are byproducts of lipolysis. They dissociate to acetoacetate and β-hydroxybutyrate, respectively, releasing a proton and thus producing an anion gap metabolic acidosis.

CLINICAL PEARL

The nitroprusside tablet test for ketones only detects acetone and acetoacetate. Because β-hydroxybutyrate is usually the predominant ketone body at presentation in patients with DKA, the initial serum or urine ketone test may be negative.

The physical manifestations of DKA are directly related to the cellular mechanisms for the cardinal biochemical features of DKA—hyperglycemia, ketosis, and acidosis. The kidney is very effective in reabsorbing glucose in the proximal convoluted tubule (PCT) to the point at which, at physiologic levels, 100% of glucose filtered at the glomerulus is reabsorbed by the tubules. Once the serum glucose level is >200 mg/dL, the PCT can no longer absorb all the glucose, and therefore the excess glucose remains in the renal tubule. This creates an osmotic gradient that drags water and other electrolytes into the tubule. Because of this osmotic diuresis, the patient can become severely dehydrated and can have profound electrolyte disturbances. They tend to complain of excess thirst (polydipsia) and excessive urination (polyuria). Signs of volume depletion, such as dry mucous membranes, resting tachycardia, orthostatic hypotension, and hypovolemic shock, are reflections of the severity and duration of the osmotic diuresis.

In addition to volume depletion from glycosuria, the metabolic acidosis that is produced from ketogenesis also produces symptoms. Acidosis, along with electrolyte abnormalities, can produce anorexia and abdominal pain along with nausea and vomiting. Sometimes, a paralytic ileus may even occur. Vomiting is ominous because it precludes the patient from maintaining hydration with oral fluid intake. The metabolic acidosis stimulates the medullary respiration center, which causes deep and rapid respirations (Kussmaul breathing) in order to provide a compensatory respiratory alkalosis. If the patient can keep up with rehydration, the symptoms from the acidosis are usually the reasons why the patient comes to the hospital.

Acetoacetate spontaneously converts to acetone. Acetone cannot be converted back to acetyl-CoA, so it is excreted in the urine and through exhalation. The exhalation of acetone is responsible for a "fruity" smell on the patient's breath (similar to the odor of nailpolish remover).

HHS is similar in pathogenesis to DKA except that it occurs due to relative, rather than absolute, insulin deficiency. Although ketogenesis is the not the predominant feature, it can occur at low levels. Hyperglycemia is much more severe in HHS because patients tend to go longer without symptoms in the absence of severe acidosis. Because of the severe hyperglycemia that is common to HHS, a hyperosmolar state occurs and may cause neurologic complications due to intracellular fluid shifts from the brain into the blood.

Epidemiology

Based on population-based studies, the annual incidence of DKA in diabetic patients is 4.6 to 8 episodes per 1,000 patients (1,2). The incidence of HHS is difficult to determine due to the lack of population-based studies.

Etiology

The cause of these hyperglycemic crises is a net reduction in effective insulin coupled with a concomitant elevation in counterregulatory hormones (glucagon, catecholamines, cortisol, and growth hormone). The two most common reasons for this are (a) omission and/or undertreatment with insulin and (b) infection. These account for approximately 80% to 90% of cases. Other important triggers to consider include myocardial infarction and stroke. A good history and physical exam can usually lead you toward the diagnosis without an expensive workup.

ACUTE MANAGEMENT AND WORKUP

DKA and HHS are medical emergencies that require prompt recognition and treatment. Despite aggressive treatment, mortality rates are 5% for DKA and 15% for HHS. The timely administration of intravenous fluids and insulin, the correction of electrolyte abnormalities, and the detection and treatment of the precipitating illness is critical.

Initial Assessment

Early on, it is important to perform a targeted history and physical exam with special attention to (a) patency of the airway, (b) mental status, (c) cardiovascular status, (d) renal status, (e) sources of infection, and (f) volume status.

The First 15 Minutes

The initial attention should be placed on the ABCs. Assess the patient's mental status and determine if airway protection with an endotracheal tube is needed. In patients with severe acidosis or hemodynamic instability, intubation and mechanical ventilation should also be considered. Restoring intravascular volume in patients with hemodynamic instability is crucial. Another immediate issue is to correct life-threatening electrolyte abnormalities.

The patient in our encounter has evidence of a severe metabolic acidosis with appropriate respiratory compensation as well as likely severe dehydration. He will need aggressive fluid resuscitation and the initiation of an insulin drip in order to avoid impending hemodynamic collapse and respiratory failure.

Admission Criteria and Level of Care Criteria

Every patient with either DKA or HHS needs to be admitted to the hospital for inpatient management. Patients should be admitted to the intensive care unit (ICU), especially if there is hemodynamic instability or neurologic manifestations. All patients will require frequent monitoring (every 1 to 2 hours) of vital signs, glucose levels, and the level of serum electrolytes. In some tertiary care hospitals, this can be accomplished in a step-down unit or an intermediate care unit.

The First Few Hours

After addressing the initial life-threatening concerns, one must be prepared to closely monitor and titrate fluids, insulin, and electrolyte replacement solutions.

History

Given that the most common cause of hyperglycemic crises is underdosing and/or the omission of insulin and infection, these need to be ruled out before exploring other possible causes. It is important to get a good history from the patient regarding insulin administration. Sometimes the patient may not be alert enough to give a history and, in these cases, you may need to talk to family or friends. You should ask if the patient ran out of his or her prescription, if his or her dose has changed recently, or if he or she ran out of syringes or needles. In patients with an insulin pump, you need to make sure that the pump is functioning.

Symptoms of fevers, night sweats, shaking chills, shortness of breath, pleuritic chest pain, dysuria, recent wounds, tooth pain, headache, or a stiff neck may indicate that the patient has an underlying infection. Other precipitants for DKA or HHS include myocardial infarction, stroke, pulmonary embolism, pancreatitis, and thyrotoxicosis. Finally, it is important to ask about other medication changes besides insulin because certain medications can worsen glucose control in diabetic individuals (e.g., steroids, beta-blockers).

Physical Examination

The physical examination pertaining directly to hyperglycemic crises should include an assessment of volume status, neurologic function, and respiratory status. In addition to skin turgor and observation of the mucous membranes, volume status assessment needs to include measurement of the patient's resting heart rate, supine blood pressure, orthostatic blood pressure, and jugular venous pressure. The neurologic exam, especially in those with HHS, should be performed to assess for signs of obtundation, coma, seizures, and even hemiparesis due to the hyperosmolar state. Finally, the respiratory exam should be performed to look for signs that the patient is "tiring out" from the Kussmaul breathing and may need ventilatory support. The rest of the physical exam should focus on identifying the precipitating cause, especially infection.

Labs and Test to Consider

Laboratory evaluation is the mainstay of the diagnosis, management, and treatment of hyperglycemic crises, but is also needed to help elucidate the precipitating cause.

Key Diagnostic Labs and Tests

The initial labs in a patient with suspected DKA should include a basic metabolic panel, measures of serum magnesium and phosphate, arterial blood gas (ABG) testing, and a measure of serum ketones and serum osmolality. These tests will help you gauge the severity of DKA and HHS and will also provide you with initial results that may need immediate attention. Because infection is a common precipitant, all patients should have a complete blood count with differential, a urinalysis with urine culture, two sets of blood cultures, and a chest radiograph. A baseline electrocardiogram should be obtained in all patients because electrolyte abnormalities occur commonly and myocardial ischemia can precipitate these crises. Other labs (e.g., measures of cardiac enzymes and amylase/lipase) should be obtained if there is something in the patient's history that leads you to suspect another precipitating cause.

> ### CLINICAL PEARL
>
> *Ketones can interfere with the Jaffe reaction, the most common method for measuring serum creatinine. As a result, creatinine may be falsely elevated at presentation in a patient with DKA.*

Imaging

Imaging can be important for discovering the precipitating cause of DKA, especially infection. A chest radiograph should be routinely ordered to evaluate for pneumonia. Other imaging should be considered if there are signs or symptoms that suggest pathology (e.g., stroke, abscess). Be wary of ordering a study with the use of intravenous iodinated contrast because it can cause contrast nephropathy in patients with acute renal failure, which is frequently present in these patients.

Treatment

The treatment of hyperglycemic crises requires very frequent assessment of the patient's physical exam and laboratory data before deciding on the next intervention. Although this sounds daunting, the use of a flowsheet for the documentation of clinical parameters, fluids and electrolytes, laboratory values, insulin therapy, and urine output can make managing the care of these patients much easier. Although many aspects of treatment of a hyperglycemic crisis occur simultaneously, an easy way to manage it is by thinking of different physiologic disturbances individually and treating them as separate entities.

Fluid Administration

One very common mistake in DKA and HHS is not administering enough fluids. Patients with DKA, like our patient in the encounter, typically have 5 to 6 liters of volume depletion, while those with HHS may require more than 10 liters of intravenous hydration. The reason why HHS requires more fluid is twofold: First, patients with HHS tend to have higher serum levels of glucose and therefore have a greater degree of osmotic diuresis; second, these patients tend to have hyperglycemia and/or glycosuria for longer periods because they present to the hospital later. Initially, 1 liter of normal saline should be given within the first hour.

The type of fluid to administer subsequently is dependent on the patient's hemodynamic status and his or her measured sodium level. If a patient is in hypovolemic shock, he or she should continue to receive 0.9% NaCl solution until this resolves. Once the patient is no longer in shock, the next type of fluid used is dependent on the patient's corrected sodium level. Recall that in the setting of hyperglycemia, excess glucose will cause the level of a patient's serum osmolality to increase, which pulls water from the intracellular space into the intravascular space, thus diluting the serum sodium. You can predict what the sodium level would be if the glucose level was normal by adding 1.6 mEq to the measured serum sodium level for every 100 mg of plasma glucose above the normal serum glucose level (which is 100 mg/dL). After the initial volume resuscitation mentioned previously is administered, if the patient has a normal or high corrected serum sodium level, 0.45% normal saline (half-normal saline) should be used. If the patient's corrected sodium level is low, 0.9% normal saline should be used until the corrected sodium level is in the normal range.

Insulin Administration

It is important to recognize that the main purpose of insulin in treating DKA is to halt ketogenesis and the resulting anion gap metabolic acidosis.

There are many protocols for managing DKA, although they usually take on some form of the following protocol for insulin administration: 10 units of regular insulin can be given intravenously (IV) initially, followed by a continuous insulin drip. The concentration of the drip can be started at 0.1 units/kg/hour with the goal of decreasing the glucose level by 50 to 70 mg/dL/hour. If the glucose is corrected more quickly than that, fluid shifts will occur too rapidly and can cause neurologic complications. If the patient's glucose level does not decrease at this rate, the dose of the drip should be doubled until this rate is achieved. One can make the assumption that if the anion gap is not normal, ketogenesis is still occurring. If the patient's anion gap has not normalized but his or her serum glucose level has reached 250 mg/dL, you must add dextrose to the IV fluids to prevent hypoglycemia while the insulin drip is continued. Once the anion gap closes and the serum bicarbonate is above 17, administer long-acting insulin (NPH or glargine) subcutaneously 1 hour before stopping the drip. The half-life of IV insulin is approximately 5 minutes and the patient will reinitiate ketogenesis unless a basal level of insulin is in his or her system before the insulin drip is discontinued. The patient's glucose level needs to be checked every hour while he or she is being treated for a hyperglycemic crisis. In addition, basic metabolic panels need to be checked approximately every 2 hours to monitor the anion gap acidosis.

CLINICAL PEARL

The administration of normal saline should occur prior to insulin administration, especially in those with severe hyperglycemia, because in patients who are severely dehydrated and hemodynamically unstable, insulin will drive glucose into cells and, due to osmosis, will drag water with it. This can cause cardiovascular collapse.

Potassium Management

Through the osmotic diuresis that occurs during hyperglycemia, the patient's total body potassium level is usually low and will require repletion. But due to the initial acidosis, potassium gets shifted from the intracellular space into the extracellular space and the initial serum potassium measurement is usually elevated. The acidosis will resolve with the insulin drip and drive potassium back into cells, thus producing hypokalemia. The management of potassium is rather straightforward but requires that levels be checked every 1 to 2 hours, with adjustments made. A simple rule of thumb is that if the patient's potassium level is >5.5 mEq/L, no additional potassium should be given. If the value is between 3.3 and 5.5 mEq/L, the patient should receive 20 mEq/L of fluid administered. Potassium should only be added once good urine output has been established (50 to 100 mL/hour) as hyperkalemia may occur in the setting of renal failure and potassium repletion. If the patient's initial potassium level is low (<3.3 mEq/dL), potassium should be repleted before administering insulin because insulin will shift potassium into cells, creating the potential for life-threatening complications of hypokalemia.

Phosphate Administration

Similar to potassium, the serum phosphate level is usually low due to the renal tubular osmotic load pulling phosphate in and thus inappropriately excreting it. Phosphate is a crucial electrolyte in the production of adenosine triphosphate (ATP). The concern about phosphate levels becoming too low is that skeletal muscle will no longer have ATP and will not be able to contract properly. This is extremely concerning because respiratory muscles need to be continuously working to exchange oxygen and carbon dioxide. As such, it is recommended that patients with DKA and HHS have their serum phosphate levels measured every 2 hours and have it repleted once the level is <1.0 mg/dL.

Bicarbonate Administration

Patients with an arterial pH level <7.0 should be supplemented with 50 mEq/hour of intravenous bicarbonate until the level is >7.0. A pH level >7.0 generally does not require IV bicarbonate administration.

EXTENDED IN-HOSPITAL MANAGEMENT

Once the patient's mental status is near baseline, glucose control is stable, and anion gap is closed, he or she can be moved to a regular hospital bed before being prepared for discharge.

DISPOSITION

Discharge Goals

Because many homeostatic disturbances occur in patients with hyperglycemic crises, many factors need to be considered in deciding when it is appropriate to send a patient home. In general, a patient can be discharged home once he or she is on a stable oral or insulin-based regimen and his or her underlying cause for admission has been treated. The patient should be clear about his or her outpatient regimen and should know how to use a glucometer to measure his or her glucose levels at home. Finally, if a patient is taking medication that can cause hypoglycemia (e.g., insulin or sulfonylureas), he or she needs to be educated about the symptoms of hypoglycemia and what to do when this occurs.

Outpatient Care

Most patients can follow up with their primary care physician within 1 to 2 weeks following hospitalization. It is important to note that approximately 50% of hospitalizations for DKA and HHS can be prevented. This prevention begins with effective communication and education. It is important for both inpatient and outpatient providers to ensure that patients understand how to manage their glucose during exercise, fasting, and illness in addition to being able to identify the signs and symptoms of early hyperglycemic crises.

 WHAT YOU NEED TO REMEMBER

- DKA and HHS are medical emergencies that have relatively high mortality rates. Admission to an ICU is usually necessary.
- DKA and HHS are biochemical abnormalities caused by insulin deficiency, but a precipitating cause must always be identified. Recall that underdosing of insulin and infection are the two most common underlying causes.
- Organizing a flowsheet in order to follow the patient's electrolytes, volume status, and vital signs is crucial in preventing any omissions of care.

REFERENCES

1. Kitabchi AE, Nyenwe EA. Hyperglycemic crises in diabetes mellitus: diabetic ketoacidosis and hyperglycemic hyperosmolar state. *Endocrinol Metab Clin North Am.* 2006;35(4):725–751, viii.
2. Umpierrez GE, Smiley D, Kitabchi AE. Narrative review: ketosis-prone type 2 diabetes mellitus. *Ann Intern Med.* 2006;144(5):350–357.

SUGGESTED READINGS

Kitabchi AE, Umpierrez GE, Murphy MB, et al. Management of hyperglycemic crises in patients with diabetes. *Diabetes Care.* 2001;24:131–153.
Inzucchi S, Sherwin R. Type 1 diabetes. In: Goldman L, ed. *Cecil Medicine.* 23rd ed. Philadelphia: Saunders Elsevier; 2009.

Management of Hospitalized Patients with Diabetes Mellitus

A 58-year-old man with type 2 diabetes complicated by peripheral neuropathy presents to your clinic with complaints of left foot pain. A large ulcer with green-gray discharge is discovered on the plantar surface of his left foot. He is directly admitted to the medicine service for debridement and antibiotic management.

OVERVIEW

Definition

Diabetes is a chronic disease characterized by hyperglycemia, absolute or relative insulin deficiency, and variable degrees of peripheral insulin resistance. The diagnosis is made when one of three criteria is fulfilled: (a) a fasting plasma glucose level ≥126 mg/dL, (b) an oral glucose tolerance test with a 2-hour plasma glucose value ≥200 mg/dL, and (c) diabetes symptoms plus a random plasma glucose level ≥200 mg/dL.

Diabetes can be divided into three major classes: type 1, which is caused by pancreatic β-cell destruction that leads to insulin deficiency; type 2, which results from a combination of insulin resistance and β-cell dysfunction; and gestational diabetes, which is due to insulin resistance induced by placental hormones and increased caloric consumption during pregnancy.

In the hospital setting, hyperglycemia may be secondary to (a) preexisting diabetes, (b) illness-related stress in individuals without diabetes, or (c) previously undiagnosed diabetes.

This chapter will deal with the management of patients with diabetes admitted to the hospital for other medical conditions. See Chapter 43 for a discussion of diabetic ketoacidosis and hyperosmolar hyperglycemic state.

Pathophysiology

While β-cell dysfunction is the main culprit in type 1 diabetes, genetic and environmental factors (diet, obesity) affect the likelihood of developing type II diabetes. Once type II diabetes is diagnosed, a dangerous cycle of insulin resistance and β-cell dysfunction ensues with hyperglycemia, which leads to further impairments in β-cell function and insulin sensitivity.

Hyperglycemia impairs the normal functioning of numerous body systems, including the immune, cardiovascular, and neurologic systems. Leukocyte dysfunction that leads to immunosuppression has been linked to elevated blood glucose levels. Hyperglycemia can increase infarct size following acute myocardial infarction, elevate blood pressure, and prolong the QTc interval. In addition, increased neuronal damage following brain ischemia has been documented in hyperglycemic patients.

Epidemiology

Prevalence

In the United States today, 7% of the population or approximately 20.8 million people have diabetes. One in three diabetics is unaware of the diagnosis. The prevalence of diabetes in hospitalized patients is high, modestly estimated at 12.4% to 25%. When undiagnosed diabetes, illness-induced hyperglycemia, and medication-induced hyperglycemia are considered, the prevalence approaches 30% (1).

Incidence

In 2005, 1.5 million new cases of diabetes in people age 20 or older were diagnosed. The estimated total health care cost of diabetes in the United States in 2002 was $132 billion (1).

Etiology

Diabetic individuals are hospitalized two to four times more frequently than people without diabetes. Risk factors for hospitalization include advanced age, high-glycosylated hemoglobin (HbA1c), the use of insulin, the presence of diabetic complications, and poor glycemic control.

ACUTE MANAGEMENT AND WORKUP

Your initial management should focus on the patient's chief complaint.

The First 15 Minutes

While your patient may not be admitted for a direct complication of diabetes, it is very likely that his or her current illness is in some way modified by his or her underlying diabetes.

Initial Assessment

It's not uncommon for patients with diabetes to present with subtle complaints that signify serious disease. For example, diabetics with acute coronary syndrome may not present with chest discomfort. As a result, it is important to have a high index of suspicion for potentially life-threatening disorders. A foot ulcer, such as the one seen in our patient encounter, may seem like a fairly straightforward issue but it may be the result of limb-threatening peripheral arterial disease, or it may lead to osteomyelitis that may require surgical treatment.

Admission Criteria and Level of Care Criteria

The presence of systemic inflammatory response syndrome, blood pressure disturbances (hypotension/hypertension), electrolyte abnormalities (hypokalemia/hyperkalemia, hypoglycemia/hyperglycemia, anion gap acidosis), acute renal failure, and cardiac ischemia warrant early intervention and more intensive care. Any patient who requires intravenous insulin should also be transitioned to at least a step-down level of care.

The First Few Hours

Once the patient's primary complaint is addressed and therapy is initiated, you can turn your attention to the management of his or her diabetes.

History

Types 1 and 2 diabetes behave differently; ask the patient about the type of diabetes he or she has and how long he or she has been diagnosed with diabetes. In particular, ask the patient what diabetes medications he or she takes at home. Medication noncompliance results in a number of diabetes complications, so ask the patient about his or her medicine adherence as well. In addition, inquire about microvascular (retinopathy, nephropathy, and neuropathy) and macrovascular (coronary artery disease, cerebrovascular disease, and peripheral arterial disease) complications of diabetes. Diabetes increases cardiovascular risk, so determine if the patient has other risk factors such as hypertension, tobacco abuse, dyslipidemia, and a family history of heart disease.

A focused review of systems can effectively screen for acute complications of diabetes including diabetic ketoacidosis (DKA) and hyperosmolar hyperglycemic state (HHS) (see Chapter 43). Hypoglycemia results in autonomic activation that leads to sweating, palpations, and tremor. Generalized symptoms (fatigue, weakness) or specific neurologic symptoms (double vision, slurred speech, behavior disturbances) may also be observed.

Evaluating the patient's nutrition status and his or her ability for oral intake will affect management of inpatient diabetes. Nausea, vomiting, and a decrease in appetite are signs that the patient may require less insulin. However, remember that insulin-deficient patients (those with type 1 diabetes, a pancreatectomy, or insulin-requiring type 2 diabetes) will still require basal insulin when NPO or eating poorly.

Physical Examination

Cardiovascular, ophthalmologic, and neurologic examination can identify microvascular and macrovascular complications of diabetes. Make sure to perform a complete skin examination, paying particular attention to the feet and lower extremities. Many patients may develop ulcers, cellulitis, or skin changes (e.g., diabetic dermopathy, necrobiosis lipoidica diabeticorum, or acanthosis nigricans) without their knowledge. Palpate pedal pulses to determine if occult peripheral arterial disease may be present. Atrophic changes, such as hair loss and pale extremities, may be another sign of impaired circulation.

Labs and Tests to Consider

Laboratory testing should focus on the patient's presenting complaint and his or her underlying diabetes. A measure of glycosylated hemoglobin and a fasting lipid profile may be beneficial in assessing disease severity and comorbid conditions.

CLINICAL PEARL

If a patient receives a blood transfusion prior to measuring his or her glycosylated hemoglobin, it will be inaccurate as it will reflect the glycemic control of the blood donor and not the patient. Hemolysis will lead to a falsely low glycosylated hemoglobin level, as reticulocytes and early red blood cells will not have yet been glycosylated.

Key Diagnostic Labs and Tests

Glucose monitoring is essential in the management of inpatient diabetes. Insufficient data exist on the optimal frequency of bedside glucose testing. Experts and consensus panels recommend the following glucose testing times: (a) premeal and at bedtime for patients who are eating, (b) every 4 to 6 hours for patients who are not eating, and (c) every 1 to 2 hours for patients on continuous intravenous insulin.

Be aware that bedside glucose testing is affected by certain patient characteristics and can lead to erroneous results. Low hematocrit, hyperbilirubinemia, and severe hyperlipidemia can cause an artificially high reading. High hematocrit, dehydration, and hypoxia, as well as certain drugs (e.g., acetaminophen overdose, ascorbic acid, dopamine, mannitol, and salicylate), can produce low bedside glucose results. If a result is in question or the patient is deteriorating, send a confirmatory serum sample for glucose testing.

Electrocardiography, serum electrolytes, blood urea nitrogen, creatinine, and urine analysis are important diagnostic tests in diabetic patients. In addition, checking urine and serum ketones and serum osmolality is helpful in diagnosing DKA and HHS.

Imaging

Imaging studies should be used in conjunction with the history, the physical exam, and laboratory testing to diagnose and guide patient therapy.

Treatment

Hyperglycemia in the hospitalized patient increases the risk of inpatient mortality, postoperative infections, intensive care unit admission, and a longer length of stay. Treating hyperglycemia along with the patient's presenting problem leads to improved outcomes. The patient in the encounter is presenting with an acute infection and will certainly benefit from tight glycemic control while in the hospital.

Limited data exist on the inpatient use of oral diabetes agents. All drug classes have a significant side effect profile, and the long-acting nature of these medicines prevents rapid titration. In general, oral agents should be discontinued and insulin should be used to manage hospitalized patients with diabetes.

Insulin dosing should replicate the body's normal insulin pattern. With this in mind, two types of insulin are required: basal insulin, which is the amount of insulin needed to prevent excessive gluconeogenesis and ketogenesis, and nutritional insulin, which is the amount of insulin needed to cover discrete meals, total parenteral nutrition, enteral feedings, and intravenous dextrose. Correctional, or supplemental, insulin should be used to treat hyperglycemia between meals but should rarely be used as the sole insulin therapy during hospitalization.

CLINICAL PEARL

Basal, nutritional, and correctional insulin regimens are superior to sliding scale insulin in achieving glycemic targets in hospitalized patients.

When designing an inpatient insulin regimen, the total daily insulin requirement should be calculated. A useful estimate is 0.5 to 0.7 units/kg/day for type 1 diabetes and 0.4 to 1.0 units/kg/day for type 2 diabetes. Approximately 40% to 50% of the total daily insulin requirement should be given in the form of basal insulin (Table 44-1). Typically, NPH is given twice daily (morning and bedtime), while glargine and detemir are given once every 24 hours. The remaining daily insulin should be given in the form of nutritional insulin, usually before meals. While regular insulin can be used for nutritional coverage, the rapid-acting insulin analogs aspart, lispro, and glulisine are preferred for nutritional insulin administration due to their rapid onset of action and shorter half-life, which results in less hypoglycemia. Because nutritional intake may be poor in hospitalized patients, the onset of action of the rapid-acting analogs is such that they can be administered after meals, ensuring that the patient has consumed the majority of carbohydrates on the tray (see Table 44-1).

TABLE 44-1
Overview of Insulin Products

Insulin	Onset of Action	Peak (hr)	Duration of Action (hr)
Lispro	5–15 min	1	4–5
Aspart	5–15 min	1	4–5
Glulisine	0.2–0.5 hr	0.5–1.5	3–4
Regular	0.5–1 hr	2–4	6–10
NPH	1–3 hr	5–7	10–20
Detemir	3–4 hr	6–8	6–23
Glargine	1–2 hr	Flat	24

Hospitalized patients often do not eat, secondary to nausea and vomiting or based on the recommendation of their medical team. Although they are not eating, insulin-deficient patients still require basal insulin to prevent ketoacidosis. Patients with known type 1 diabetes, pancreatic dysfunction or pancreatectomy, a history of diabetic ketoacidosis, type 2 diabetes with insulin use for more than 5 years, or a history of type 2 diabetes for more than 10 years are classified as insulin deficient.

The optimal levels for glycemic control in the hospital are not entirely clear at this time. The American Association of Clinical Endocrinologists and the American Diabetes Association recommend a preprandial glucose of 110 mg/dL and maximal glucose of 180 mg/dL for patients in noncritical care units. In intensive care units, the recommended goal is 80 to 110 mg/dL, although these guidelines are likely moving targets.

Hypoglycemia is a serious, yet preventable, consequence of insulin therapy. Comorbid conditions, such as heart failure, malignancy, infection, and renal or liver disease, place diabetic patients at an increased risk of hypoglycemia. In addition, the development of new emesis, a reduction in intravenous dextrose or corticosteroid dose, a change in or discontinuation of enteral or parenteral nutrition, or altered mental status can result in hypoglycemia. The key to reducing the complications of hypoglycemia is prevention. Recognizing factors that place patients at high risk of hypoglycemia and good communication among nursing, pharmacy, and physician staff are important.

EXTENDED IN-HOSPITAL MANAGEMENT

The extended hospital management of the diabetic patient will depend on the particular reason for admission. However, his or her hospital stay can provide an excellent opportunity for diabetic education and optimization of his or her medical regimen.

DISPOSITION

Discharge Goals

Once the patient's underlying condition has been appropriately addressed and he or she is at or close to baseline health status, he or she should be able to go home. Careful thought should be given to constructing an antihyperglycemic outpatient regimen, especially in patients who are at increased risk of hypoglycemia. Social workers are an invaluable asset and may be able to help patients by assessing their insurance status and providing information on inexpensive community medication programs.

Outpatient Care

In general, diabetes patients should have follow-up with their primary care provider or endocrinologist within 1 month after discharge. Patients without a prior diabetes diagnosis with a random blood glucose >125 mg/dL during hospital admission should get tested for diabetes as an outpatient because up to 60% of these patients will be diagnosed with diabetes.

WHAT YOU NEED TO REMEMBER

- Hyperglycemia in the hospitalized patient increases the risk of inpatient mortality, postoperative infections, intensive care unit admission, and length of stay.
- Treating hyperglycemia along with the patient's presenting problem leads to improved outcomes.
- In general, insulin should be used to manage hospitalized diabetes patients.
- Hypoglycemia is a serious, yet preventable, consequence of antihyperglycemic therapy.
- Inpatient diabetes self-management education, medication reconciliation, and assessing a patient's ability to pay for medication and supplies are important discharge goals.

REFERENCES

1. Centers for Disease Control and Prevention. National Diabetes Fact Sheet: General Information and National Estimates on Diabetes in the United States, 2005. Atlanta: US Department of Health and Human Services, Centers for Disease Control and Prevention; 2005.

SUGGESTED READINGS

Clement S, Brauthwaite SS, Magee MF, et al. Management of diabetes and hyperglycemia in hospitals. *Diabetes Care.* 2004;27(2):553–591.

Garber AJ, Moghissi ES, Bransome ED Jr, et al. American College of Endocrinology position statement on inpatient diabetes and metabolic control. *Endocr Pract.* 2004;10(1):77–82.

Malmberg K. Prospective randomised study of intensive insulin treatment on long term survival after acute myocardial infarction in patients with diabetes mellitus. DIGAMI (Diabetes Mellitus, Insulin Glucose Infusion in Acute Myocardial Infarction) Study Group. *BMJ.* 1997;314(7093):1512–1515.

Umpierrez GE, Smiley D, Zisman A, et al. Randomized study of basal-bolus insulin therapy in the inpatient management of patients with type 2 diabetes (RABBIT 2 trial). *Diabetes Care.* 2007;30(9):2409–2410.

van den Berghe G, Wilmer A, Hermans G, et al. Intensive insulin therapy in the medical ICU. *N Engl J Med.* 2006;354(5):449–461.

Endocrine Emergencies

THE PATIENT ENCOUNTER

A 30-year-old woman who recently underwent elective surgery is now having nausea, vomiting, and abdominal pain in the setting of severe hypotension and volume depletion. She also describes a more chronic history of malaise, fatigue, weakness, weight loss, and anorexia. Further investigation reveals that the patient has signs of hyperpigmentation and her labs demonstrate a low early morning cortisol level with hyponatremia and hyperkalemia.

OVERVIEW

Definition

Adrenal insufficiency (AI) is a failure of the adrenal glands to produce appropriate amounts of adrenocortical hormones. Primary AI (Addison disease) is caused by dysfunction of the adrenal cortex, secondary AI is caused by dysfunction of the anterior pituitary gland with decreased secretion of adrenocorticotropic hormone (ACTH), and tertiary AI is caused by dysfunction of the hypothalamus with decreased secretion of corticotropic-releasing hormone (CRH). Adrenal crisis, or acute AI, is a severe attack of a chronic adrenocortical disorder caused by insufficient amounts of adrenocortical hormones during periods of physiologic stress.

Pathophysiology

The adrenal cortex produces three steroid hormones: glucocorticoids (cortisol), mineralocorticoids (aldosterone), and androgens. Cortisol and aldosterone are the main hormones involved in AI and adrenal crisis. Cortisol is part of the stress response that promotes gluconeogenesis and acts as an immunosuppressive agent. Aldosterone is part of the renin-angiotensin system and acts on the distal tubules and collecting ducts in the kidneys to cause potassium excretion and sodium and water retention, which leads to increased blood pressure.

During an episode of acute adrenal crisis, mineralocorticoid deficiency clinically manifests as volume depletion and hypotension, while glucocorticoid deficiency decreases vascular tone, thereby further contributing to hypotension as well as leading to electrolyte abnormalities. Because mineralocorticoid deficiency is not a prominent part of secondary or tertiary AI, acute AI occurs less often in patients with these disorders.

Epidemiology

Addison disease typically presents in adults between the ages of 30 and 50 years old. Women outnumber men with a ratio of 4:1. Secondary AI and tertiary AI are equally common between men and women.

Etiology

The most common cause of AI is suppression of the hypothalamic-pituitary-adrenal axis due to the use of chronic exogenous steroids (i.e., prednisone or hydrocortisone). Other causes include autoimmune disorders (i.e., Addison disease), infiltrative diseases, infections, hemorrhage, metastatic disease, and numerous others (Table 45-1). Worldwide, the most common cause of AI is tuberculosis.

TABLE 45-1
Etiology of Adrenal Insufficiency

Primary Adrenal Insufficiency	Secondary and Tertiary Adrenal Insufficiency
Autoimmune (Addison disease)	Following discontinuation of exogenous glucocorticoids
Infiltrative: Sarcoidosis, amyloidosis, hemochromatosis, Wilson disease	After curing Cushing syndrome
Infectious: tuberculosis, fungal	Tumors
Metastatic disease	Autoimmune
Congenital adrenal hyperplasia/hypoplasia	Inflammation
AIDS	Infections
Adrenoleukodystrophy (X linked)	Trauma
Bilateral adrenalectomy	Granulomatous infiltration
Drugs: steroid synthesis inhibitors (i.e., ketoconazole), glucocorticoid antagonists (i.e., mifepristone)	Pituitary-hypothalamic radiation/surgery/ hemorrhage (apoplexy)
	Acquired ACTH deficiency

ACTH, adrenocorticotropic hormone; AIDS, acquired immunodeficiency syndrome.

Adrenal crisis most often occurs in bilateral adrenal gland infarction and hemorrhage and in primary AI during periods of physiologic stress (such as infection or surgery). This occurs both in previously undiagnosed patients and in patients with known primary AI who do not supplement their regular steroid dose. Less often, acute AI can occur in patients with secondary or tertiary AI who undergo severe stress or in patients who are rapidly withdrawn from high doses of exogenous steroids.

> ### CLINICAL PEARL
>
> *Patients who are going to be on supraphysiologic doses of exogenous steroids (roughly 7.5 mg of prednisone daily) for an extended period of time (more than 2 to 3 weeks) need to be tapered off to avoid precipitating acute AI.*

ACUTE MANAGEMENT AND WORKUP

Acute AI is a life-threatening emergency that demands immediate intervention. Looking for important clues in the history, physical, and laboratory data can help make the correct diagnosis earlier and enable the physician to start treatment as soon as possible.

The First 15 Minutes

The primary presentation of adrenal crisis is volume depletion and hypotension, as seen in our patient encounter. As with any etiology of hypotensive shock, the patient must be rapidly assessed and resuscitated.

Initial Assessment

After the airway and breathing have been assessed and are stable, attention should be given to the circulation. First establish good intravenous (IV) access and draw blood for the evaluation of serum cortisol, ACTH, electrolyte, and glucose levels. Next, aggressively perform volume resuscitation in the patient while watching closely for any signs of volume overload, especially if the patient has known heart, kidney, or liver dysfunction.

Once the patient's volume status has been addressed, initiate treatment with glucocorticoids. In a patient without a previous history of AI, dexamethasone (4-mg IV bolus) is the treatment of choice because it is not measured in serum cortisol assays and therefore will not interfere with diagnostic tests (if drawn within a short period of time after administering the dexamethasone). In patients with a known diagnosis of AI, either dexamethasone or hydrocortisone (100-mg IV bolus) may be used.

During this critical time period, the patient must also be evaluated for any concurrent causes of hypotension, such as sepsis, or life-threatening precipitants of the adrenal crisis.

Admission Criteria and Level of Care Criteria

Most patients with acute AI will require admission to an intensive care unit.

The First Few Hours

Once the patient is stabilized, attention can be focused on determining if the patient has underlying AI with an acute precipitant or if this is an acute presentation of AI.

History

During an acute adrenal crisis, the predominant manifestation is shock, occasionally complicated by confusion or coma. If patients are communicative, they may also complain of nonspecific symptoms, such as nausea, vomiting, abdominal pain, lethargy, anorexia, fatigue, and fever. The patient should also be questioned regarding any acute stressors, including symptoms of infection, recent surgery, and trauma.

Further questioning may help to elucidate whether the AI has been long-standing (e.g., Addison disease, infiltrative diseases, acquired immunodeficiency syndrome [AIDS]) or more acute (e.g., bilateral adrenal hemorrhage, bilateral adrenal infarction, withdrawal of exogenous steroids). Symptoms of chronic adrenal insufficiency may include a prior history of weight loss, amenorrhea, weakness, fatigue, gastrointestinal symptoms, postural dizziness, myalgias/arthralgias, and salt craving. Acute causes of adrenal insufficiency may have additional symptoms based on the etiology, such as back pain in bilateral adrenal hemorrhage and infarction or severe headache and visual loss in pituitary apoplexy.

Physical Examination

Findings in acute AI primarily involve signs of hypoperfusion, such as low blood pressure and dusky extremities. Attention should also be paid to looking for precipitants, such as fever, which suggests infection or abdominal rigidity, which in turn suggests adrenal hemorrhage or infarction. Additionally, the patient may exhibit stigmata of underlying AI, which mainly consist of postural hypotension and hyperpigmentation. This is often most noticeable in areas with the greatest light exposure and those exposed to chronic pressure or friction from clothing, such as at the elbows or the waistline. Occasionally, hyperpigmentation can be seen in the mucous membranes of the mouth or the palmar creases. Lastly, the patient may have signs relating to the primary cause of AI.

Labs and Test to Consider

Patients with a suspected diagnosis of acute AI should have ACTH and cortisol levels checked. Because the syndromes of sepsis and acute AI can overlap, blood and urine cultures are usually taken as well. In patients with suspected chronic underlying AI, special attention should be given to their electrolyte levels as hyponatremia and hyperkalemia are often seen. Consideration should also be given to the evaluation of thyroid function as the clinical manifestations of hypothyroidism can have significant overlap with AI.

Key Diagnostic Labs and Tests

The hallmark of AI is a low cortisol level, usually measured in the early morning (around 4 to 8 a.m.) as this is when the serum cortisol concentration is normally highest. An early morning serum cortisol concentration of <3 μg/dL is diagnostic of AI, whereas a level <10 μg/dL is suggestive. To confirm suspected AI, a cortisol stimulation test can be performed by administering parenteral synthetic ACTH (cosyntropin) and measuring serum cortisol levels at 0, 30, and 60 minutes. The standard, high-dose, ACTH stimulation test uses 250 μg of cosyntropin to induce pharmacologic levels of ACTH. An increase in cortisol concentration to a peak of 18 to 20 μg/dL is considered a normal response. There is a low-dose ACTH stimulation test that uses 1 μg/1.73 m^2 that is theoretically more sensitive in identifying chronic partial AI or early secondary/tertiary AI as this dose of cosyntropin results in more physiologic levels of ACTH.

Primary AI can be distinguished from secondary/tertiary AI by measuring early morning cortisol and ACTH concentrations simultaneously; in primary AI, the cortisol level is low and the ACTH level is high, while in secondary/tertiary AI, the levels of cortisol and ACTH are both low. A CRH stimulation test can be performed to further distinguish between secondary (high CRH) and tertiary (low CRH) AI. Additional testing regarding the etiology of the AI can then be pursued as appropriate.

Imaging

There are no standard imaging studies for adrenal crisis, but imaging can be directed at confirming a suspected cause of the AI, such as an abdominal computed tomography (CT) scan for adrenal hemorrhage or infarction or a head CT scan or magnetic resonance imaging for pituitary apoplexy.

Treatment

As in our patient encounter, the initial treatment is high-dose parenteral glucocorticoid replacement therapy. This should be tapered over 3 to 4 days as oral replacement therapy is initiated. The treatment of primary AI requires both long-term glucocorticoid and mineralocorticoid replacement, whereas secondary and tertiary AI only necessitate glucocorticoid replacement. Androgen replacement for women with primary AI is being studied as the adrenal cortex is its primary source.

EXTENDED IN-HOSPITAL MANAGEMENT

Once the patient's acute electrolyte and volume abnormalities have been addressed, the focus of admission should transition to treating any underlying etiologies or concurrent stressors.

DISPOSITION

Discharge Goals

In addition to treating the acute and underlying abnormalities, the goals of care should include transitioning the patient to an oral glucocorticoid replacement therapy and educating the patient and family members about adrenal insufficiency/crisis and the rationale behind treatment. Also, appropriate endocrine follow-up should be arranged to monitor the patient for signs of adrenal insufficiency or excess so that the glucocorticoid dose may be adjusted. Lastly, if the underlying adrenal insufficiency was determined to be due to another disease process, such as AIDS, malignancy, or another cause, then additional follow-up with the appropriate specialist should be arranged.

Outpatient Care

In addition to monitoring the chronic maintenance regimen of oral medication, one of the most important components of outpatient treatment is making sure the patient knows how to escalate his or her glucocorticoid dose to cover himself or herself in times of stress. During a minor febrile illness or stress, such as an upper respiratory infection, the patient should increase his or her glucocorticoid dose two- to threefold during the first few days of the illness. During severe stress or trauma, the patient should inject intramuscular dexamethasone and present to a physician as soon as possible. The patient may also need to use intramuscular dexamethasone if he or she is unable to tolerate oral medications due to nausea and vomiting. No dose escalation is needed for most uncomplicated, outpatient procedures under local anesthesia, but any larger procedures that require general anesthesia or IV sedation should be done in a hospital setting with endocrine consultation. As part of emergency treatment education, the patient should be shown how to inject dexamethasone intramuscularly, be instructed how to obtain a Medic-Alert bracelet/emergency medical information card, and be supplied with prefilled syringes containing 4 mg of dexamethasone in 1 mL of saline.

OTHER ENDOCRINE EMERGENCIES

In addition to acute adrenal insufficiency and diabetic ketoacidosis and hyperosmolar nonketotic coma (see Chapter 43, which addresses these conditions), there are less common endocrine emergencies that deserve brief mention, such as thyrotoxic storm and myxedema coma.

THYROTOXIC STORM

THE PATIENT ENCOUNTER

A patient presents to the emergency department after a minor motor vehicle accident. She is complaining of shortness of breath, nausea, vomiting, diarrhea, abdominal pain, and shaking. On examination, she is noted to be diaphoretic, severely tachycardic, and hyperthermic and to have pulmonary edema. She mentions that she has a history of Graves disease.

Discussion

Thyrotoxic storm is an acute, life-threatening exacerbation of thyrotoxicosis with a substantial mortality rate. Often, thyroid storm is precipitated by a stressor, such as surgery, burns, trauma, or infection, but it can also occur in patients with long-standing untreated hyperthyroidism. Pathophysiologically, it is thought that thyroid storm is a result of acute surges of thyroid hormone, coupled with an exaggerated response to the surge of catecholamines associated with the precipitating event. It accounts for 1% to 2% of hospital admissions for thyrotoxicosis. Depending on the severity, patients can present with hyperthermia, diaphoresis, tachycardia, atrial fibrillation, congestive heart failure, nausea/vomiting/diarrhea, abdominal pain, jaundice, tremulousness, agitation/delirium/psychosis, seizure, and/or coma. Some patients may also have signs and symptoms of underlying hyperthyroidism, such as a goiter or exophthalmos. The diagnosis is based on the clinical presentation, but can sometimes be seen in the laboratory with elevated levels of thyroid hormones (serum thyroxine [T_4], free T_4, triiodothyronine [T_3]) and suppressed thyroid-stimulating hormone (TSH). Other laboratory abnormalities may include hyperglycemia, leukocytosis, hypercalcemia, transaminitis, and an elevated level of alkaline phosphatase (from increased bone turnover).

Patients with thyrotoxic storm are critically ill, so the acute management centers on stabilizing the patient, particularly from a cardiac standpoint. The patient is often admitted to an intensive care unit for full supportive therapy, including volume management, cardiac monitoring, and antipyrexia treatment. Pharmacologic treatment usually consists of multiple medications that work to blunt the effects of the thyroid hormones while blocking further synthesis and secretion. Intravenous beta-blockers (e.g., propranolol) help to decrease adrenergic tone, digoxin is used to treat atrial fibrillation or heart failure, a thionamide (e.g., methimazole) blocks de novo hormone synthesis, an iodide solution (e.g., Lugol solution) blocks further secretion of thyroid hormone, cholestyramine or colestipol bind T_4 in the gut and bring down circulating levels, and glucocorticoids (e.g., dexamethasone) additionally inhibit conversion of T_4 to T_3 while providing adrenal support and possibly treating underlying Graves disease. In severe cases, plasmapheresis and dialysis have been used to acutely reduce levels of circulating hormones.

Any potential exacerbating factors, such as infection, need to be treated as well.

CLINICAL PEARL

Iodide administration decreases the release of thyroid hormone from the gland. In normal individuals, iodide also results in a transient decrease in iodine organification, called the Wolff-Chaikoff effect. In the case of thyroid storm, iodide solutions should be administered after thionamides to prevent the use of this iodine as a substrate for organification and production of additional thyroid hormone.

Dramatic clinical improvement with the appropriate treatment often occurs within 12 to 24 hours. Extended inpatient management centers around treating the precipitant and appropriately managing the patient's chronic hyperthyroidism. Upon discharge, the patient should be scheduled to follow up with an endocrinologist who can continue to manage his or her hyperthyroidism.

MYXEDEMA COMA

THE PATIENT ENCOUNTER

An elderly, obese woman is brought in by her family members because she has become progressively withdrawn, lethargic, and unresponsive. On examination, the patient is hypothermic, bradycardic, and hypotensive with coarse, dry skin and a delayed reflex relaxation phase. Upon further questioning, the family recalls that the patient had been treated with radioactive iodine in the past.

Discussion

Myxedema coma is a rare presentation of severe hypothyroidism with a high mortality rate. It is most often seen in patients with severe long-standing untreated or undertreated hypothyroidism or in patients with known hypothyroidism who have an acute illness or who receive sedatives. Pathophysiologically, severe hypothyroidism causes a slowing of many metabolic pathways and a decrease in the function of various organ systems. It follows that the main signs of myxedema coma are progressive confusion, lethargy, and, ultimately, coma with hypothermia, hypotension, bradycardia, hypoventilation, and possibly pericardial/pleural/peritoneal effusions and ileus. Rarely, patients may present with psychotic features or seizures.

Because the patient may not be able to give an adequate history, family members must be questioned about a history of hypothyroidism or radioiodine treatment. Also, they may be able to provide a history of hypothyroid symptoms followed by a decreased mental status. On examination, in addition to the aforementioned acute signs, the patient may have evidence of underlying hypothyroidism, such as dry skin, thinning hair, nonpitting edema, macroglossia, reflexes with a slow reflex relaxation phase, a hoarse voice, or a thyroidectomy scar. There may also be evidence of a precipitating cause. The diagnosis is based on the patient's history and clinical presentation, but can sometimes be seen in the laboratory evaluations, with a low level of free T_4 and an abnormal TSH; the latter is usually elevated in patients with primary hypothyroidism but is occasionally decreased if the patient has hypothalamic or pituitary dysfunction (10% of cases). Other laboratory abnormalities may include hyponatremia, hypoglycemia, and a low cortisol level, which can be seen with associated adrenal insufficiency or hypopituitarism.

Patients with myxedema coma usually require an intensive care unit admission for full supportive therapy, possibly including mechanical ventilation, volume management, correction of hyponatremia and hypoglycemia, correction of hypothermia, and empiric antibiotic therapy. Pharmacologic treatment mainly consists of rapidly increasing serum thyroid hormone levels with T_3 and/or T_4, although controversy exists as to the ideal thyroid hormone replacement regimen. During this time, the patient must be carefully monitored because myocardial infarction or atrial arrhythmias could be precipitated by treatment. Until coexisting AI can be excluded with a cosyntropin stimulation test, the patient must also receive treatment with stress-dose glucocorticoids. As with other endocrine emergencies, the patient must be evaluated and treated for any underlying precipitants.

The mortality rate of myxedema coma is 20% to 40%, with persistent hypothermia and bradycardia carrying a poorer prognosis. If the patient survives, extended inpatient management again centers around treating the precipitant and appropriately managing the patient's underlying chronic hypothyroidism. Upon discharge, the patient should be scheduled to follow up with an endocrinologist who can continue to manage the patient's hypothyroidism.

WHAT YOU NEED TO REMEMBER

- Adrenal crisis can occur in the setting of preexisting adrenal insufficiency or can result from acute adrenal insufficiency. The main clinical presentation is volume depletion and hypovolemic shock.
- Thyrotoxic storm often occurs in patients with underlying hyperthyroidism during periods of stress. The main clinical presentation is cardiac instability, hyperpyrexia, gastrointestinal symptoms, and neurologic signs.
- Myxedema coma occurs with untreated or undertreated severe hypothyroidism or with known hypothyroidism in the setting of acute stress. The main clinical presentation is of depressed mental status, hypothermia, bradycardia, hypotension, and hypoventilation.
- Adrenal insufficiency, thyrotoxic storm, and myxedema coma are all life-threatening medical emergencies that require rapid identification, stabilization, and treatment, most often in an intensive care unit.

SUGGESTED READINGS

Dorin RI, Qualls CR, Crapo LM. Diagnosis of adrenal insufficiency. *Ann Intern Med.* 2003;139:194–204.

Jiang YZ, Hutchinson KA, Bartelloni P, et al. Thyroid storm presenting as multiple organ dysfunction syndrome. *Chest.* 2000;118:877–879.

Oelkers W, Diederich S, Bahr V. Therapeutic strategies in adrenal insufficiency. *Ann Endocrinol.* 2001;62:212–216.

Ringel MD. Management of hypothyroidism and hyperthyroidism in the intensive care unit. *Crit Care Clin.* 2001;17:59–74.

Wall CR. Myxedema coma: diagnosis and treatment. *Am Fam Physician.* 2000;62: 2485–2490.

Anemia

THE PATIENT ENCOUNTER

A 19-year-old college freshman presents to the emergency department with severe fatigue. Over the past 2 months, she has noted increasing fatigue and went to her student health center. A complete blood count was drawn due to her complaint and the finding of pallor on examination. The results are the following: hematocrit, 18%; hemoglobin, 6 g/dL; white blood cells, 7,800/mm^3; platelets, 675,000/mm^3; mean corpuscular volume, 59.3; mean corpuscular hemoglobin, 18.3; mean corpuscular hemoglobin concentration, 30.7; red cell distribution width, 17.

She has noted no change in bowel habits or excess menses. She reports that she had a normal blood count 6 months prior when she underwent a college preadmission physical. Over the past 6 weeks, she reports a craving for crushed ice (pagophagia). She reports no family history of anemia. Her physical is remarkable only for pallor, blue-tinged sclera, and mild epigastric tenderness. A rectal exam is negative for occult blood. She is admitted to the hospital for a new diagnosis of severe anemia.

OVERVIEW

Definition

Anemia is defined as a reduction below normal in the number of red cells in the circulation of blood. Anemia is being recognized earlier in its presentation because of automated cell counters and the routine evaluation of the complete blood count in almost all patients that we see. Men typically have more red cells and higher hematocrit and hemoglobin values than do women, due largely to androgen production in men. The normal hematocrit and hemoglobin levels have a wide normal range, and of course changes in plasma volume can result in significant changes in the hematocrit level. The World Health Organization defines anemia as a hemoglobin level of <13 g/dL in men and <12 g/dL in women (1).

Pathophysiology

There are many ways to morphologically describe anemias. The most common is to characterize anemias according to four categories: (a) microcytic, which suggests iron deficiency or thalassemia; (b) normocytic, which suggests a production defect or a destruction defect; (c) macrocytic, which suggests vitamin B_{12} or folate deficiency; and (d) sideroblastic, which may suggest a myelodysplastic syndrome.

It may be more useful to evaluate anemia based on four parameters that are important in the production of red cells:

1. The erythron, which is the marrow's ability to produce red cells
2. Gastrointestinal (GI) absorption, which is the ability to absorb iron through diet or supplemental iron intake
3. The reticuloendothelial system, in which red cells are taken out of the circulation after their lifespan. This primarily occurs in the spleen, but in the absence of the spleen this can take place in the liver and bone marrow.
4. Iron stores, in which nonerythroid iron is stored for potential use

The Erythron

The erythron represents the bone marrow's ability to produce red cells. Red cell lifespan is 120 days; therefore, the daily production of red cells must average about 1%. Red cell mass is dependent on weight. Total blood volume is 70 mL/kg, red cell mass averages 30 mL/kg, and plasma volume averages 40 mL/kg. Therefore, for a 70-kg man, his red cell mass would be 70 kg × 30 mL/kg, or 2,100 mL. His plasma volume would be 40 mL/kg × 70 kg, or 2,800 mL. If you add those two together, it gives you about 5 liters of whole blood volume. Each day, 1% of the red cells is replenished; therefore, 1% of 2,000 mL gives you 20 mL of red cells produced each day. The normal maximum reticulocyte response is 3%. Thus, the maximum amount of blood you could make each day would be 60 mL. Because it takes 1 mg of iron to make 1 mL of blood, this would require 60 mg of iron.

The Reticuloendothelial System

The reticuloendothelial (RE) system represents the system in the body that is responsible for removing aged red cells from the circulation, that is, red cells that are 120 days old or damaged. The primary organ for this is the spleen, but there are also RE cells in the liver and the bone marrow. Each day, approximately 1% of your red cell mass is 120 days old and therefore 20 mL of red cells is destroyed. The 20 mg of iron that is scavenged from these red cells by the RE system is then transported back to the erythron for incorporation into new red cells.

Gastrointestinal Absorption

The normal American diet contains 10 to 15 mg of elemental iron. This is typically in the ferric state. In the stomach, this ferric iron is changed into ferrous iron and is absorbed primarily in the duodenum. The duodenal cell interface with the vascular compartment allows the iron to be transformed back into the ferric state to be bound to transferrin and taken into the erythron or the storage compartment where the iron is needed. The typical individual loses about 1 mg of iron per day insensibly through the GI tract and the sloughing of skin. Women who are menstruating lose about twice this amount. The requirement for normal men is about 1 mg absorption per day from the diet, and for women, about 2 mg/day from the diet. The maximum that your GI tract can absorb is 40% of what is presented. Therefore, a person with a normal diet who is iron deficient could potentially absorb 4 to 6 mg/day. Individuals who have hemochromatosis have altered regulation of absorption and, independent of their iron status, they absorb iron excessively, resulting in iron overload.

Iron Stores

Iron is stored in the bone marrow in the form of ferritin; there is also some hemosiderin iron that is stored there. Men have about 750 mg of storage iron; women have somewhat less than that, depending on their menstrual history and their childbirth history, usually somewhere in the range of 250 to 500 mg. This storage iron is available to augment hematopoiesis during periods of excessive blood loss.

Epidemiology

Anemia affects approximately 2% to 15% of the American population. The incidence and prevalence are higher in underdeveloped countries. Anemia is about twice as common in women as in men.

Etiology

Most anemia is caused by iron deficiency. In developed countries, peptic ulcer disease is the primary etiology. In developing countries, infections are the primary etiology. Other causes include sickle cell disease, thalassemia, G6PD deficiency, malaria, and other parasitic infections. African Americans have a higher incidence of sickle cell anemia and G6PD deficiency. Other ethnic groups are at higher risk for certain hemoglobinopathies.

ACUTE MANAGEMENT AND WORKUP

Any patient with hemodynamic instability from blood loss, manifested first by tachycardia and only much later by hypotension, should be admitted to the hospital. Most workups of anemia can be done in the outpatient setting.

The First 15 Minutes

Evaluating and assessing the vital signs in anemia due to blood loss are the first steps in triage.

Initial Assessment

Assessing for acute blood loss includes taking a quick history and evaluating for the source of bleeding (this will be readily apparent in acute blood loss). Acute replacement of intravascular volume with isotonic fluids is the quickest way to stabilize a patient with hemorrhagic shock. At the same time, the blood bank can be called to transport unmatched type O blood (trauma blood) in instances of shock. If time allows and in the optimal situation, a type and crossmatch is needed to reduce the risk of transfusion reactions.

Admission Criteria and Level of Care Criteria

Patients with hemodynamic instability or recent episodes of active blood loss need to be admitted to the hospital. Hospitals frequently admit patients with unexplained new-onset severe anemia (hematocrit level of <20%) as in our patient from the encounter. However, most cases of anemia are safely worked up in the outpatient setting.

The First Few Hours

After the patient is deemed hemodynamically stable, a thorough history and physical exam is needed to help elucidate the cause of anemia.

History

Once an anemia has been identified, then it is useful to go back and take additional history to see if there is an obvious source of blood loss. In men, blood loss usually occurs from one of three sites: (a) hemoptysis, which is always obvious; (b) hematuria, which is usually obvious; and (c) GI blood loss, which is often not clinically apparent. In women of menstrual age, blood loss from menses is an additional source. Defining excess menses in women is often very difficult. Extended days of menses (i.e., >7 days in a month), more than two cycles per month, and clots during the menstrual cycle suggest excessive bleeding.

Historically, it is also interesting to see if there is a history of pica (an unrealistic craving for nonnutritional foods), which is usually a marker for iron deficiency. Pica can take many forms. Patients may eat clay, topsoil, Argo starch (amylophagia), ice (pagophagia), or other rarer substances. Much of the craving seen during pregnancy for ice cream, celery, match heads, and other items probably relates to iron deficiency and is a form of pica.

Physical Examination

The physical exam may vary widely, depending on the etiology of anemia. The depletion of total body iron results in the fatigue, weakness, and exercise intolerance out of proportion to the anemia. This relates to depletion of metabolic enzymes that produce energy and contain iron. Pallor is the most common finding with iron deficiency. Other findings of iron deficiency include glossitis (sore tongue) and cheilosis (breakdown of the mouth corners). Nail findings include spoon nails (koilonychia), which may be seen with minimal anemia. Blue sclerae have also been observed in iron deficiency. Difficulty in swallowing may be due to an esophageal web (Plummer-Vinson syndrome). Tachycardia and exercise intolerance are relatively late findings and are seen with dramatic falls in the hematocrit level. The rapidity of the onset of the reduced hematocrit level will also determine the symptoms and signs that are seen.

Labs and Tests to Consider

Essentially, all patients admitted to a medical service will get a complete blood count (CBC). The automated multichannel analyzers utilized to do CBCs directly assess the following parameters: the red blood count, the mean corpuscular volume, red cell distribution width (reflecting the degree of variation in red cell size), and the hemoglobin level (the concentration of hemoglobin in the whole blood after lysing the red cells). The machine then calculates the hematocrit, mean cell hemoglobin, and mean cell hemoglobin concentration from the directly measured parameters. You can get falsely abnormal results in these measurements with certain situations, such as high white blood cell count, dyslipidemias, monoclonal proteins, cold agglutinins, and hyperglycemia.

CLINICAL PEARL

Any time that the hemoglobin and the hematocrit levels are not proportionate (i.e., the hemoglobin level should be approximately one third of the calculated hematocrit level), you should consider the presence of a confounding factor.

The workup of anemia usually entails "iron studies," including the iron, iron-binding capacity, and ferritin. A reticulocyte count, corrected for the hematocrit level, is frequently helpful. Cases in which the diagnosis is not readily apparent from the history, the physical exam, and lab tests may require a bone marrow biopsy. Table 46-1 provides a basic interpretation of these tests.

Cases of acute blood loss and unexplained iron deficiency anemia need an evaluation for the source of bleeding. This most often takes the form of a colonoscopy and/or an esophagogastroduodenoscopy (EGD). In cases of hemoptysis, a bronchoscopy is usually helpful, and in cases of hematuria, cystoscopy is indicated.

Key Diagnostic Tests and Labs

A reticulocyte count is technically performed by staining peripheral blood with new crystal violet or Methylin blue, which stains residual RNA in young red

TABLE 46-1

Interpretation of Laboratory Results in Common Causes of Anemia

Type of Anemia	Blood Smear	Fe/TIBC	Marrow Iron	Reticulocyte Count
Normal	Normocytic/ normochromic	100/300 one-third saturation	+	1%
Iron ↓	Microcytic hypochromic	↓/↑ <16% saturation	Absent	<1%
B₁₂ ↓	Macrocytic	↑/nl >50% saturation	Microaggregated iron	↓
Hemolytic anemia	Variable	↑/nl >50% saturation	↑	↑
Sideroblastic anemia	Dimorphic population	↑/nl >50% saturation	↑ (ringed)	↓
Anemia of chronic disease	Normocytic to microcytic	↓/↓ 10%–16% saturation	↑	↓

nl, normal; TIBC, total iron-binding capacity.

cells (within 24 hours from release into the circulation) with a blue stippled color. If you count 500 red cells and five of those cells contain residual RNA, the reticulocyte response is 1%. A reticulocyte count should reflect the daily production index of red cells and it is therefore dependent on the hematocrit level. If a normal hematocrit level is 45% and one is anemic with a hematocrit level of 22% and the daily production of red cells is stable, when you measure the reticulocyte index, it would be 2%, but corrected for the degree of anemia, it would once again be 1%. In the same mode, the other correction that has to be taken into consideration is that under situations of hypoxemic stress, red cells leave the bone marrow early and appear on a routine blood smear as big polychromatophilic cells. You must correct your reticulocyte count for those cells as well. That requires looking at multiple smears or having someone with expertise help you do that. If you correct for the hematocrit level and shift, the maximum normal reticulocyte response is 3%. The bone marrow has the capability to increase production six- to eightfold, so there are situations in which one could see reticulocyte responses that would be in the range of 6% to 8%. The factor that limits normal individuals to a reticulocyte response of 3% is iron transport. Individuals who have a reticulocyte response above 3% have evidence of intravascular hemolysis in which iron is available to the erythron without being transported bound to transferrin. Examples of that are individuals with autoimmune hemolytic anemia with intravascular hemolysis, individuals with sickle cell anemia, or individuals with any chronic intravascular hemolytic process. If you correct for shift and for the degree of anemia and you obtain a corrected reticulocyte response of >3%, you should think of some process that causes intravascular hemolysis. See Figure 46-1 for some characteristic blood smear findings of anemia.

Imaging

Direct imaging for the source of blood loss is usually the first step in evaluating bleeding. Computed tomography scans can be helpful in identifying retroperitoneal or intra-abdominal bleeds. Other nuclear medicine tests can occasionally be helpful, such as a tagged red cell scan for GI bleeding not apparent by colonoscopy or EGD.

Treatment

The treatment of anemia depends on the cause. Iron deficiency anemia is frequently encountered in the hospital and should be corrected by iron replacement either by mouth or intravenously (IV). Vitamin B_{12} or folate should be replaced accordingly after a diagnosis of this condition is made. Anemia of chronic disease may be treated in certain cases by erythropoietin analogs. This is most commonly encountered in patients with chronic renal failure. The treatment for hemolytic anemias is supportive and aimed at treating the underlying cause of hemolysis. The patient in our encounter appears to have severe iron deficiency anemia based on her symptoms, her

A

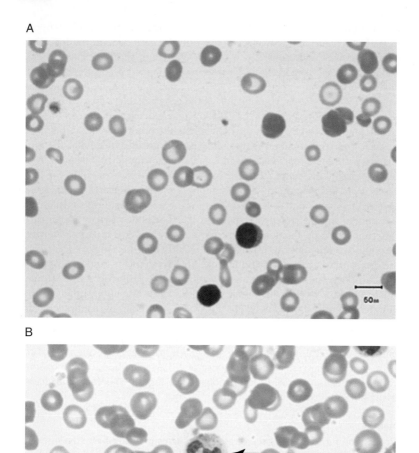

B

FIGURE 46-1: Characteristic blood smear findings in anemia. **A:** Microcytic, hypochromic red blood cells (*arrows*) with poikilocytosis (*different shapes*) and anisocytosis (*different sizes*), suggestive of iron deficiency. **B:** Hypersegmented neutrophils (*arrows*) suggestive of vitamin B_{12} deficiency.

C

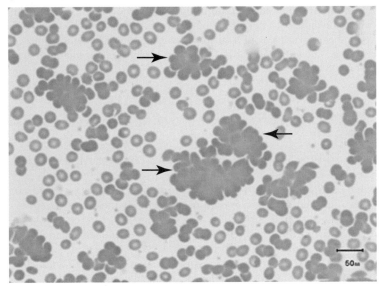

FIGURE 46-1: (Continued) **C:** Autoagglutination (*arrows*) characteristic of IgM-mediated (cold) hemolytic anemia. (*courtesy of Alison Moliterno, MD, Division of Hematology, The Johns Hopkins Hospital.*)

physical exam findings, and her CBC. The search for the cause will be important for long-term management but she should be started on iron repletion during her admission.

EXTENDED IN-HOSPITAL MANAGEMENT

Most patients with newly diagnosed iron deficiency anemia will need to be started on a regimen of oral iron replacement. Patients who receive IV iron need to be observed as adverse reactions to the IV infusions are possible (although are less common now with newer compounds). Patients with acute GI bleeds should have a stable hematocrit level before leaving the hospital. The source of bleeding should be ascertained during the hospitalization in most cases.

DISPOSITION

Discharge Goals

Once a patient's cause for anemia has been ascertained and there is no further active bleeding, he or she is ready for discharge from the hospital. The patient should be educated on the reason for his or her anemia and should be counseled, as appropriate, about taking his or her medications.

Outpatient Care

The timing of follow-up visitation depends on the reason for admission. With iron deficiency, a period of about 4 to 6 weeks is needed to get a feel for whether replacement of iron stores is improving the hemoglobin concentration. The initiation of B_{12}, folate, and erythropoietin therapies should be followed on a similar schedule.

 WHAT YOU NEED TO REMEMBER

- The first step in evaluating anemia is to ascertain the defective compartment of hemoglobin production or destruction.
- The peripheral smear, the iron and iron-binding capacity, the serum ferritin, and a reticulocyte response can classify most anemias appropriately.
- The marrow ferritin is helpful in unclear cases of anemia and gives a reflection of the amount of marrow iron.
- All patients with a diagnosis of iron deficiency anemia and an unclear source of bleeding should undergo colorectal cancer screening.

REFERENCE

1. World Health Organization. *Worldwide Prevalence of Anaemia Report 1993–2005. WHO Global Database on Anaemia.* Geneva: World Health Organization; 2008.

SUGGESTED READINGS

Borthwell TH, Charlton RW, Cook JD, et al. *Iron Metabolism in Man.* Oxford, London, Edinburgh, Melbourne: Blackwell Scientific Publications; 1979.

Crosby WH. Food pica and iron deficiency. *Arch Intern Med.* 1971;127:960–961.

Crosby WH. Pica. *JAMA.* 1976;235(25):2765.

Hillman RS, Ault KA, Rinder HM. *Hematology in Clinical Practice.* 4th ed. New York: McGraw-Hill; 2005.

Ioannou GN, Spector J, Scott K, et al. Prospective evaluation of a clinical guideline for the diagnosis and management of iron deficiency anemia. *Am J Med.* 2002; 113:281–287.

Thrombocytopenia

THE PATIENT ENCOUNTER

A 45-year-old woman with a history of epilepsy presents to the emergency room with a 3-day history of lightheadedness, nosebleeds, and bleeding from the gums. She has no history of previous episodes of bleeding. She was recently started on valproic acid for a seizure disorder. Her initial labs demonstrated a platelet count of 15,000 platelets/μL.

OVERVIEW

Definition

Thrombocytopenia is defined as a platelet count <150,000/μL. The differential diagnosis for thrombocytopenia is broad, and management will depend on both the etiology and the severity of the thrombocytopenia. This chapter will focus on the approach to and management of inpatients with thrombocytopenia.

Pathophysiology

Megakaryocytes give rise to platelets by cytoplasmic shedding within the bone marrow. Once platelets are released into the circulation, approximately one third are sequestered in the spleen. The remainder survive in the circulation for approximately 8 to 10 days, until they are removed by the monocyte-macrophage system or are consumed in hemostasis. Thrombocytopenia can arise from three potential mechanisms: (a) the decreased production of platelets, (b) the increased destruction of platelets, or (c) increased splenic sequestration.

Epidemiology

The incidence of thrombocytopenia is not well defined and will depend in large part on the underlying etiology.

Etiology

Impaired platelet production occurs when the bone marrow lacks growth factors and nutrients or is damaged or suppressed. Etiologies of suppression and damage include viral infections (varicella, parvovirus, Epstein-Barr virus, human immunodeficiency virus [HIV]), neoplastic disease, myelofibrosis, drugs, and vitamin deficiencies (i.e., B_{12}, folate). Rare causes of inherited thrombocytopenia include congenital bone marrow aplasias, such as Fanconi anemia.

A number of conditions can lead to the accelerated destruction of platelets. In immunologically mediated thrombocytopenia, platelets are coated with antibodies and then destroyed via the complement system or monocyte-macrophages. Etiologies include infections (cytomegalovirus infectious mononucleosis, hepatitis C), drugs (e.g., heparin, carbamazepine, methyl-dopa), systemic lupus erythematosus, or idiopathic thrombocytopenic purpura (ITP). ITP, which is an autoimmune disorder, is a diagnosis of exclusion.

Nonimmunologically mediated thrombocytopenia occurs in the setting of intravascular prostheses, thrombi, or abnormal vessels, all of which can shorten the survival of platelets. Hemolytic uremic syndrome (HUS), thrombocytopenic purpura (TTP), vasculitis, intra-aortic balloon pumps, and disseminated intravascular coagulation (DIC) are all examples of this phenomenon. The most common condition associated with DIC is sepsis.

Typically, one third of platelets are sequestered in the spleen. When the spleen enlarges, the platelet count drops as the fraction of platelets sequestered in the spleen increases. Causes of splenomegaly include portal hypertension, malignancies (myeloproliferative or lymphoproliferative disorders), or storage disorders (Gaucher disease).

Dilutional thrombocytopenia can be seen in patients who have suffered blood loss and have received a large number of transfusions with packed red blood cells. Occasionally, thrombocytopenia is a laboratory artifact in which platelets clump or adhere to leukocytes; this occurs if ethylenediaminetetraacetic acid (EDTA) is used as an anticoagulant in the collection tube and the patient has an antibody that results in platelet clumping.

ACUTE MANAGEMENT AND WORKUP

As you assess your patient, you should start to think about the differential diagnosis for his or her thrombocytopenia because your intervention will differ depending on the etiology.

The First 15 Minutes

Bleeding is the most common symptomatic presentation of thrombocytopenia. For an actively bleeding patient, it is critical to evaluate for hemodynamic instability because this warrants rapid intervention with intravenous fluids and blood products, including red blood cells, fresh frozen plasma, and platelets, depending on the situation. Our patient's dizziness in the encounter could be a sign of either orthostasis or severe anemia and deserves immediate attention.

Initial Assessment

Any signs of neurologic impairment in the thrombocytopenic patient should warrant immediate assessment of the ability to protect the airway, followed by radiographic evaluation (i.e., a noncontrast computed tomography [CT] scan of the head) to rule out an intracranial bleed.

Admission Criteria and Level of Care Criteria

In general, actively bleeding patients with hemodynamic instability will need intensive care unit–level care. Patients with evidence of intracranial hemorrhage should have neurosurgical evaluation immediately. In both cases, rapid intervention with the transfusion of blood products should be initiated to prevent ongoing bleeding.

The First Few Hours

It is important to start thinking about the possible etiology of thrombocytopenia as soon as you meet the patient because management differs depending on the cause of the thrombocytopenia.

History

Assess the patient's history of bleeding. Try to understand the timing and severity of the bleeding. Does the patient have a history of nosebleeds or bleeding from the gums? Has the patient noticed melena, bright red blood from the rectum, or hematuria? Does the patient have a history of excessive bleeding after surgeries or dental procedures? For women, inquire about the presence of menorrhagia or metrorrhagia. Patients with platelet counts between 30,000 and 50,000 may develop ecchymoses with even minor trauma. Those with counts between 10,000 and 30,000 are at risk for spontaneous petechiae and ecchymoses. Platelet counts less than 10,000 put patients at risk for spontaneous internal bleeding. Thrombocytopenic patients may also have systemic systems such as nausea, lightheadedness, and vomiting.

It is important to ask about recent infections, a prior history of hematologic disease, alcohol abuse, and risk factors for HIV, hepatitis C, and liver disease.

Fevers can be associated with TTP, though a higher fever (>38.9°C [102°F]) suggests an infection. Along with fever, the classic pentad of TTP is renal failure, thrombocytopenia, microangiopathic hemolytic anemia, and neurologic abnormalities. You may elicit a history of seizures, confusion, or focal neurologic deficits. Patients with TTP may also commonly complain of nausea, vomiting, and abdominal pain.

Review the list of medications and the history of exposures, and compare these to the timing of symptom onset. Common agents include anticonvulsants such as carbamazepine and valproic acid, and antibiotics such as trimethoprim-sulfamethoxazole. Drug-induced thrombocytopenia typically presents 1 week after the onset of the sensitizing drug, but occasionally symptoms may begin as early as 1 to 2 days after the initial drug exposure. Heparin-induced thrombocytopenia (HIT) usually occurs 5 to 10 days after the start of heparin. Remember to inquire about recent vaccines, over-the-counter medications, and herbal remedies.

Physical Examination

The physical examination should focus on any evidence of bleeding. Examine the mucosa for evidence of gingival bleeding or epistaxis. Perform a thorough skin exam to look for evidence of petechiae, purpura, or ecchymoses. For bedridden patients, the presacral area should be carefully examined for ecchymoses. A rectal exam should be performed for occult blood. Examine the abdomen to look for splenomegaly, as this can suggest splenic sequestration. Also search for stigmata of end-stage liver disease. A complete neurologic examination (including funduscopy) is also important to assess for deficits that could suggest a central nervous system event such as a bleed.

In the case of HIT, the risk of thrombosis is substantial. Careful examination for evidence of clots is critical. Look for asymmetric leg swelling and heparin-induced skin necrosis. Limb ischemia resulting in amputation occurs in 5% to 10% of patients with HIT.

Labs and Tests to Consider

A complete blood count (CBC) and a peripheral smear are essential to the evaluation of thrombocytopenia.

Key Diagnostic Labs and Tests

The blood smear is probably the most important test to help with your diagnosis. Large platelets with large granules may be suggestive of a congenital thrombocytopenia. Platelet clumps could suggest a pseudothrombocytopenia. Fragmented red blood cells (schistocytes, helmet cells) are present in a thrombotic microangiopathic process such as TTP or HUS (Fig. 47-1). The fragmentation occurs as the red blood cells try to pass through areas of the circulation that are occluded by platelet clumps. Spherocytes are suggestive of hypersplenism. Blasts are suggestive of a hematologic malignancy.

A CBC to look for other cytopenias is important, as is comparison to previous values to help establish the chronicity of the thrombocytopenia. In cases of bone marrow suppression, usually all cell lines will be affected, with a resulting leukopenia and anemia. An elevated creatinine level may be present in TTP/HUS. Hemolysis is suggested by an elevated reticulocyte count, an elevated lactate dehydrogenase (LDH) level, and a decreased haptoglobin level. A urinalysis may show hemoglobinuria or hemosiderinuria. A direct Coombs test will be negative in a microangiopathic hemolytic anemia, whereas it will be positive in an autoimmune hemolytic anemia.

DIC will present with elevated prothrombin time, partial thromboplastin time (PTT), D-dimer, and fibrin degradation products, as well as with an elevated level of LDH, the presence of schistocytes, and a decreased haptoglobin level.

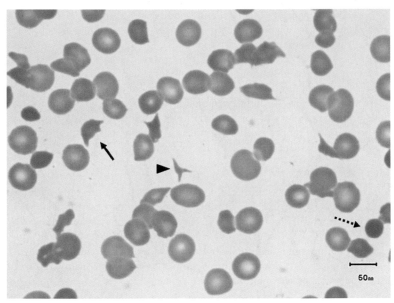

FIGURE 47-1: Blood smear of a patient with thrombotic thrombocytopenic purpura showing schistocytes (*solid arrow*), red cell fragments (*arrowhead*), and microspherocytes (*dashed arrow*). (*Courtesy of Alison Moliterno, MD, Division of Hematology, The Johns Hopkins Hospital.*)

CLINICAL PEARL

A newer test used in the evaluation of thrombocytopenia is the immature platelet fraction (IPF), which measures the percent of reticulated platelets. A higher immature platelet fraction is suggestive of increased thrombopoiesis that may be a response to increased platelet destruction.

Other lab tests will depend on the suspected etiology of the thrombocytopenia. Consider testing for viruses such as HIV and hepatitis C, especially in patients with risk factors. If you suspect a vitamin deficiency, check vitamin B_{12}, folate levels, and even iron levels. To confirm the diagnosis of HIT, serologic assays to look for heparin-dependent antibodies are available. Given the high sensitivity and relatively low specificity of this assay, the negative predictive value is quite high, but the positive predictive value of this assay may be lower. The serotonin release assay is a more specific test for HIT, which is often used for confirmation in the setting of a positive HIT antibody.

Some hospitals have tests to identify antibodies to specific drugs. However, these tests are expensive, technically demanding, and may not be helpful in the immediate care of a patient. Deficiency of the protease ADAMTS13 has been reported in TTP; however, assays for ADAMTS13 deficiency are time consuming and are not yet widely available. Waiting for the results should not delay initiating the treatment of TTP.

In cases of severe thrombocytopenia for which the diagnosis is not evident from the patient's history and the tests noted previously, a bone marrow aspirate and biopsy is usually indicated. A bone marrow biopsy is also warranted if you suspect a hematologic malignancy.

Imaging

The decision to image the patient will largely depend on the patient's symptoms and history. For patients with neurologic symptoms or with changes in mental status, the ability to protect the airway should be assessed, followed by a noncontrast head CT scan. In an alcoholic patient in whom you suspect portal hypertension, obtaining an abdominal CT scan may reveal splenomegaly. A CT scan may also be helpful in cases of severe abdominal pain to rule out intra-abdominal or retroperitoneal hemorrhage.

Treatment

Bleeding patients with severe thrombocytopenia should be aggressively managed with platelet and red blood cell transfusions. In bleeding patients, the antifibrinolytic aminocaproic acid can also be used to help stabilize clot formation.

More definitive treatment will depend on the etiology. For drug-induced thrombocytopenia, in which there is no evidence of bleeding, discontinuation of the suspected agent may suffice. Platelets will usually recover within a few days. In the setting of sepsis, treatment is with appropriate antibiotics and other measures of supportive care. TTP/HUS is treated with immune suppression and prompt plasmapheresis; some clinicians also use immunosuppressive agents such as steroids. Platelet transfusions are contraindicated in TTP/HUS given the increased risk of thrombosis with transfusions. HIT is treated by discontinuation of all heparin sources, and by anticoagulation with a direct thrombin inhibitor, such as argatroban or bivalirudin. The treatment of DIC begins with managing the underlying illness. Fresh frozen plasma, cryoprecipitate, and platelets are supportive measures that may be used in the bleeding patient.

Idiopathic thrombocytopenic purpura is treated with corticosteroids. However, in severe cases of ITP, intravenous methylprednisolone is given with intravenous immune globulin and an infusion of platelets. In extreme cases, more aggressive immunosuppression or even splenectomy may be required.

The patient in our encounter likely has a drug-induced thrombocytopenia from the recent initiation of valproic acid. Valproic acid should be stopped immediately and consideration should be given to administering aminocaproic acid because she is having mucosal bleeding on presentation. Further interventions will depend on her platelet count response to stopping the drug as well as on the severity of her bleeding while she is thrombocytopenic.

EXTENDED IN-HOSPITAL MANAGEMENT

Prolonged hospitalization for thrombocytopenia is not uncommon. A poor response to treatment warrants re-evaluation of both the diagnosis and the treatment plan. A change in mental status or other new neurologic symptom warrants reimaging of the head to rule out a bleed. Bone marrow biopsy is a necessary diagnostic test when there is not a clear etiology to the thrombocytopenia or if treatment is not yielding expected improvement.

DISPOSITION

Discharge Goals

Discharge depends on whether the underlying illness has responded to treatment. Prior to discharge, a comprehensive plan for follow-up and further evaluation with specialists should be arranged on an as-needed basis.

Outpatient Care

Outpatient care will again depend on the etiology of the thrombocytopenia. Patients should follow up with their primary care physician within a few days. Repeat blood tests should be obtained to follow the platelet count, and patients will often require follow-up with a hematologist.

WHAT YOU NEED TO REMEMBER

- Thrombocytopenia can arise from one of three mechanisms: (a) the decreased production of platelets, (b) the increased destruction of platelets, or (c) increased splenic sequestration.
- The examination of the peripheral smear is critical for the evaluation of any patient who presents with thrombocytopenia.
- Patients with platelet counts <10,000 are at risk for spontaneous bleeds.
- Neurologic symptoms in a thrombocytopenic patient warrant an assessment of the ability to protect the airway followed by evaluation for an intracranial bleed and/or TTP.
- Thrombotic thrombocytopenic purpura is a medical emergency that requires prompt intervention with plasma exchange.
- Idiopathic thrombocytopenic purpura is a diagnosis of exclusion.

SUGGESTED READINGS

Arepally GM, Ortel TL. Clinical practice. Heparin-induced thrombocytopenia. *N Engl J Med.* 2006;355(8):809–17.

Aster RH, Bougie DW. Drug-induced immune thrombocytopenia. *N Engl J Med.* 2007;357(6):580–587.

Cines DB, Blanchette VS. Immune thrombocytopenic purpura. *N Engl J Med.* 2002;346(13):995–1008.

George JN. Clinical practice. Thrombotic thrombocytopenic purpura. *N Engl J Med.* 2006;354(18):1927–1935.

Moake JL. Thrombotic microangiopathies. *N Engl J Med.* 2002;347(8):589–600.

Moake JL. Thrombotic thrombocytopenic purpura and the hemolytic uremic syndrome. *Arch Pathol Lab Med.* 2002;126(11):1430–1433.

CHAPTER

Alcohol Intoxication and Withdrawal

48

THE PATIENT ENCOUNTER

A 55-year-old man is brought to the emergency room after a witnessed stumble and fall on an icy sidewalk outside the local bar. His clothes and breath smell of alcohol, and he is quite animated but confused. Serum volatile testing reveals a blood alcohol level of 400 mg/dL.

OVERVIEW

Definition

Alcohol intoxication and withdrawal are the short- and long-term effects of the consumption of alcoholic beverages. Legally, all 50 states have adopted a blood alcohol content (BAC) level of 0.08% (1 g of alcohol per 500 g of blood) as the limit above which driving is illegal. However, there is no specific alcohol level that medically defines intoxication. Clinically, alcohol intoxication is manifest by disinhibited behavior, a slowed reaction time, and poor coordination. Alcohol withdrawal, usually seen only in patients with chronic alcohol use or dependence, is defined as a cluster of symptoms that occur at various time points after consumption of the last alcoholic beverage. The clinical course will vary and symptoms cover a wide range, including nausea and vomiting, tremors, seizures, hallucinations, delirium, and autonomic instability.

Pathophysiology

Chronic ethanol use down-regulates the effect of γ-aminobutyric acid (GABA) at the GABA-A inhibitory receptor. Therefore, when alcohol is removed, inhibition is reduced, producing increased excitability. Additionally, alcohol inhibits N-methyl D-aspartate (NMDA) receptors, which are excitatory. Chronic alcohol use up-regulates the number of NMDA receptors, so when alcohol is abruptly withdrawn, there is an abrupt increase in NMDA activity and, therefore, excitability. The overall effect in withdrawal is to increase excitatory and decrease inhibitory neurotransmission.

Epidemiology

Alcohol use is widespread. In 2006, 61% of U.S. adults reported drinking alcohol; one third of those adults said they had consumed five or more alcoholic beverages on at least one occasion in the last year (1). In 2005, there were more than 4 million visits to the emergency room for alcohol use, resulting in more than 1.2 million hospitalizations (2).

Etiology

Alcohol intoxication can occur in anyone—in an alcoholic or a first-time user. Alcohol withdrawal, however, occurs in those who use alcohol chronically. While it is easy to recognize a heavy drinker, even those with "milder" habits can be at risk for withdrawal if they drink chronically.

ACUTE MANAGEMENT AND WORKUP

Alcohol withdrawal is potentially fatal, but it is preventable if it is recognized and managed early.

> ### CLINICAL PEARL
>
> *Patients may feel like they will die when withdrawing from narcotics, but they could actually die from alcohol withdrawal.*

The First 15 Minutes

The goal of your initial encounter with the intoxicated or withdrawing patient is to determine the risk of developing complications in the next minutes to hours.

Initial Assessment

The most important questions to ask are the following: (i) "How much alcohol do you consume on a daily basis?" (ii) "How long has it been since your last drink?" and (iii) Have you ever experienced withdrawal symptoms, particularly 'DTs,' (delirium tremens) or 'the shakes,' when you aren't drinking?" This should give you an idea of how much alcohol your patient consumes.

Next, evaluate the patient's vital signs. Tachycardia (heart rate >90 bpm) and hypertension are early signs of the autonomic instability of alcohol withdrawal. Hypoxia (SpO$_2$ <90%) or a substantially decreased respiratory rate in an intoxicated patient could indicate suppressed respiratory drive and may warrant intubation. Fever >38°C (>100.4°F) should raise suspicion for aspiration pneumonia. Conversely, hypothermia (<35.5°C [<95.9°F]) and bradycardia (heart rate <50 bpm) can often occur after prolonged exposure and should be managed acutely. In the case of a suspected fall, as in our patient encounter, be sure to look for signs of intracranial hemorrhage or other posttraumatic complications.

A quick physical exam should look for the following signs of active withdrawal: hand or tongue tremors, disorientation/confusion, and witnessed hallucinations or seizures.

Admission Criteria and Level of Care Criteria

Depending on the practice of your hospital, many times an intoxicated patient will not be admitted but rather will "sleep it off" in the emergency room. Patients who are likely to be admitted to a general medicine service are those with a coexisting medical condition. Vigilance is therefore crucial because "alcohol withdrawal" will likely not be the chief complaint or admitting diagnosis, but rather something that will develop while a patient is hospitalized.

Once admitted, the level of care will be determined by vital signs, medication requirements, and monitoring requirements. For example, a patient experiencing severe withdrawal, requiring infusions of benzodiazepines, will be sent to the intensive care unit.

The First Few Hours

Alcohol withdrawal is an active and ongoing process throughout a patient's hospitalization. A patient's condition, and therefore treatment strategy, can change on an hour-to-hour basis.

History

It is important to get a detailed history of the patient's alcohol use—how much, how often, what type, and any history of withdrawal. Keep in mind that substances of abuse often track together, and intoxication/withdrawal from other substances can change management.

- *Quantity.* When trying to quantify a patient's daily alcohol consumption, ask specific questions. If the patient says he or she drinks four beers per day, ask what size can. If the patient says he or she drinks "often," ask if that means once per weekend or all day long. Familiarize yourself with the local vernacular—if you don't know what a "double deuce" (22 oz.) or a "forty" (40 oz.) is, ask.
- *Duration of use.* Although we do not report alcohol consumption in pack-years as we do for tobacco, it is helpful to know how long a patient has been drinking. Many patients are quite literal—if you ask, "do you drink," they will say, "no." But if you ask when the patient's last drink was, he or she might say that he or she quit yesterday.
- *Withdrawal symptoms.* One useful way to obtain a history of withdrawal is to ask for the longest amount of time a patient has gone without alcohol. The follow-up question should focus on what symptoms the patient experienced when he or she abstained. Patients who have experienced alcohol withdrawal seizures, or who have a history of DTs, are at higher risk for

subsequent development of DTs. If your patient has previously experienced withdrawal, ask if he or she is having any similar symptoms now. Be sure to ask about prior hospital admissions and past intubations and, if possible, try to obtain records about the quantity of benzodiazepines that were previously required to treat the patient's withdrawal syndrome.

• *Associated conditions.* Abdominal pain could be from pancreatitis, hepatitis, or gastritis. Midline chest pain, hemoptysis, and subcutaneous emphysema might indicate esophageal rupture (Boerhaave syndrome). Remember that your patient will likely be admitted to the hospital for something other than alcohol, and coexisting conditions can cloud the picture. While it's important to maintain a high suspicion for alcohol withdrawal, it is just as important to entertain alternative diagnoses for the signs and symptoms you observe.

Physical Examination

Look carefully for the stigmata of chronic alcohol use, such as muddy sclerae, lacrimal gland hypertrophy, and parotid swelling. The cardiovascular exam should focus on evaluating for any signs of heart failure associated with an underlying alcohol-induced cardiomyopathy. When listening to the lungs, evaluate for focal consolidation that might be secondary to aspiration. A thorough neurologic evaluation should include questions about orientation and a mini-mental exam. It is useful at this point to compare the patient's current mental state to his or her baseline, particularly if family or friends are available. Focus on evaluating for tongue/hand tremors and any focal neurologic deficits that might indicate intracranial pathology (i.e., hemorrhage after falling).

Your initial assessment of the patient—vital signs, tremulousness, degree of agitation—should be repeated at regular intervals throughout the hospital stay. Alcohol withdrawal is a condition that evolves, so vigilant observation is the mainstay of management. There are several clinical tools that are useful in the frequent evaluation of the severity of alcohol withdrawal symptoms. Probably the best studied is the Clinical Institute Withdrawal Assessment for Alcohol (CIWA). Symptoms such as nausea and vomiting, tremors, sweats, anxiety, hallucinations, headaches, and confusion are assigned a point value. The total score can be used to diagnose the syndrome of alcohol withdrawal but can also be used to help guide treatment with benzodiazepines. Note that tachycardia and hypertension are not included in this scoring system as they represent much later stages of alcohol withdrawal symptoms (3).

Labs and Tests to Consider

While there is no laboratory test that can indicate alcohol withdrawal, basic lab work is important in the assessment of concurrent illness.

Key Diagnostic Labs and Tests

Initial basic labs should include a complete blood count and a complete metabolic panel. An elevated white blood cell count could indicate aspiration pneumonia or other infection. A low hematocrit can indicate hemorrhage or anemia from chronic alcohol use. Low platelets are likely a complication of either liver disease or alcohol itself. If you see acute renal failure in conjunction with an elevated serum creatine kinase, particularly in a patient who was "found down," rhabdomyolysis should be high on your list of differential diagnoses. An anion gap metabolic acidosis might indicate alcoholic or starvation ketoacidosis, or that a patient has ingested another substance, such as methanol or polyethylene glycol. Elevated liver enzymes, particularly in a 2:1 ratio of aspartate aminotransferase to alanine aminotransferase, could indicate acute alcoholic hepatitis.

Beyond these basic labs, a toxicology screen of urine and serum, as well as serum volatiles and osmolal gap, can provide useful information about any other ingested substances. In any alcoholic patient with abdominal pain or nausea/vomiting, amylase and lipase should be ordered to evaluate for pancreatitis. In a patient with suspected alcoholic cirrhosis, coagulation studies provide information about the degree of liver dysfunction.

Imaging

As in most hospitalized patients, a chest radiograph can provide valuable information. Evidence of focal consolidation or an infiltrate, particularly in the right lower or middle lobe, could indicate aspiration pneumonitis or pneumonia. A widened mediastinum or pneumomediastinum in a vomiting patient should raise concern for Boerhaave syndrome. Other imaging should be dictated by the patient's symptoms and clinical presentation.

Treatment

Remember that the patient from our encounter will be at the highest risk for alcohol withdrawal 24 to 48 hours into his or her hospital admission. Benzodiazepines are the drugs of choice for treating alcohol withdrawal. Two approaches have been described for dosing benzodiazepines: the fixed dose-interval taper method, and the load and redose method. In the taper method, a relatively intermediate-acting drug (such as oxazepam or lorazepam) is given at an initial dose and frequency, and gradually the dose is decreased and the dose interval is increased until the patient no longer has active circulating metabolites. In the load and redose method, a long-acting benzodiazepine (such as diazepam or chlordiazepoxide) is given in an initial loading dose (chosen based on tolerance and the history of withdrawal), and patients are monitored frequently for signs of withdrawal. When a patient reaches a threshold on the withdrawal scale, he or she will receive another bolus of a long-acting drug. This method requires more frequent monitoring, either by nursing staff who are trained in assessment or by a member of the physician team. In either method, short-acting drugs, such as lorazepam, can be given for breakthrough symptoms. Studies comparing these methods head to head found no difference in the mortality or complication rate, but they did note a smaller overall dose of drug and a shorter hospital stay with the load and redose approach (4). Some patients will be refractory even to the high doses of benzodiazepines provided in these methods and will require a continuous infusion of a benzodiazepine such as lorazepam to control their symptoms. Such patients need to be carefully monitored in an intensive care unit or step-down unit setting. Also in your arsenal are adjunctive therapies such as clonidine (central α-adrenergic blocker) and haloperidol (antipsychotic). Studies have shown repeatedly that benzodiazepines are the superior treatment, but these additional medications may help to lower the overall dose of benzodiazepines required to control symptoms of withdrawal.

> ### CLINICAL PEARL
>
> *In patients receiving high doses of lorazepam (usually >8 mg/hour), a new anion gap acidosis and renal failure may be signs of propylene glycol toxicity from the carrier solution.*

Beyond treating withdrawal symptoms alone, electrolyte and fluid disturbances must be corrected. Remember that many of these patients are malnourished and specifically thiamine deficient.

> ### CLINICAL PEARL
>
> *Thiamine should be administered before glucose in order to avoid precipitating Wernicke encephalopathy.*

EXTENDED IN-HOSPITAL MANAGEMENT

Remember that alcohol withdrawal is an ongoing and dynamic process. The course of withdrawal is extremely variable; the general progression is presented in Table 48-1.

Those who develop seizures, or those with a history of DTs, are at higher risk of subsequently developing DTs. This dreaded complication can be fatal secondary to cardiovascular collapse. The hallmark of DTs is delirium and altered cognition. However, it can often be challenging to distinguish the delirium of DTs with a more nonspecific delirium from the patient's other conditions.

TABLE 48-1
Time Course of Alcohol Withdrawal

Symptom Complex	Time Since Last Drink	Examples
Minor abstinence syndrome	0–6 hr, up to 48 hr Peak 12–24 hr	Tremors, anxiety, nausea, vomiting, sweating, headache
Alcoholic hallucinosis	12–24 hr	Visual, auditory, or tactile hallucinations, but sensorium intact
Withdrawal seizures	2–48 hr Peak 24 hr	Generalized tonic-clonic seizure, can progress to status epilepticus
Delirium tremens	48–96 hr, up to 1 week	Delirium, sympathetic surge

DISPOSITION

Discharge Goals

Different physicians have different thresholds for keeping patients in the hospital; many times, if a patient has no desire to quit drinking and has no other conditions warranting admission, he or she will be allowed to go home and "self-treat" his or her withdrawal. For those patients who are hospitalized throughout the course of their withdrawal, they are ready for discharge when they have been tapered off benzodiazepines and are oriented.

Persistent and direct substance abuse counseling, on multiple occasions by multiple people, is of utmost importance. While your patient may not be motivated today, repeated counseling has been shown to increase the likelihood of cessation in the future. The CAGE questions are a validated screening tool for alcohol abuse; the four questions are (a) "Do you feel the need to **cut back** on your alcohol use?" (b) "Do you get **annoyed** when people talk to you about your drinking?" (c) "Do you feel **guilty** about your habit?" and (d) "Do you ever need an '**eye-opener**' drink when you wake up in the morning?" (5). This is a powerful tool for understanding a patient's degree of alcohol abuse and willingness to quit (6).

Outpatient Care

Patients will ideally follow up with a local substance abuse program. Some motivated patients can be prescribed Antabuse (disulfiram), a medication that produces nausea and vomiting when alcohol is ingested. This should be done under the direction of a primary care physician or substance abuse specialist.

Chronic alcohol abuse puts patients at risk for other illnesses beyond alcohol withdrawal. Alcohol-induced pancreatitis, cirrhosis, thrombocytopenia and anemia, malnutrition, cerebellar dysfunction, and gastritis are just a few of the long-term consequences of alcohol that will require close outpatient follow-up.

Oftentimes, patients will be misdiagnosed with essential hypertension or a primary seizure disorder and will be treated with antihypertensives or neuroleptics. A long-term relationship with a patient can help to distinguish whether these only occur in the setting of alcohol abuse and withdrawal.

WHAT YOU NEED TO REMEMBER

- Alcohol withdrawal is not only uncomfortable for a patient; it is potentially fatal.
- Alcohol withdrawal can be separated into the early phase (8 hours to 2 days) of minor abstinence syndrome, hallucinations, and seizures and the late phase (2 to 3 days or longer) of DTs.
- Alcohol-dependent patients who are hospitalized for other medical conditions are at great risk for withdrawal if the potential is not recognized. This risk is greatest *not* when they first present, but approximately 48 hours into their hospitalization.
- Patients who develop alcohol withdrawal seizures, or who have had DTs in the past, are at higher risk for subsequently developing DTs.
- Benzodiazepines, whether on a tapered schedule or load plus symptom-based bolus schedule, are the drugs of choice for treatment of alcohol withdrawal.

REFERENCES

1. National Centers for Health Statistics. Centers for Disease Control and Prevention. http://www.cdc.gov/nchs/fastats/alcohol.htm
2. National Centers for Health Statistics. Centers for Disease Control and Prevention. http://www.cdc.gov/alcohol/quickstats/general_info.htm
3. Sullivan JT, Sykora K, Schneiderman J, et al. Assessment of alcohol withdrawl: The revised Clinical Institute Withdrawl Assessment for Alcohol Scale (CIWA-Ar). *Br J Addict.* 1989;84;1353–1357.

4. Daeppen JB, Gache P, Landry U, et al. Symptom-triggered vs fixed-schedule doses of benzodiazepine for alcohol withdrawal. *Arch Intern Med.* 2002;162:1117–1121.
5. Bush B, Shaw S, Cleary P, et al. Screening for alcohol abuse using the CAGE questionnaire. *Am J Med.* 1987;82(2):231–235.
6. Ewing JA. Detecting alconolism. THe CAGE questionnaire. *JAMM.* 1984;252(14): 1905–1907.

SUGGESTED READINGS

Baynard M, Mcintyre J, Hill KR, et al. Alcohol withdrawal syndrome. *Am Fam Physician.* 2004;69(6):1443–1450.

Kosten TR, O'Connor PG. Management of drug and alcohol withdrawal. *N Engl J Med.* 2003;348(18):1786–1795.

Mayo-Smith MF, Beecher LH, Fischer TL, et al. Management of alcohol withdrawal delirium. *Arch Intern Med.* 2004;164:1405–1412.

Toxic Ingestions

THE PATIENT ENCOUNTER

A 58-year-old woman was brought to the emergency room after being found down in a bathtub. She is lethargic, confused, and oriented only to person. Emergency medical service providers found an empty bottle of nortriptyline on the bathroom floor. She is tachycardic, with unremarkable pupils, and moves all extremities spontaneously. Her daughter says she has a history of depression, insomnia, alcohol abuse, and chronic pain. She has not spoken with her in 3 days, and is unaware of her recent activities.

OVERVIEW

Definition

Toxic ingestions include any of a number of intentional, unintentional, iatrogenic, or other exposures that may destroy life or impair health.

Pathophysiology

The pathophysiology of a particular toxic ingestion will depend on the substance in question as well as the medical comorbidities of the patient.

Epidemiology

The American Association of Poison Control Centers received 2,354,160 reported total human exposures in 2006, with 77% being ingestions. Approximately 60% of these were unintentional, including environmental, occupational, foodborne, and iatrogenic exposures. Eight percent were intentional, including suicide attempts, drug abuse, and other misuse. While less than one third of exposures occurred in adults, more than 90% of the 1,229 fatalities occurred in those older than age 19. Of these fatalities, analgesics, alcohols, sedatives, hypnotics, antipsychotics, cardiovascular drugs, and stimulants were the most commonly reported sources (1).

Etiology

Table 49-1 lists common toxidromes and the substances commonly implicated.

TABLE 49-1

Common Toxidromes and Their Causes

Toxidrome	Manifestations	Causes
Sympathomimetic	Tachycardia, hypertension, agitation, mydriasis, seizures	Amphetamines, caffeine, cocaine, ephedrine, pseudoephedrine, theophylline
Cholinergic	Salivation, lacrimation, urination, gastrointestinal distress, emesis, bradycardia, bronchospasm, miosis	Organophosphates, bethanechol, physostigmine, pilocarpine
Anticholinergic	Tachycardia, hypertension, fever, dry skin, flushing, psychosis, urinary retention, ileus, mydriasis	Atropine, antihistamines, phenothiazines, tricyclic antidepressants
Sedative/narcotic	Central nervous system depression, respiratory depression, bradycardia, hypotension, miosis	Anticonvulsants, antipsychotics, benzodiazepines, barbiturates, opiates, ethanol, dextromethorphan
Extrapyramidal	Rigidity, tremor, trismus, choreoathetosis	Haloperidol, prochlorperazine, phenothiazines, atypical antipsychotics
Serotonergic	Fever, irritability, flushing, diarrhea, diaphoresis	Selective serotonin reuptake inhibitors, tricyclic antidepressants, meperidine

ACUTE MANAGEMENT AND WORKUP

Depending on the clinical scenario, the first few hours can be critical in dealing with a toxic ingestion. As soon as ingestion is suspected, be sure to notify your local poison control center because it provides a wealth of clinical knowledge and practical experience.

The First 15 Minutes

A focused history and physical with only limited initial labs may give invaluable information as to what and how much was ingested and how long ago the ingestion occurred. Oftentimes, however, specifics will not be available but timely executed advanced cardiac life support (ACLS) care is paramount. Securing a stable airway prevents aspiration. A palpable pulse with cardiac monitoring suggests a perfusing rhythm. These measures, along with reliable intravenous access, allow rapid response to any hemodynamic instability. Cervical spine precautions should also be in place until trauma can be ruled out.

Initial Assessment

The presentation of a patient with a toxic ingestion can range from a detailed self-reported exposure to the limited history of an obtunded, delirious, or agitated patient. A quick focused history and physical as well as some basic laboratory testing will help to narrow your differential diagnosis. This will allow the timely administration of interventions to prevent further absorption, enhance elimination, and, when appropriate, administer antidotes. This information also helps predict a clinical course and allows you to separate those who need reassurance from those who require inpatient admission or intensive care unit (ICU)–level care.

Don't forget the value of simple observation. Is the patient agitated and unarousable or calm, alert, and oriented? Note any obvious unintentional movements or neurologic deficits. Remember to consider other causes of altered mental status, such as seizures or cerebrovascular events, that require very different but equally emergent interventions.

Admission Criteria and Level of Care Criteria

While some patients will need admission for frequent vital signs, laboratory monitoring, or observation, other patients can be sent home with reassurance. In general, if a toxin can be identified, the patient's safety can be guaranteed, a benign course can be predicted, and a patient or his or her caregiver is deemed reliable, then outpatient management is acceptable.

The need for specialized nursing care, frequent labs, continuous infusions, hemodialysis, specific antiarrhythmics, invasive cardiac monitoring, and ventilatory support may require admission to the ICU.

The First Few Hours

Now is the time to gather additional history, review initial laboratories and imaging, and execute time-sensitive interventions.

History

A good history may make diagnosis, management, and prognosis routine, but frequently such information will not be available. When necessary, history can be gathered from the patient's family, friends, health care providers, and pharmacists. Where the patient was found and what was found on the scene is important and can often be obtained from emergency medical service providers. The finding of an empty nortriptyline bottle in our patient encounter strongly suggests that tricyclic antidepressant (TCA) toxicity is playing at least a part in our patient's current toxidrome.

Knowing the time of ingestion is important when deciding on the appropriateness of therapy and predicting the clinical course. For example, a relatively recent ingestion may benefit from gut decontamination via gastric lavage, activated charcoal, or whole bowel irrigation. Also, being able to predict what complications may occur and when, including increased somnolence, respiratory depression, hemodynamic instability, agitation, seizure, or major organ failure, may allow for early interventions and appropriate triage. Next, some idea of the level of exposure may be helpful, as the harmful or even lethal doses of many substances can be quite high.

Knowledge of the patient's comorbidities may point to specific toxic exposures (i.e., prescription drugs) and complicating factors to consider. Particular attention should be paid to those with renal and hepatic disease as drug metabolism can become significantly altered. A history of psychiatric illness and, most importantly, suicidal attempts or gestures should be considered. Finally, a history of substance abuse can help guide the search for likely ingestions.

Physical Examination

When examining a patient with a presumed toxic ingestion, looking for a classic presentation or toxidrome can be helpful (see Table 49-1). When a specific toxidrome is not obvious, vital signs and a limited physical exam can narrow your differential diagnosis. Hyperthermia can be seen with exposure to sympathomimetics, anticholinergics, and salicylates. Malignant hyperthermia, neuroleptic malignant syndrome, and serotonin syndrome also deserve particular attention in these patients. Hypothermia, while less common, can be seen with opiates, alcohols, and barbiturates. Upon further examination of the patient, note pupil size, as miosis can be seen with alcohols, cholinergics, narcotics, barbiturates, and antipsychotics. Mydriasis more likely suggests exposure to anticholinergics or sympathomimetics. In your general physical exam, your goal should be to identify underlying cardiovascular, pulmonary, hepatic, or renal disease that may complicate or contribute to the patient's presentation.

Labs and Tests to Consider

The basic metabolic panel may provide the most valuable objective data.

Key Diagnostic Labs and Tests

Electrolyte abnormalities, such as hypo- or hyperglycemia, hypo- or hypernatremia, and hypo- or hyperkalemia may be responsible for a patient's presentation or may be the clue to help identify the specific ingestion. Elevated liver function tests may suggest toxins such as salicylates, acetaminophen, or concomitant liver disease. Tests of hepatic synthetic function, such as the international normalized ratio, may also provide prognostic information.

It is critical to calculate an anion gap in all patients, even when the serum bicarbonate appears to be "normal" (see Chapter 40). An elevated gap suggests toxic ingestions such as methanol, ethanol, ethylene glycol, methanol, formaldehyde, salicylates, and iron. Additionally, an osmolal gap should be calculated (see Chapter 40). The normal osmolal gap is 10 mOsm, with an elevated gap suggesting the presence of unmeasured, nonionized compounds such as ethanol, ethylene glycol, methanol, isopropanol, propylene glycol, or formaldehyde.

> ### CLINICAL PEARL
>
> *Isopropyl alcohol will cause an elevated osmolal gap but not an elevated anion gap.*

A serum and urine toxicology screen may be helpful, although it is estimated that it only changes management in about 5% of cases. Toxicology screens for specific compounds, including tricyclic antidepressants, lithium, phenytoin, valproic acid, digoxin, and salicylates, should be considered when appropriate. An acetaminophen level should be drawn in most cases, given the benign nature and overwhelming response rate to its antidote, *N*-acetylcysteine. Acetaminophen is also commonly added to other analgesics and over-the-counter remedies so that patients may not even realize they have ingested potentially toxic amounts. Remember that as many as 10% of ingestions involve more than one substance, so a positive toxicology screen does not exclude the presence of a coingestion.

An arterial blood gas should be sent in all patients with an anion or osmolal gap or in any patient with altered mental status. Remember that hypoxia can present with agitation, hyper- or hypotension, and dyspnea. Hypercapnia can present with lethargy, bradycardia, hypotension, and dyspnea.

Imaging

Radiographic imaging may help provide prognostic information or uncover an alternative diagnosis. A chest radiograph may be useful when respiratory failure is apparent and may uncover evidence of aspiration in patients with altered mental status. In particular, infiltrates in the superior segment of the right lower lobe and middle lobe are common in those who aspirate supine, but depending on the patient's positioning at the time of aspiration, infiltrates can appear in other lobes as well.

Treatment

In most cases, the management of patients with a toxic ingestion will be watchful waiting and reassurance. When interventions are considered, they include methods to prevent absorption, increase elimination, provide hemodynamic and respiratory support, or provide the administration of specific antidotes.

All forms of gastric decontamination require a protected airway, the known ingestion of a noncorrosive substance, and an exposure that poses a serious toxicity. Ipecac-induced emesis is generally not recommended in the inpatient setting. Gastric lavage with either a nasogastric or orogastric tube remains largely controversial due to the risks of gastrointestinal tract perforation and aspiration but is probably most useful within an hour of exposure. Single-dose activated charcoal with its large absorptive surface area is the most commonly used form of gastric decontamination. The drug is most beneficial when used within 1 hour and may not absorb particular toxins, including alcohols, alkalis, hydrocarbons, iron, and lithium. Finally, whole bowel irrigation with a bowel-cleansing solution such a polyethylene glycol can be considered in toxic ingestions with delayed-released or enteric-coated drugs, transdermal patches, and other drugs not absorbed by activated charcoal.

Methods to enhance elimination of a toxin fall largely into the categories of corporeal (including forced diuresis and urinary alkalinization) and extracorporeal (most notably, hemodialysis and hemoperfusion). These methods require an understanding of the pharmacokinetic properties of individual drugs and go beyond the scope of this chapter, but they should be considered when gut decontamination is determined futile or inefficient and a serious toxicity is suspected. In general, substances with low molecular weight, low protein binding, low volume of distribution, and high water solubility are candidates for hemodialysis-enhanced elimination. Examples include lithium, alcohols, and salicylates.

The application of supportive measures including intravenous fluids, vasopressors, and mechanical ventilation may be required in some patients.

One final therapy to consider is the use of antidotes (Table 49-2).

The patient in our encounter should most likely be administered activated charcoal because the timing of her ingestion is unknown. Because TCA toxicity is highly suspected, she may benefit from sodium bicarbonate administration as alkalinization has been shown to decrease the fraction of unbound

TABLE 49-2
Common Toxins with Associated Antidotes

Toxin	Antidote
Acetaminophen	N-acetylcysteine
Anticholinergic, organophosphate	Atropine, physostigmine, pralidoxime
Beta-blocker	Glucagon
Benzodiazepine	Flumazenil
Digoxin	Antidigoxin Fab
Ethylene glycol	Ethanol, dialysis
Methanol	Fomepizole, dialysis
Iron	Deferoxamine
Lead	Ethylenediaminetetraacetic acid, succimer, dimercaprol
Opiates	Naloxone
Warfarin	Vitamin K, fresh frozen plasma

TCAs and helps to reverse cardiovascular side effects such as QRS prolongation and hypotension. Because of the large volume of distribution, hemodialysis is not effective in the treatment of TCA toxicity and she will require close monitoring for both cardiovascular and central nervous system complications.

EXTENDED IN-HOSPITAL MANAGEMENT

All patients should be screened for depression or suicidal intent once they are able to provide a history. While toxic ingestions are often unintentional, it is important to determine the patient's safety both in the hospital and when considering discharge.

The inpatient course will be short for most patients with toxic ingestions, as toxins are eliminated and their effects reversed. It is largely end-organ damage and nosocomial complications that prolong a patient's stay.

DISPOSITION

Discharge Goals

In general, patients are ready to go home when serious toxicities are reversed or avoided, the anticipated course is benign, or it is deemed that permanent complications can be safely managed outside of the hospital. The patient must return to a safe environment where future exposures, either purposeful or accidental, can be avoided.

Outpatient Care

Most patients can follow up with their primary physician in 1 to 2 weeks. Other follow-up, including psychiatry and subspecialty services, should be arranged on a case-by-case basis.

WHAT YOU NEED TO REMEMBER

- The American Association of Poison Control Centers (1-800-222-1222 or www.aapcc.org) is a resource for patients and clinicians to prevent and manage toxic ingestions.
- Approximately 10% of toxic exposures include more than one substance.
- Expect patients with comorbidities to have a more complicated course.
- Frequently the source of ingestion will not be known, but through a limited history, physical exam, and standard admission labs, your differential diagnosis can be quickly narrowed.
- Remember that cerebrovascular events, seizures, and infections are important alternative causes of altered mental status.
- Acknowledged or suspected suicidal attempts require one-on-one monitoring in the hospital, urgent psychiatric evaluation, and guided discharge planning.
- Antidotes receive a lot of attention, but initial supportive care, monitoring, and thoughtful reassurance will prove the most valuable in managing the majority of toxic ingestions.

REFERENCE

1. Bronstein AC, Spyker DA, Canilena LR, et al. 2006 annual report of the American Association of Poison Control Centers; poison data system (NPDS). *Clin Toxicol.* 2007;45(8):815–917.

SUGGESTED READINGS

Brett AS, Rothschild N, Gray R, et al. Predicting the clinical course in intentional drug overdose: implications for the use of the intensive care unit. *Arch Intern Med.* 1987;1:133–137.

Brok J, Buckley N, Gluud C. Intervention for paracetamol (acetaminophen) overdose. *Cochrane Database Syst Rev.* 2006;2.

de Pont AC. Extracorporeal treatment of intoxications. *Curr Opin Crit Care.* 2007; 12(6):668–673.

Greene S, Harris C, Singer J. Gastrointestinal decontamination of the poisoned patient. *Pediatr Emerg Care.* 2008;24(3):176–186.

Mokhlesi B, Leiken JB, Murray P, et al. Adult toxicology in critical care: part I: general approach to the intoxicated patient. *Chest.* 2003;123(2):577–592.

Mokhlesi B, Leiken JB, Murray P, et al. Adult toxicology in critical care: part II: specific poisonings. *Chest.* 2003;123(3):897–922.

The Hospitalized Elderly Patient

OVERVIEW

Elderly patients are a special group that you are going to regularly encounter during your medical career. This chapter will focus on the assessment and management of older individuals and their passage through our medical care.

Today in the United States, there are 35 million people who are older than the age of 65. By the year 2030, this number will double due to the baby boomer population and the improved diagnosis and treatment of chronic conditions. The older individual has to be viewed with a slightly different perspective to avoid common pitfalls. Just like pediatric patients, the elderly have a distinct group of diseases that are very common in their population; they have a different physiology, and they may react differently to medications that are commonly prescribed to younger patients.

WORKUP

When approaching a patient that is elderly, take a few moments to prepare yourself for some of the differences you may encounter. To begin with, you should remind yourself of the changing times that these patient have been through. They have experienced many forms of medicine, and may find it difficult and distressing to open up to and be examined by a young physician. More than any other time in medicine, you really need to listen to these patients and hear what they are saying—often, it may not be what you expect, and your goals of care should address the patient's complaint as much as the disease process itself.

One problem that physicians run into with older adults is the failure to realize that patients do not always present with the usual "textbook" symptoms. For example, a myocardial infarction in an older patient can and will present as acute confusion or possibly even a fall. The common thread is that older patients may not have adequate physiologic reserve, so even minor insults can have profound systemic effects.

History

It is important to make sure that you have time to establish a good rapport and gain your patient's trust. Older individuals may have concerns over losing their independence or being unable to return home, which is not something we usually encounter with our younger patients. It is important to remember that most elderly patients are not frail and disabled. The majority of people older than age 75 still live independently and enjoy an active and fulfilling life. Many of their symptoms are not a normal consequence of aging and need to be investigated thoroughly rather than being chalked up to just being "old."

Taking a good history in elderly patients should include all of the points that we have discussed in previous chapters. However, there are certain areas that deserve more focus. Along with the details of the presenting complaint, it is important to find out how this complaint affects their life and their ability to perform activities of daily living. Symptoms such as dizziness or incontinence can be very distressing; they can cause patients to be frightened to be on their own or can cause them to reduce their social activities due to embarrassment. Getting a history from family members, friends, or caregivers either in person or by making a phone call can be extremely helpful as it can often fill in the details of the problem. A review of systems can often yield details that the patient may not have deemed important. An elderly person (just like his or her physician) may attribute key symptoms to "old age," so it is important to be thorough. It is also important to screen for depression. For example, weight loss, poor appetite, and a reduction in activities could be a sign of an underlying malignancy, but they might also be a sign of unrecognized depression.

A full medication list from a pharmacy, along with all the bottles of medications from home, can help with assessing interactions of polypharmacy. It is not unusual for a patient to be taking medications from many different practitioners, or to continue old medications from the same practitioner. The patient might even be taking different formulations of the same medication. You should also ask about tonics, herbal medications, and over-the-counter medications.

The family history usually does not have the same implications compared to younger patients, but the social history is extremely important. Where and how patients spend their time, their activities, and their ability to live and perform independently are crucial in your assessment. Include questions about how they mobilize, cook, dress, and get to the store. You should also ask about the support of family and friends. Be sure to ask about alcohol and illicit drug use—it is more common than you think and can impair stability, interact with medications, and lead to life-threatening accidents and falls.

Physical Examination

An older adult may not want to let you know how long a problem has been going on. Attention to the general overall appearance, state of nutrition, and evidence of weight loss may help you understand the chronicity of the presentation, even if it is denied. A good inspection of skin, including bruising and sores, is paramount. Pressure sores or sacral decubitus ulcers can lead to an immense amount of morbidity. As a physician taking care of older adults, you must always look for evidence of elder abuse. Unexplained injuries or very poor nutrition in a patient who is being taken care of by family, home nursing, or a facility should be investigated because elder abuse is, unfortunately, not uncommon.

The physical exam should pay attention to the signs of conditions that are common, such as diastolic heart failure, peripheral vascular disease, systolic hypertension, and cerebrovascular disease. Malignancy is also common in this population so the appropriate exam, including a breast and rectal exam, may be necessary. As always, be respectful when examining a patient. It is important to remember that elderly people may not be comfortable undressing and exposing themselves to a young physician, so awareness and appropriate interaction can put patients at ease.

Key Diagnostic Labs and Tests

An older adult may present with a range of nonspecific symptoms, so routine basic laboratory testing can reveal an unexpected diagnosis. One common problem that has been estimated to occur in 40% of older adults presenting to the emergency room is delirium. Remember that elderly patients do not always present with "textbook" signs and symptoms, so searching for common infectious causes of delirium such as urinary tract infection or pneumonia should be included in the delirium assessment. The incidence of delirium increases during a hospital admission and is often due to iatrogenic causes. Obviously, we are under pressure to find the diagnosis and manage a patient in the least amount of time. However, keeping an elderly individual up all night going to imaging studies can often cause even the most astute patient to become delirious.

> ### CLINICAL PEARL
> *Try to limit studies to the work day and try to maintain a normal wake–sleep cycle. Although it may hinder your workup in the beginning, managing a delirious patient on a later day can be far more challenging.*

One other point of advice about ordering studies is that you should know what the next step will be when the result is known. For example, if the patient has expressed very strong wishes to not undergo a surgical procedure, you may want to reconsider ordering a test to diagnose a disease for which surgery is the only potential treatment option. You may still eventually order the test, but you should talk about the test's implications with your patient before doing so.

MANAGEMENT

The management of each individual patient should be tailored to his or her problems. Side effects of medications are more common in older adults, and dosing should be adjusted to account for factors such as volume of distribution and hepatic and renal clearance. You should try to eliminate any medications that are not necessary to achieve your goals of treating an illness, improving the quality of life, and, if appropriate, improving life expectancy. The longer the list of medications, the more likely the patient is to be noncompliant. Try to remember why the patient initially came to you and how you are going to achieve that goal.

More than in any other specialty, the care of the older adult requires intimate relationships with a multidisciplinary team. Do not be afraid to ask the patient about his or her wishes and goals—you will be surprised how many older adults have thought about these issues, and they may have quite strong views. A discussion on resuscitation status should be a relaxed and thorough process, and should be done when you can still discuss these issues with the patient himself or herself. If you let the patient know the discussion is a normal part of hospital admission, it can be viewed as routine. Nothing can substitute knowing the true wishes of your patient when decisions need to be made.

Discharge Goals

Discharge should be planned well in advance and the whole team should feel comfortable about the process. When the planning is rushed and not well thought out, it often results in early readmission. The patient should be transferred to home or a facility when the primary problems have been addressed and it is safe for the patient to be discharged. A good history of the home environment will come in handy as you will know what is needed to achieve a smooth transition. It may even be appropriate to perform a home health/safety evaluation to make sure that the home environment is appropriate for the patient's needs. Temporary rehabilitation facilities play a crucial role during this time as even a minor illness can result in a reduced capacity to perform activities of daily living. A discussion with the patient and family so that all members are prepared for discharge is ideal so that any issues not previously realized can be brought to the attention of the medical staff.

Outpatient Care

All older adults should be seen by their primary care physician within 1 to 2 weeks after discharge. It is beneficial to have these appointments made and details given to the patient before he or she leaves, along with an accurate list of medications. Many hospitals have a transition program for older patients that involves a follow-up telephone call and a nurse/care provider visit after hospitalization. Transitions of care are the times when most mistakes and misunderstandings occur and should be approached with the same meticulous care that is applied to the search for the initial diagnosis.

WHAT YOU NEED TO REMEMBER

- Elderly patients may manifest disease differently than younger patients, in part due to a smaller physiologic reserve.
- Beware of polypharmacy in your elderly patient.
- Delirium is a common problem in elderly patients and can often be avoided by reducing polypharmacy and attempting to maintain normal sleep–wake cycles.
- Transitions of care are a dangerous time—communication and careful planning are critical to ensuring a safe discharge.

Index

Page numbers followed by f indicate figure; those followed by t indicate table.